T0135875

Studien zur Mustererkennung

herausgegeben von:

Prof. Dr.-Ing. Heinrich Niemann

PD Dr.-Ing. Elmar Nöth

Bibliografische Information der Deutschen Bibliothek

Die Deutsche Bibliothek verzeichnet diese Publikation in der Deutschen Nationalbibliografie; detaillierte bibliografische Daten sind im Internet über http://dnb.ddb.de abrufbar.

ISBN 978-3-8325-1769-4

ISSN 1617-0695

Logos Verlag Berlin GmbH
Comeniushof
Gubener Str. 47
10243 Berlin
Tel.: +49 030 42 85 10 90
Fax: +49 030 42 85 10 92
INTERNET: http://www.logos-verlag.de

Automatic Evaluation of Tracheoesophageal Substitute Voices

Der Technischen Fakultät der
Universität Erlangen–Nürnberg

zur Erlangung des Grades

DOKTOR–INGENIEUR

vorgelegt von

Tino Haderlein

Erlangen — 2007

Als Dissertation genehmigt von der
Technischen Fakultät der
Universität Erlangen-Nürnberg

Tag der Einreichung:	27.06.2007
Tag der Promotion:	31.10.2007
Dekan:	Prof. Dr.-Ing. habil. J. Huber
Berichterstatter:	Prof. em. Dr.-Ing. H. Niemann
	Prof. Dr. med. Dr. rer. nat. U. Eysholdt

Acknowledgments

This thesis is the result of a cooperation between the Institute of Pattern Recognition (formerly "Chair for Pattern Recognition") with two other institutes at the University of Erlangen-Nuremberg, namely the Department of Phoniatrics and Pedaudiology (head: Prof. Dr. Dr. Eysholdt) and the research group for Audio Communications and Computational Acoustics (head: Prof. Dr. Kellermann) at the Chair of Multimedia Communications and Signal Processing. Hence, there are many colleagues I would like to thank for their fruitful cooperation.

First of all, I wish to thank my supervisors, Prof. Dr. Heinrich Niemann and Prof. Dr. Dr. Ulrich Eysholdt, for their reviews of this thesis, and also Prof. Dr. Walter Kellermann for being the external examiner, and the chairman of the exam, Prof. Dr. Wolfgang Schröder-Preikschat.

The working group of Prof. Dr. Kellermann supported us during the experiments on speech in reverberated environment. Just as an example, I would like to mention the great support of Dipl.-Ing. Herbert Buchner when we had to design and record the EMBASSI corpus within a few days, and the software for artificial reverberation that we received from Dr. Wolfgang Herbordt.

Our cooperation partner for the evaluation of substitute voices was the Department of Phoniatrics and Pedaudiology. The colleagues there recorded patients and control groups and prepared the human evaluation of these data. I would like to thank Prof. Dr. Frank Rosanowski who put a great deal of effort in the application for funding and for chairing the project, PD Dr. Maria Schuster for organizing the recording sessions and data acquisition, Dr. Hikmet Toy for recording the speech data, and the "human raters" Prof. Dr. Peter Kummer, PD Dr. Jörg Lohscheller, and Prof. Dr. Dr. Ulrich Hoppe.

In the name of all participants of the research project, I would like to thank the Deutsche Krebshilfe (German Cancer Aid) for their funding of the project.

All the members of the speech group at the Institute of Pattern Recognition supported my work by answering many questions or providing me with programs and scripts. I wish to thank PD Dr. Elmar Nöth for his proof-reading of this thesis and many helpful hints, Dr. Georg Stemmer, Dipl.-Inf. Christian Hacker, and Dipl.-Inf. Stefan Steidl for their help with the speech recognizer, Dipl.-Inf. Viktor Zeißler for his help with the prosody module, and especially Dipl.-Inf. Andreas Maier for supporting my entire work on pathologic voices. I would also like to thank all the other current and former "pattern recognizers" for being just great colleagues, and our students Korbinian Riedhammer, Tobias Bocklet, and Martina Bellanova for their assistance in maintaining all the data we produced.

Finally, I would like to thank my parents who supported me as much as only they could and kept a lot of work at home away from me.

Abstract

In 20 to 40 percent of all cases of laryngeal cancer, total laryngectomy has to be performed, i.e. the removal of the entire larynx. For the patient, this means the loss of the natural voice and thus the loss of the main means of communication. A popular method of voice restoration involves a shunt valve ("voice prosthesis") between trachea and pharyngoesophageal segment which establishes the tracheoesophageal (TE) substitute voice. From time to time, the substitute voice has to be evaluated by the therapist for the purpose of reporting therapy progress. This evaluation is subjective; it is therefore dependent on the particular expert's experience and similar factors. In the frame of this thesis, it was examined how automatic methods can be used in order to provide an objective means of the evaluation of substitute voices.

There are some established objective measures which are, however, restricted to the evaluation of sustained vowels. In this thesis, the step from the automatic analysis of vowel recordings to text recordings is done. For judging speech quality objectively in a real communication situation, the analysis of entire words and sentences is necessary because the intelligibility of a substitute voice in a dialogue is a substantial criterion for evaluation. Automatic word recognition methods were applied to a standard text that was read out by the test persons. Information on the intelligibility of the individual speakers was gained by the comparison of word recognition rates with reference evaluation data from human experts. The use of a prosody module allowed to extract not only acoustic information on the speaker's voice, but it also measured individual speaking characteristics.

The inter-rater variability among humans was compared to the automatic analysis results, and the main finding was that the correlation between human and automatic ratings was as good as the agreement among the human rater group.

The automatic recognition could be slightly improved on distant-talking recordings by the use of μ-law features which are modified Mel-Frequency Cepstrum Coefficients (MFCC). Artificially reverberated training data for the recognizer is another possibility to achieve better recognition rates even when the reverberation in the test data does not match the acoustic properties of the training data. This is a step towards a therapy session where the patients will not be required to wear a headset any more.

Contents

List of Figures

List of Tables

Chapter 1

Introduction

In 20 to 40 percent of all cases of laryngeal cancer, total laryngectomy has to be performed, i.e. the removal of the entire larynx [TMF01]. For the patient this means the loss of the natural voice and thus to lose the main means of communication. For all affected persons, this is an outstanding stigma [DSK94]. Dependent on the oncological therapy, different methods of voice restoration can be applied. Some of them involve rarely used surgical methods, the esophageal substitute voice and electronic aids. Besides these, the use of shunt valves ("voice prostheses") in order to create a substitute voice has become more and more popular in the USA in the last 25 years; for Germany there was a delay of about one decade [AS92, HAA+90, Rob84].

Today, voice rehabilitation with shunt valves is regarded "state-of-the-art" [BHIB03, Blo00]. But although speech rehabilitation has been improved substantially, many problems and complications associated with laryngectomy, like the loss of nasal function (smelling, humidification of the airstream), poor cough, swallowing difficulties and changes in lung function are still present. After getting a shunt valve, patients have to undergo therapy in order to learn speaking again. From time to time, the substitute voice is evaluated by the therapist for the purpose of reporting therapy progress. This thesis will introduce methods for objective, automatic voice and speech evaluation. It is based upon the cooperation of the Chair of Pattern Recognition at the University of Erlangen-Nuremberg (Technical Faculty) with two other research institutes at the same university. The first one is the Department of Phoniatrics and Pedaudiology of the University Hospital[1] in Erlangen which was the partner for the analysis of substitute voices. The second one, for the field of recognition of reverberated speech, is the Chair of Multimedia Communications and Signal Processing[2].

1.1 The Need for Objective Evaluation

The evaluation of the substitute voice by the patient and by other persons is subjective at first. This holds also for the therapists because the currently available technical methods for objective voice analysis, like the Hoarseness Diagram (Chapter 2.5.4), have not been adapted to substitute voices yet. This means that the medical personnel must rely on its experience. In this thesis, the correlation between subjective evaluation by humans and objective automatic means of evaluation will be examined.

---

[1]http://www.phoniatrie.uni-erlangen.de
[2]http://www.lnt.de/lms

The raters' experience has a very large influence on the inter-rater agreement. Professional backgrounds and experience or knowledge of the patient's history may result in high intra- and inter-rater variability [FPB$^+$05]. Professionals, even more when they are closely working together, may show a much higher concordance on the same rating criteria than semi-professionals, such as speech therapy students or even naïve listeners [MMB$^+$06, DRF$^+$96]. Sometimes the inter-rater variation is avoided by a "forced" consensus of the raters before the final score is further processed [PJ01]. This, however, requires the involvement of more than one expert which is exactly the opposite of the desired quick and inexpensive evaluation.

For the development of automatic methods, subjective evaluation data have to be collected as a reference first. This holds for the rating of speech criteria, like e.g. the use of prosody by the patient, but also for acoustic parameters like the intensity of the voice or the maximum phonation time. However, comparison between different former studies on this topic is almost impossible since many researchers had a very restricted amount of data because of a low number of patients. In the literature, many contributions can be found based upon speaker groups of single-digit size. A lot of researchers developed their own rating criteria for speech and voice quality (see Chapter 2) which makes it complicated to find analogies among them. The speech data used for evaluation is very different, too. For measuring voice parameters, many studies use sustained vowels only, others employ words or sentences. The analysis of these data becomes more complicated because researchers measure different quantities. Whereas maximum phonation time, for instance, is a quite common measure, some other groups prefer parameters like the duration of an arbitrarily chosen sentence or even the "intensity in millimeters" on some analog output which might be very hard to reproduce. In order to reduce the variability in speaker groups and to get an impression what speech quality is possible in substitute voices, Bellandese et al. suggested that a study on this task should only involve speakers that were rated as excellent [BLG01]. The result of such a study, however, cannot be generalized to non-excellent speakers and would not support the search for real objective analysis methods.

The setup of evaluation studies is also very important for their universal validity. During intelligibility tests, for example, the amount of data presented to the listeners should be large enough to prevent playing back the same data more than once in order to avoid learning effects with the listeners. In a study with 50 college students as listeners, the intelligibility of normal and tracheoesophageal (TE) substitute voices (Chapter 2.2.5) in noisy conditions were compared [MFP$^+$98]. The test persons were one normal speaker and one TE speaker reading a sentence pair from a standard text [Fai60]. The background noise was multi-voice babble from the Speech Perception in Noise test (SPIN, [KSE77]). The test recordings were presented to the listeners once without noise and after that with added noise at different intensities. During each session, the listeners had to judge how intelligible the speech sample was. Although the study yielded interesting results, the evaluation may have been highly affected by the fact that all listeners heard the same two sentences by the respective speaker all the time. It seems to be very unlikely that the findings reveal independent or even "objective" measures.

The given examples show that there is a real need for a compact set of automatically computable, objective evaluation criteria in speech therapy, even more since several researchers just define "objective" evaluation as the average or consensus of several subjective ratings. With the large amount of studies on small data, this might not be a consistent and valid definition. The standardization of voice evaluation must already begin at the time of data acquisition. This procedure, however, is dependent on the goal of the speech therapy as the next section will point out.

1.2 Towards Screening in Natural Settings

For the purpose of comprehensive documentation of a voice, the European Laryngological Research Group (ELRG) recommended five essential items in voice assessment [DBC+01]:

- videostroboscopy

- acoustic analysis

- aerodynamic measures

- perceptual ratings

- self-evaluation, i.e. ratings by the patient him- or herself

The physically most unpleasant assessment for the patient is the videostroboscopy because it means bringing an endoscope into the mouth and recording the glottis or – in the case of substitute voices – the pseudoglottis (see Chapter 2.2.2).

The goal for the future of voice assessment must be to reduce the effort or even pain for the patient as far as possible. Another important point is to reduce the psychological pressure on the patient. The ideal situation for the test person would be one where the patient can act freely and does not have the impression of being watched or controlled. For the case of the perceptual ratings, this thesis tries to give some solutions. In the ideal case, the patient would be able to speak without wearing a headset during recording. If the recording is done by a distant-talking microphone, then the awareness of the currently running evaluation would be reduced enormously. Speech recognition in reverberated environment is an important topic in this thesis. Furthermore, the subject should be able to speak spontaneously, i.e. there is a normal dialogue between patient and therapist which serves as the audio data for later analysis. However, completely free speech is not suitable for automatic evaluation due to several reasons, like the out-of-vocabulary problem or varying average word duration due to different words used by different speakers, for instance. For this reason, a phonetically rich standard text with a defined vocabulary was read out by the test speakers and analyzed afterward. Nevertheless, this is a large enhancement of established objective measures which are restricted to the evaluation of sustained vowels. Typical features in objective analysis are automatically computed from frequency (e.g. jitter) or amplitude (e.g. shimmer) of parts of the voice signal, or they can be gained from time-determined measures, like the duration of words and sentences, or the maximum phonation time [BLG01, PFKB89, Rob84]. The position of the formants [CMG01] and the voice onset time [RCK86, SKA00, SC02] are also taken into account. While the computation of the acoustic parameters from jitter, shimmer, etc. is done automatically, determining the duration of a text or phrase is often still done by listening to the recording.

In the case of vowel durations, viewing the voice or speech signal graphically on a monitor and then measuring the wanted times by hand was very common at the beginning of the 1990s. The staff expense is very high in these experiments, even more if more than one rater is consulted in order to reach a certain degree of objectivity [GW83].

For judging speech quality objectively in a real communication situation, the analysis of entire words and sentences is necessary because the intelligibility of a substitute voice in a dialogue is a substantial criterion for its self-evaluation and evaluation by experts [AS92, MFP+98, SKA00]. Especially the communication via telephone is affected here [MZ96, MMG93, ZP86] because due to the band-limitation of the telephone channel the voice is deteriorated even more, and no possibility of supporting the communication by facial or hand gestures is available.

The analysis of telephone calls is an aspect that might ease the situation for the patients. The telephone is a crucial part of social life. Laryngectomees are often older than 70 or even 80 years (see Chapter 4.4), and it is necessary for them to have a means of communication that does not require them to leave their home. And when these persons need some kind of help, they will very likely use the telephone to call the doctor or their relatives. Another aspect that has to be considered is that their social companions are often older persons, too, which may lead to problems on the listener's side [Cla85]. Therefore, the voice evaluation over a telephone reflects a communication situation which is important for the patient. If an objective rating of the intelligibility of telephone speech could be part of the clinical evaluation of voice rehabilitation, this would be very comfortable for the affected persons, and it would be a step towards a more global evaluation of post-laryngectomy speech.

Perceptual voice evaluation is subjective in the first place since it is performed by a human expert. Furthermore, the experiments described in the literature assume a certain kind of listening experience with substitute voices [DDRS98] which does primarily not reflect the patient's everyday situation. The subjective and objective methods for measuring the voicing function that are currently used in speech therapy mostly do not correspond to the standard of the technically possible voice and speech analysis. In the frame of this thesis, it was examined how such methods can be used in order to provide an objective means of the evaluation of substitute voices. The next section gives an overview of approaches that were examined.

1.3   Contributions Made in this Thesis

In this thesis, the step from the automatic analysis of vowel recordings to text recordings is done. The new methods require only a standard computer and microphone; they are also designed for internet-based evaluation. It was examined

- whether automatic measures can be obtained that can objectively describe and evaluate tracheoesophageal substitute voices,

- whether the objective parameters correlate well with evaluation criteria of human raters,

- and whether the objective evaluation is also possible via telephone or using a distant-talking microphone.

The speech recognizers for the experiments with TE speakers were trained with normal-speaking persons because it was important for the evaluation that the system simulates a naïve listener, i.e. a human being that never heard TE speech before. This is the situation that the patients face in their daily life. Nevertheless, the effect of the interpolation of the acoustic models with TE speech recordings was examined.

Human rating criteria in speech therapy are usually intelligibility, vocal tone, quality, use of prosody during speaking, etc. The correlations of these human scores to the word accuracy of the speech recognizers were determined for a set of TE speech files. They were also obtained for automatically computed prosodic features which represent voice onset time or word and pause durations, for instance.

For several experiments, the intelligibility rating was focused since it is the most important criterion in voice evaluation by humans. An automatic version of the Post-Laryngectomy Telephone Test (PLTT) is introduced. This test was originally developed for human listeners in order to represent the communication situation via telephone. Additionally, the word accuracy and the prosodic features were processed together by leave-one-speaker-out multi-correlation/regression analysis in order to determine the measures that represent the intelligibility criterion best.

For speech therapists, it might be very helpful to get a graphical visualization of pathologic speech. The Sammon mapping performs a topology-preserving reduction of data dimension. It minimizes a "stress function" between the topology of the low-dimensional Sammon map and the high-dimensional original speech data. In this thesis, the ability of Sammon maps to express human rating criteria was examined.

For the speech recognition in reverberated environment, speech corpora of normal speech were employed which contain synchronously recorded close-talking and distant-talking portions. Different methods were tested in order to enhance the recognition results of reverberated test data. The main difference to most other studies is that the target environment was assumed to be unknown at training time, i.e. the test data were recorded in another environment than all of the training data. In order to create a "universal" recognizer for close-talking and reverberated test data, the training sets were partially or entirely reverberated artificially using many different room characteristics.

Mel-Frequency Cepstrum Coefficients (MFCC) were the features used for the baseline recognizer. However, the logarithmic compression of the filterbank coefficients may be disadvantageous on noisy data. Therefore, alternative features were tested. The root cepstrum and the "μ-law features" which are based upon a compression method used in telecommunications replace the logarithm by other functions that are supposed to avoid these problems.

As no distant-talking data from laryngectomees were available, the root cepstrum and the μ-law features were tested on artificially reverberated TE speech signals in order to simulate a therapy session where no headset is used. These features were also tested with simulated telephone speech.

Synchronous recordings of the test data were combined by delay-and-sum beamforming as a preprocessing step in order to create a new signal with less noise. This test set was processed by recognizers using different features and artificially reverberated training data.

1.4 Overview

This thesis is organized as follows:

Chapter 2 introduces different ways for establishing a substitute voice, like e.g. surgical methods or the esophageal voice. The focus is on tracheoesophageal (TE) voices. The properties of several voice restoration approaches are compared, and subjective evaluation methods that are used in speech therapy are introduced. Objective measurements for voice quality will be discussed in detail including commercial applications.

Chapter 3 describes measures that are used to determine the agreement between human raters or between a human rater and the automatic evaluation of a speech signal. Namely, the correlation coefficients by Pearson and Spearman are compared to Cohen's κ and its extensions, and Krippendorff's α is introduced as a powerful alternative.

Information about the speech corpora used for the experiments in this thesis can be found in Chapter 4. The EMBASSI corpus and the Fatigue corpus are available in different signal qualities and were therefore used for improving the recognition in reverberated environment. Parts of the VERBMOBIL corpus served as training data for all speech recognizers. For the recordings of the laryngectomized test speakers, also human evaluation results were obtained as reference for the automatic evaluation. The respective information is also summarized in this chapter.

An important topic of the work on the speech recognition system was the search for speech features that are more robust against reverberation than Mel-Frequency Cepstrum Coefficients in order to improve the automatic recognition of distant-talking speech data. Adaptation of Hidden Markov Models to TE speech was performed in order to improve the recognition results of substitute speech. The graphical representation of speech data from the phone model adaptation and the prosodic analysis were further essential aspects for the evaluation. For the theoretical principles of these methods, see Chapter 5.

In Chapter 6, the results on the speech recognition in reverberated environments are summarized. This includes experiments with artificially reverberated training data in order to cover as many unknown test environments as possible. The improvements of the results by modified MFCC as features are described as well as the combination of signals from more than one microphone (beamforming) in order to eliminate noise in the respective test signals.

The experiments on automatic evaluation of substitute voices are described in Chapter 7. The agreement between human evaluation and the automatically obtained measures is pointed out in detail for the intelligibility criterion which is represented best by the word accuracy of the speech recognizer, and for the prosodic analysis of TE speech data. The intelligibility on the telephone is measured by the automatic version of the Post-Laryngectomy Telephone Test. The effects of reverberation in the test signals and recognizer adaptation on the recognition results are also explained. Finally, the visualization of substitute voices by the Sammon transform is presented.

Major findings of other research groups and their comparability with this thesis are summarized and discussed in Chapter 8. Future work and possible extensions of the evaluation methods are presented in Chapter 9. Chapter 10 summarizes the entire thesis.

Chapter 2

Tracheoesophageal Substitute Voices

This chapter gives an overview on voice rehabilitation after total removal of the larynx. Different kinds of substitute voice will be introduced. The focus is on tracheoesophageal voices which restore the original functionality better than earlier approaches. Their acoustic properties and measures for automatic evaluation will be discussed in detail.

2.1   Laryngectomy

The production of speech uses three main functional components. The first one is respiration, i.e. breathing. The initiation of an airstream is followed by the second component known as phonation: the airstream causes cyclic opening and closing of the vocal folds which in this way produce pulses – the actual voice. The third component is the articulation which means that the organs of the upper vocal tract, like the tongue or the lips, modify the pulse train. After total laryngectomy, all of the mentioned aspects are altered. With a healthy person, the larynx is positioned between the trachea and the pharynx (see Figure 2.1). It is located in the neck where the pharynx branches off into the digestive part (esophagus) and the airway (trachea). It has got two main functions [Loh03]:

- Working like a valve, it allows a connection of the pharynx either to the esophagus or to the trachea. In this way, it controls the airflow during breathing and prevents aspiration during swallowing, i.e. nutrition will not get into the airway.

- It is the voicing generator of a "normal", *laryngeal* voice.

The primary voice generator are the two parallel vocal folds. The gap between them is called the glottis. An airstream exceeding a certain threshold sets them into vibration which in turn modulates the airstream [Tit76, TS97, Ber58]. The specific vibration behavior of the vocal folds is caused by their histology which is explained in detail e.g. in [Hir74, Loh03]. Irregularities are perceived as hoarse, creaky or dry voice sound [Loh03, p. 9].

During laryngectomy the larynx is removed, and the trachea is connected to a new opening for breathing in the front of the neck, the *tracheostoma*. After the procedure, the trachea and the esophagus stay separated (see Figure 2.1). The consequences are manifold. Problems with breathing occur because the respiratory resistance is much lower than before which leads to less blood oxygen saturation. The inspiratory air is no longer filtered, moistened and warmed causing

7

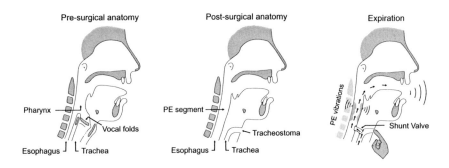

Figure 2.1: Anatomy of a person with intact larynx *(left)*, anatomy after total laryngectomy *(middle)*, and the substitute voice *(right)* caused by vibration of the pharyngoesophageal segment (pictures after [Loh03, Chapter 2])

higher rate of infects and irritation. The psychic consequences, like the loss of social contacts and depressions, have to be considered as well [HAA$^+$90, AHAB94, TMP$^+$84].

By restoring the ability to communicate by voice, the quality of life will be enhanced. Some approaches to achieve this to a certain extent are described in the following sections. Together with laryngectomy, more surgery can be done in order to improve the substitute voice [DDRS98, BPC91, WBJR94]. This may be necessary when also partial or total removal of the pharynx (pharyngectomy) was required due to advanced stages of cancer.

2.2   History of Substitute Voices

After laryngectomy the first means of communication is pseudo-whisper. It corresponds to "real" whisper, but because of the missing airstream from the lungs only the small air volume in the mouth can be used for speaking. The different phonemes have to be formed accurately in order to get an intelligible result at all. Furthermore, the surroundings have to be very quiet [Zen93].

2.2.1   Different Kinds of Voice Rehabilitation

The first laryngectomy was performed by Billroth in Vienna in 1873, and already at that time voice rehabilitation was regarded very important. For the very first patient, a kind of voice replacement was introduced by Billroth's assistant Gussenbauer [Gus74]. However, the mortality rate after surgery was high, and the later on established separation of the ways for air and nutrition brought a quick end of such substitute voice approaches. From the beginning of the 20th century onwards, mainly three different kinds of voice restoration were developed [Hag97]:

- The *esophageal substitute voice*: The patient learns to swallow air and release it back through the pharynx where the tissue vibrations can be used for voicing (see Chapter 2.2.2).

- Surgical methods creating a stable and open connection between trachea and pharynx with the body's own tissue: These artificial fistulae have the same purpose as a shunt valve (see below), but they avoid the dependence of material that has to be brought into the body (see Chapter 2.2.4).

- Methods using extrinsic material: This covers mechanical sound generators which are brought in the nose or mouth, and electrical sound generators (Chapter 2.2.3) which are hand-held and placed at the outside of the neck in order to amplify vibrations and thus produce a hearable voice [Sch97a]. Also shunt valves between the tracheostoma and the pharynx belong to this group. The resulting *tracheoesophageal (TE)* substitute voice, caused by tissue vibrations in the pharyngoesophageal segment (see Figure 2.1), is the object of interest in the experiments described in this thesis. For details on this kind of voice rehabilitation, see Chapter 2.2.5.

2.2.2 The Esophageal Substitute Voice

At the beginning of the 20th century, the esophageal[1] substitute voice became the only kind of voice restoration because it does not need any technical support [Gut09]. Still today, it is very common in many countries, also in the USA and in Germany [Hag90b, SD01, Zen93].

In the esophageal voice, the cervical esophagus serves as *pseudoglottis*, and the pharynx and stomach can be used as air reservoir [See22]. Vibration – and thus the voicing source – has its origin in the pharynx at the level between the fourth and sixth cervical vertebra ([BHIB03], cf. Chapter 2.3.1). The patients either press air back into the pharynx and esophagus with their tongue (injection method) or produce a pressure in the esophagus that is lower than the atmospheric pressure and causes air to flow to this area (inhalation method). Another possibility is to swallow air into the stomach which, however, often causes stomach problems. The controlled relief of the air back past the pharyngoesophageal segment is then used for voicing and causes a low-pitched, guttural sound (ructus). No aspiration is possible due to the complete separation of trachea and esophagus, and the patient does not need a finger to close the tracheostoma as it is the case with the tracheoesophageal voice (Chapter 2.2.5). However, it takes several months or even years until laryngectomees can control this kind of voice, and as the air volume in the mouth is only about 80 ml on average while the vital capacity of the lung reaches about 3 liters, only short syllables can be uttered [BMD58, Die68, CFM92]. Some physical parameters and other evaluation measures for the esophageal voice and other voice types are summarized in Table 2.1 and presented in detail in Table 2.5, 2.6 and 2.7.

2.2.3 Electrical Sound Generators

The voicing function of the larynx can be replaced by a sound generator. In most cases it is electrically operated and is therefore called *electrolarynx*. The device is either held to the outside of the neck, to the floor of the mouth or placed intraorally. The sound can then be modulated by the tongue, lips, or the teeth [SD01, WM95]. An important feature of this kind of voice rehabilitation is that the voice production is completely independent from breathing. This has consequences mainly for uttering consonants, because only the small air volume in the mouth can be used to form them. The quality of these voices is often, however, not satisfactory as it sounds very "robot-like" and monotone. Furthermore, the patient is always dependent on some (electrical) device for speaking. The intelligibility of the voices is about at the same level as for

---

[1]In British English, the spelling "oesophageal" is used.

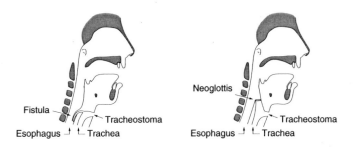

Figure 2.2: Surgical voice rehabilitation methods by Conley [CAP58] with a mucosa tunnel between trachea and esophagus *(left)* and Staffieri [Sta81] featuring a slit-shaped neoglottis *(right)*

esophageal voices (see Table 2.1). By 1990, both in the USA and in Germany 28% of all laryngectomees used this kind of external electronic vibrators, like e.g. the Servox® device[2] [Hag97]. A German study of 1999 [Hum99] reports that only 18% preferred the electrolarynx in communication compared to 11% using esophageal (Chapter 2.2.2) and 71% using tracheoesophageal speech (Chapter 2.2.5). For an overview of the available devices, see e.g. [BHIB03].

2.2.4 Surgical Methods

Several different surgical methods tried to allow the redirection of expiratory air from the trachea into the pharynx by means of fistulae or similar ways, sometimes also establishing a neoglottis which is a surgically provided replacement for the glottis. This has the advantage that the voicing pressure is lower in comparison to shunt valves ([Hag97], cf. Table 2.1) and that the voice fistulae are made from the body's own material. However, all these approaches faced the problem of aspiration. When the patient eats or drinks, it is often not possible to close the way to the larynx completely which can have serious consequences. Spontaneous closure or inflammation of the natural links are further problems. Application of these methods reached its summit in the third quarter of the 20th century ([CAP58, Asa65, Ars72, Sta81]; see examples in Figure 2.2). Further methods were developed in Germany after 1980 [Hag90b, EWP+85, MW94], but the purely surgical methods were not a breakthrough in voice rehabilitation, and so by 1989 less than one percent of the patients in Germany (Federal Republic) and 15% in the USA underwent this kind of treatment [Hag90a]. More than two thirds of the patients in Germany (69%) learned to use the esophageal voice, in the USA this portion already had gone down to 49% due to the introduction of shunt valves (30%, Chapter 2.2.5) which were still rarely used in Germany by then (6%).

2.2.5 The Tracheoesophageal (TE) Substitute Voice

The idea of connecting the trachea and the esophagus for diverting air into the esophagus and thus cause voicing was described first by Guttman in 1932 [Gut32, Gut35]. However, problems by infections and fistula stenosis prevented the spread of this technique. The first commercialized voice prosthesis was developed by Taub et al. [TS72, Tau75]. It was an external

---

[2]http://www.servox.com

voicing time	duration (s)	average (s)
laryngeal voices	15–25	20
esophageal voices	1–5	3
surgical shunt methods	2–20	10
voice prostheses	7–18	11
voice intensity	volume (dB)	intra-individual dynamics (dB)
laryngeal voices	50–100	$\leq$50
esophageal voices	50–70	$\leq$20
surgical shunt methods	55–90	$\leq$30
voice prostheses	64–95	$\leq$28
tracheal pressure	pressure (kPa)	flow resistance (Pa·s/ml)
laryngeal voices	0.8–2	$\approx$4
esophageal voices	n/a	n/a
surgical shunt methods	0.5–6	$\leq$20
voice prostheses	2–8	$\leq$50
intelligibility	PLTT (%, Chapter 7.4)	one-syllable test [SH87] (%)
laryngeal voices	>90	87
good esophageal speakers	$\approx$65	43
Servox® device	$\approx$65	40
voice prostheses	79	44

Table 2.1: Physical parameters and other evaluation measures of different voice types [Hag97]

prosthesis connected to both the trachea and an esophago-cutaneous fistula and could only be used for patients who had not undergone radiotherapy. It was unhandy and expensive, and it was therefore forgotten again soon. The development of the so-called shunt valves by Singer and Blom [SB80, BSH82] were an important step towards a better communication skills after laryngectomy. During exhaling, the patient can divert the airstream from the lungs through the valve from the trachea into the pharyngoesophageal segment (PE segment, see Figure 2.1). In order to do so, the tracheostoma must be closed with a finger.

The time for learning to speak with a tracheoesophageal (TE) voice is much shorter than for an esophageal voice. Almost immediately after surgery, the patient may produce the first sounds. The main difficulty here is the proper closing of the tracheostoma. For over 90% of laryngectomized persons, the shunt valve means an immediate restoration of their voicing function, and 65% of the patients keep on using the TE voice permanently [BSC92, BSH86, HB93, LGM+96, Jan03]. Blom et al. examined the rehabilitation progress of 29 TE patients (19 males, 10 females). 81% of the speakers were more fluent 12 months after surgery, the mean pause time during reading decreased significantly between 3 weeks (25%) and 6 months (21%). In the same time period, the speaking rate, mean fundamental frequency (F_0), harmonics-to-noise ratio (Chapter 2.5.2), and percentage of periodic phonation during reading increased significantly [BPH95].

The TE voice has its origin in the same mechanism as the esophageal voice (see Chapter 2.2.2), but due to the valve between trachea and esophagus it is possible to use the entire lung volume for voicing. This allows a much longer maximum phonation time (see entry "MPT" in Table 2.7). The tracheoesophageal puncture can be done already during the laryngectomy, so basically no more surgery has to be performed for voice rehabilitation. Shunt valves are often also called voice prostheses, but this expression is actually not correct. A prosthesis is a replacement for a lost organ which is not the case here. The valves are no sound generators, they only serve for deviating air into the esophagus.

Shunt valves are classified into two categories (cf. e.g. [Sch97b]). The first one are the so-called *non-indwelling prostheses* which are supposed to be changed or cleaned by the doctor or rather the patient him- or herself from time to time. One popular type is the Blom-Singer prosthesis, the original version was also known as "duckbill". The modern variant basically comes in two diameters, namely a 16 french[3] and a wider 20 french valve. For good accessibility of the shunt, the diameter of the tracheostoma should be 1.5 to 2 cm [Blo95]. The original slit valve of the "duckbill" was also enhanced and is nowadays known as ESKA-Herrmann prosthesis [Her86]. Most of the other valves available feature a flap valve.

The second category are the *indwelling prostheses* which are purely clinician-maintained. Many patients do not want to change and clean their prosthesis themselves. For this reason, shunt valves are used today which do not have to be changed regularly. Popular types of these valves are:

- **The Provox® valve:** This low-resistance, indwelling device was developed at the Netherlands Cancer Institute in 1988 [HS90, HCB93]. The improved version Provox® II is available with 6 different diameters between 4.5 and 15 mm since 1997 (see Figure 2.3). Its main advantage is that it can be inserted and removed in an anterograde manner, i.e. through the tracheostoma, while the original version had to be replaced using a retrograde method, i.e. through the mouth [HAB+97, AHM+99]. The length of the indwelling prosthesis is 8 to 10 mm in most cases. Lifetime of a Provox® prosthesis was reported

---

[3]1 french = 1 Charrière = 1/3 mm

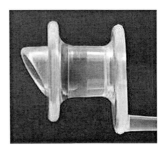 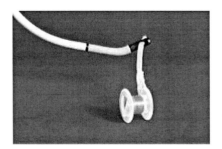

Figure 2.3: Original Provox® *(left)* and Provox® II shunt valve with guide wire for its retrograde insertion *(right)*; the flange is cut off afterward. The images are courtesy of Atos Medical AB, Sweden.

to range from 4 to 10 months (see overview in [BHIB03]), candida deposits on the valve being the main reason for replacement. All patients whose speech data are used in this thesis (see Chapter 4.4) are equipped with one of the two generations of this shunt valve.

• **The Groningen prosthesis:** This type is also called Groningen button [NASL82, NS87, SN02] and is similar to the Provox® valve, but it has an easier construction scheme.

• **The Blom-Singer indwelling prosthesis:** In use since 1994, the newest version from 2005 features e.g. silver oxide as a material preservative for longer use without being replaced [LE97, InH00].

• **The VoiceMaster prosthesis:** It was introduced in 1998 and has the advantage that it has a very low airflow resistance [VGS01, ESVB01].

An important requirement to a shunt valve is that it has to open quickly when an attempt for voicing is made and be completely closed when the patient doesn't speak. The airflow the valve has to allow for not obstructing the voicing function was reported with 350 ml/s, measured with the Groningen button [NS87].

The Department of Phoniatrics and Pedaudiology of the University Hospital in Erlangen was one of the first institutions in Germany that systematically introduced the voice restoration of laryngectomees by low-pressure shunt valve voice prostheses in 1990. The foundations were laid by a long-term cooperation with the working group of Prof. Hilgers in the Netherlands Cancer Institute at the Antoni van Leeuwenhoek Hospital in Amsterdam. About 20 patients a year have to undergo total laryngectomy in Erlangen. 283 patients had received voice prostheses, mainly of the Provox® type, by the end of 2002.

Although transplantation of an entire larynx can be performed successfully already (see e.g. [SSE⁺01]), this is not possible for persons who suffered from cancer due to the effects of radiotherapy . For this reason, shunt valves will probably stay the method of choice for voice restoration for some more years.

2.2.6 Stoma Filters and Stoma Valves

Usually tracheoesophageal speakers have to close the tracheostoma with a finger directly to divert the expiratory air into the hypopharynx. This, however, does not only draw the attention of other persons which is often inconvenient for the patients, but it also has to be done accurately which is a problem for many of the elderly patients. Furthermore it is unhygienic and not possible in situations like when driving a car.

The tracheostoma can be equipped with a heat and moisture exchanger (HME) preserving the airways from getting cold and dry [AHA+93, GBB+97]. Then the speaker touches the filter and not the stoma directly. For the Provox® system, such a filter was introduced in 1996 [HABG96]. If the tracheostoma is covered with a Provox® Stomafilter, then the digital occlusion of the stoma allows longer phonation time and a larger dynamic range than with "direct digital occlusion". No statistically significant differences between the acoustic parameters of fundamental frequency (F_0), amplitude, tremor, and harmonicity for both stoma occlusion methods were found [AHKA98].

In order to achieve real hands-free speaking, the patients can be supported by a tracheostoma valve which can either be glued onto the stoma [BSH82] or be fixated by remaining chondral tissue [Her86]. It is sensitive to variations in airflow. During normal respiration it remains open, but if the air pressure rises for speaking it will be closed and force the air to flow through the shunt valve. Except for the absence of the stoma noise, the voice properties and quality are not affected [PFKB89]. For the Provox® system, the "FreeHands HME" was developed that combines a stoma filter and a stoma valve [HAA+03]. Some of the speakers in the data collection for this thesis spoke with such a valve, some used a stoma filter during recording (Chapter 4.4).

The quality of the TE voice can be further improved by shunt valves containing a small pneumatic sound source, such as a lip reed [TMF01]. Furthermore, in case of a flaccid or hypotonic vibratory segment, the use of a neck strap to increase the tone of the PE segment can improve the voice [KD99]. These approaches were not used with the patients examined for this thesis.

2.3 Properties of Substitute Voices

2.3.1 Dynamics of the PE Segment

Videofluoroscopy and high speed video recording indicated that vibrations of the pharyngoesophageal segment (PE segment; Figure 2.1) are the primary source of substitute voice [OKNF94, SGO91, WRM+85]. A research group at the Department of Phoniatrics and Pedaudiology at the University of Erlangen-Nuremberg could objectively show for the first time that the PE segment is the origin of the substitute voice. Four different vibration patterns could be identified which can also be evaluated automatically in high speed video recordings [LDS+03, DHH+02]. The dynamics of the PE segment during phonation show a high similarity to the behavior of vocal folds [Loh03, LDR+02]. An introduced model for the latter which reduces the complexity of several aspects of voice production was developed by Ishizaka and Flanagan and is known as the Two-Mass Model (2MM, [IF72]). It describes a vocal fold as a pair of coupled oscillators vibrating due to aerodynamic forces. A simplified version of this model ([SH95a], Figure 2.4) was the basis for the model of the PE segment vibration. Whereas two 2MM are sufficient for a vocal fold model, the PE segment model places several 2MM orbitally onto a horizontal circle. The reason is that the PE segment is an elastic tube where each part of the tissue moves towards the center

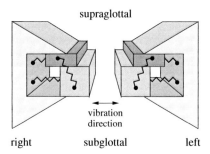

supraglottal

vibration
direction

right   subglottal   left

Figure 2.4: Cross section of the two-mass model of vocal fold vibration by Steinecke and Herzel ([SH95a], picture after [Loh03, p. 67])

	p [cm H$_2$O]	p [Pa at 20 °C]	study
subglottic pressure (normal voice)	4–8	390–780	[DDWU94]
pressure below PE segment	10–40	980–3920	[DDWU94]
trans-TE shunt pressure (without shunt valve)	1–50	100–4900	[KA86]

Table 2.2: Air pressure p in normal and substitute voices

and back more or less during voicing. This model is described in detail in [Loh03]. Due to the different anatomical conditions, the pseudoglottis is often not split-shaped. Schuster et al. identified 6 split-shaped, one triangle-shaped, and 3 circular pseudoglottides in 10 laryngectomees by high-speed video recordings [SRS+05].

2.3.2 Aerodynamic Properties

The aerodynamic properties of substitute voices were examined in several studies. An important measure is the airflow rate through the voicing source. For laryngeal voices it is up to approx. 500 ml/s [Hag97]. Trans-TE airflow rates (without a shunt valve) were measured between 20 and 400 ml/s [KA86]. More than 350 ml/s is sufficient for proper voicing [NS87]. The tracheal pressure is about 800–2000 Pa for normal and 2000–8000 Pa for tracheoesophageal voices ([Hag97], cf. Table 2.1); for further details see Table 2.2. The ratio of tracheal pressure and airflow rate is known as the airway resistance (Table 2.3). Especially for the pseudoglottis, the actual TE voice source, large inter-individual differences were reported. This holds also for the TE shunt when no valve is inserted. It may be both smaller or higher than with a valve. Interestingly, the Provox® II valve (Chapter 2.2.5) has a larger flow resistance than its competitors. In general, tracheoesophageal voice production shows increased trans-source airflow rates, similar source driving pressures and decreased airway resistances in comparison with esophageal voices. In relation to normal laryngeal voice production, it has comparable trans-source airflow rates, increased source driving pressures and increased airway resistances [MW87]. This means that speaking with TE voice takes less effort than with an esophageal voice; it is closer to a normal voice in this aspect.

	R [dyn·s/cm^5]	R [Pa·s/ml]	study
glottis (normal speaker)	30–42	3–4.2	[SH81]
glottis (normal speaker)	35–45	3.5–4.5	[ZMLS91]
esophageal source	100–1220	10–122	[KA86]
TE shunt (without shunt valve)	1–250	0.1–25	[SH81]
Blom-Singer prosthesis	45–120	4.5–12	[WHBS82]
Groningen button	≈100	≈10	[ZMLS91]
Provox® II valve	237	23.7	[STW$^+$06]

Table 2.3: Airway resistance R in normal and substitute voices

2.3.3 Acoustic and Prosodic Properties

Tracheoesophageal speech in communication is perceived as superior to esophageal speech or an electrolarynx [WW87]. The intelligibility of the TE voices is higher than for esophageal voices [DDWU94, AS92, Rob84] and electrical devices ([Hag97], cf. Table 2.1). Furthermore, the melodic, rhythmic, and dynamic accent of the individual original voice and thus the individual way of speaking are kept. Higher formant values than in normal speakers were found in esophageal and also tracheoesophageal speakers in different languages [CMG01, SW72, Kyt64]. The reason for this is the effective vocal tract length which is shorter after laryngectomy [CW76, SW72, DY66]. But still, with poor esophageal and neoglottal speakers the voice quality is so low that listeners are not able to guess even the speaker's sex [AS92, MMG93].

Laryngectomees often show unclear pronunciation without much motion of the articulatory organs. This can be due to complications after surgery, such as partial resection of the tongue, dry mucosa or the loss of teeth as a consequence of radiotherapy, and more. Therefore, the patients can produce phones like /v/, /f/, /d/, /t/, /g/ or /k/ and their combinations with other phones only to a reduced extent [SG97]. Good TE speakers can utter voiced and voiceless sounds which are perceptually distinguishable. Even in TE speakers, voice onset time (VOT) is one of the most important factors for the distinction between voiced and voiceless phones [SKA00, TKMA95]. Closure period and VOT are usually measured in recordings of syllables of the VCV type, i.e. with a voiced-closure-voiced phone sequence, such as /apa/. The voice onset time consists of both the duration of the burst wave and the time needed to restart vibration for the following vowel. Saito et al. showed that for highly intelligible TE speakers both VOT and closure duration are longer than for laryngeal speakers [SKA00]. Searl et al. examined voiced and voiceless stops and fricatives in different places of production in recordings of nonsense words [SC02]. They found that consonant intensity, consonant duration, mean vowel duration, and standard deviation are larger for TE speakers; the voice onset time is also mostly longer with TE speakers than with normal speakers. In general, the results of the few available studies are often in contrast to each other (cf. also [RCK86]) which may be caused by the different setups of the experiments and the audio material.

Gandour and Weinberg state that TE speakers are able to produce simple intonational contrast (e.g. rise vs. fall) as good as normal speakers [GW83] although laryngeal speakers differ significantly from alaryngeal speakers in F_0 (see Table 2.1 and 2.5) and intonation production due to the reduced motor control of the tissue in the PE segment [SC02, MTM00].

The properties of substitute voices that were described in this section have an influence on the perceptual impression that human beings have when listening to speech. However, humans do not describe their impressions in terms of physical measurements. For the evaluation of voice and speech pathology in the frame of speech therapy, other ways of describing a voice were defined. These will be introduced in the following.

2.4 Subjective Evaluation Methods

The voice evaluation by speech therapists and the self-evaluation by the patients often differ substantially [SKER03]. Therefore, not only the expert's opinion is considered for the individual rehabilitation concept. Nowadays, the self-evaluation plays a much stronger role in speech therapy than in earlier times. There are several tests on quality of life and coping strategies that were also applied with the test patients for this study. Some of them are presented below.

2.4.1 Subjective Evaluation Criteria

Voice evaluation by humans is usually done in the following way: The patient reads out a standard text, and the rater fills out a printed evaluation sheet. It contains several rating criteria, and each one of them gets some kind of score. These scores may be numerical or category-based, i.e. describing the criterion in words, like in the widely used Likert scales[4] [Lik32]. The range of a numerical score might be continuous with a lower and an upper bound, like in the case of the visual analog scales (VAS, [Fre23]). This means that the rater has to mark his or her decision on a line or bar of a certain length (cf. the "overall quality" criterion in Table 4.12). The distance of the mark to the beginning serves as the numerical score. This method was used with substitute voices e.g. by van Gogh et al. [GFV+05]; their scores were converted to values between 0 and 100. Many more studies evaluate on the basis of integer scores. Van As defined bipolar 7-point scales which means that the end points of the scale were denoted by "very good" and "very bad", or similar descriptions concerning the respective criterion. 19 rating criteria were defined for naïve raters and 20 scales for the trained raters [AKPH03]. However, a lot of them correlated with each other, and the evaluation was complicated for the raters due to the high number of similar criteria. For this reason, most other studies propose between 5 and 10 rating criteria. From the criteria used by van As, Moerman et al. defined a set of eight new ones in [MPM+04] which are (1) "hypotone/hypertone", (2) "fluency", (3) "voice onset", (4) "additional noise", (5) "intonation", (6) "speech rate", (7) "intelligibility" and (8) "general impression". The scores, marked on analog scales, were converted to integer values between 0 and 9. Ainsworth and Singh used 5-point scales for the criteria "normal", "intelligible", "rate" (speaking rate), "rhythm" and "intonation" [AS92]. The importance of intelligibility, "normality", and the fluency and prosody of speech for the evaluation of substitute voices are also shown in Bellandese's study where the rating criteria were named "stoma noise", "understandability", "voice quality", "rate of speech", and "speaking fluency" [BLG01]. Each of them is judged on a 4-point scale to rate speaking proficiency. That article gives also a detailed overview on the criteria used in former studies. Since the speech data used for this thesis were evaluated by experienced raters, 11 different criteria were used, most of them on 5-point Likert scales (see details in Chapter 4.4.3). For experiments with a group of naïve listeners, the number of criteria was reduced to 5. This study will not be described in detail here, it can be found in [BSH+06].

---

[4]after Rensis Likert (1903–1981), pronounced /lɪkɛt/

However, 5-point scales do not seem to be the optimum, although they are widely used in some of the common voice evaluation tests that will be introduced below [JJG+97, HS99, WS92]. Especially for experienced listeners, it is not convenient to limit their discriminative capacity to 5 grades. The reliability of the test is not necessarily reduced if there are reasonably more than 5 or 7 grades per rating category [CG00].

2.4.2 The GRBAS and RBH Scale

The GRBAS scale [Hir81] describes voice quality by five dimensions. Each one of them is rated on a 4-point scale between '0' (no abnormality) and '3' (severe abnormality) on the basis of further 4-point integer subscales. The dimensions correlate with physiologic and psychoacoustic quantities; the latter are important for the purpose of automatic evaluation as they reflect computable measures [YSAN03]:

- **"Grade (G)"**: the overall impression of abnormality in voice

- **"Roughness (R)"**: the perceived degree of pitch[5], amplitude and noise in the lower frequency regions

- **"Breathiness (B)"**: the perceived degree of noise in the mid-frequency region

- **"Asthenia (A)"**: reflects lower content of harmonic frequencies in the upper frequency region, irregularity in F_0 and amplitude, and a fading amplitude contour

- **"Strain (S)"**: probably corresponds to higher F_0, noise in the upper frequency region, increased amplitude of the higher harmonics, and increased F_0 and amplitude perturbation

However, the GRBAS scale has some drawbacks on severely pathological voices, therefore an alternative was developed by Moerman et al. [MMB+06]. It is based on the parameters "impression", "intelligibility", "noise", "fluency" and "voicing", abbreviated as "IINFVo". Each one of them was rated on a visual analog scale between 0 (very bad score) and 10 (very good score) and then converted to an integer number between 0 and 3, just like in the GRBAS scale. A high correlation ($r = 0.92$) was reported between the first two criteria which is also consistent with the findings in Chapter 4.4.4. The impression criterion was canceled, the final rating scale is called "INFVo".

An important rating system for dysphonic speech in German-speaking countries is the RBH scale [NAW94]. It allows integer scores between 0 and 3 for the three dimensions "Roughness", "Breathiness", and "Hoarseness" (in German: "Rauigkeit", "Behauchtheit", "Heiserkeit"). The basic rule for voice evaluation defined by the authors of the RBH scale is that the total hoarseness score must not be better than any of the scores for the components of the other two dimensions.

2.4.3 Self-Evaluation Scales (VHI, V-RQOL, SF-36)

For the self-evaluation of the restriction in voicing, the Voice Handicap Index (VHI) is an established method. Its original version was in English [JJG+97]; the Department of Phoniatrics

---

[5]Note that "pitch" denotes a perceptual impression; it is often used as synonym for F_0 in the literature.

and Pedaudiology at the University of Erlangen-Nuremberg adapted it for the German-speaking countries [SKER03]. The VHI consists of three 10-item subscales (functional, emotional, and physical). Typical items are e.g. the following:

- "My voice makes it difficult for people to hear me." (functional)

- "I tend to avoid groups of people because of my voice." (emotional)

- "I run out of air when I talk." (physical)

The test persons rate each of the 30 items on a 5-point scale (0 to 4) where the single points are named as "never", "almost never", "sometimes", "almost always", and "always" to indicate how frequently the subject has the respective experience. The functional, emotional, and physical subscales are calculated as the sum of the responses to the 10 items in each scale.

The total Voice Handicap Index is the sum of the scores on the three subscales, i.e. it is expressed by a numerical score between 0 (no handicap) and 120 (maximum handicap). In a study with 21 male and 2 female German TE speakers equipped with a Provox® valve, the total VHI score in the group was on average 39.3 with a standard deviation of 11.4 [SKER03]. Physical restrictions were rated higher (14.9) than functional (12.9) and emotional restrictions (11.5). Additionally, the patients rated their own voice on average with 1.6 units on a possible integer scale from 0 (normal voice) to 3 (very low quality). When the VHI ratings by the patients were compared to the ratings by 7 experts, neither between corresponding criteria like "hoarseness" or "speaking effort" nor between the global self-evaluation and evaluation by experts a significant correlation could be measured. However, single items of the expert's rating correlated with statements made by the patients about problems during telephone calls, being not understood, the avoidance of communication situations, or psychic problems due to the voice disability. For details see [SLH+04].

The *Voice-Related Quality Of Life* measure (V-RQOL, [HS99]) consists of 10 items which are rated by the patient on an integer scale between 1 ("none, not a problem") and 5 ("as bad as it can be"). The items are similar to those of the VHI. Another very important means of self-evaluation is the *SF-36®* health survey [WS92]. 36 items covering 8 dimensions are rated by integer numbers on 2-point to 6-point scales. The German version was introduced by Bullinger and Kirchberger [Bul95].

The self-evaluation of the patient's coping strategy can for instance be obtained by the TSK survey ("Trierer Skalen zur Krankheitsbewältigung") where 37 items are rated on 6-point scales and afterwards combined to express 5 dimensions describing the subject's main activities to cope with the impairment [KF93].

2.4.4   Conclusion

In general, the usability of subjective evaluation methods depends on their domain. For self-evaluation (Chapter 2.4.3), the emotional and psychic aspects are as important as the quality of the substitute voices. For evaluation by other persons, the latter is usually the only aspect that is taken into account because human raters very often evaluate by listening to recordings and have no direct contact to the patients. The criteria from the GRBAS and RBH scale (Chapter 2.4.2) are focused on voice properties rather than on speech evaluation. Since it was the topic of this thesis to extend the introduced automatic analysis methods to text recordings, criteria like intelligibility

and speech fluency had to be taken into account. They cannot be obtained from vowel recordings. Based upon the studies described in Chapter 2.4.1, a set of rating criteria was defined (see
Chapter 4.4.3). These served as a reference for the automatic text evaluation.

When evaluating speech pathology, medical sciences traditionally distinguish between impairment, disability, and handicap. "Impairment" refers to a problem with a structure or organ of
the body, "disability" is a functional limitation, and "handicap" refers to a disadvantage in filling
a particular role in daily life [WHO80]. Methods for speech evaluation are often oriented towards these categories or towards the newer revisions by the World Health Organization, respectively [WHO01, Jon01]. Automatic evaluation as described in this thesis, however, processes a
speech signal only and is therefore not able to differentiate between these aspects. It corresponds
to the perceptual evaluation of disability by human raters.

2.5 Objective Evaluation Methods

Perceptual voice analysis by humans is time-consuming and expensive [GFV$^+$05]. Furthermore,
the evaluation is dependent on the particular rater's professional experience; other persons might
not be able to understand or reproduce it. Therefore, the automation of the task by the extraction
of objective measures from voice or speech recordings is desired. Many objective measures have
already been proposed several years ago [GHSS05, QBC88, Dim89]. The "properties of substitute voices" which were introduced in Chapter 2.3 are already objective evaluation measures,
because they are gained by deterministic measuring methods. In this section, more complex
criteria will be introduced which are based on simpler approaches or combine them.

2.5.1 A Model for Alaryngeal Voices

For the mathematical description of normal voices, often the model of glottal flow by Liljencrants and Fant is used ("LF-model", [FLL85]). In the case of a pathologic or a substitute voice,
however, this model cannot be applied any more because its four parameters are not enough to
describe harsh, creaky or breathy voices, for example.

An extended model based upon five easily measurable parameters was introduced by Qi and
Weinberg [QW95]. Figure 2.5 shows the parameters obtained from the airflow function $U(t)$
and its derivative $U'(t)$, measured during sustained vowel phonation. Three timestamps on the
trajectory of the derivative are important for further computation. These are the time t_0 where
$U'(t)$ exceeds a user-defined threshold for the first time, the time t_p where $U'(t)$ crosses the zero
line, i.e. when $U(t)$ is at its maximum, and t_c where the absolute value of $U'(t)$ falls below the
threshold again at the end of the period. One of the parameters of the model is the fundamental
frequency F_0 which is computed from the measured fundamental period T. The other parameters
are the relative position of maximum flow reduction (t_e), the open quotient

$$OQ = \frac{t_c - t_0}{T} \quad , \quad (2.1)$$

the speed quotient

$$SQ = \frac{t_p - t_0}{t_c - t_p} \quad , \quad (2.2)$$

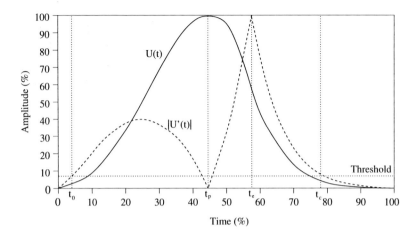

Figure 2.5: Parameters measured from the glottal airflow function $U(t)$ during sustained vowel phonation [QW95, p. 539]; the derivative $U'(t)$ is shown normalized and in absolute values.

and the relative area under the flow function

$$A = \frac{\int U(t)\,\mathrm{d}t}{U(t_p) \cdot (t_c - t_0)} \qquad . \qquad (2.3)$$

The source waves $U(t)$ of laryngeal speakers look homogeneous and show a quasi-periodic, triangular shape. The waves of esophageal speakers are not homogeneous. It was, however, possible to identify four characteristic categories with distinct patterns [QW95]. The source waves produced by the TE speakers in that study were also not homogeneous. Several speakers featured an open quotient OQ outside the range of normal speakers. For normal speakers, the distribution of the relative area A under the flow function is compact which also holds for the distribution of the TE speakers. The difference in overall voicing properties, however, showed no significant differences between normal and TE speakers while both groups significantly differed from the esophageal speakers. For the single parameters, with the exception of open quotient OQ, however, significant group effects could be measured. Significance was reached between normal and TE speakers for the mean speed quotient SQ. The properties computed on recordings of the vowel /a/ are subsumed in Table 2.4. Qi and Weinberg did not examine whether the approach is able to distinguish "good" from "bad" speakers within one specific speaker group. The results of their experiments indicate that it is not possible. Furthermore, the flow analysis has a crucial disadvantage. The volume velocity has to be measured with a tight face mask and expensive instruments while the evaluation of an audio recording does not require special hardware. For this reason, the following sections will introduce methods to obtain appropriate measurements from sound files.

measure	laryngeal	esophageal	TE
F_0 mean (/a/)	132 Hz	82 Hz	86 Hz
F_0 st. dev. (/a/)	27 Hz	48 Hz	27 Hz
open quotient OQ mean	0.62	0.50	0.63
open quotient OQ st. dev.	0.11	0.25	0.18
speed quotient SQ mean	1.40	1.02	1.01
speed quotient SQ st. dev.	0.25	0.49	0.28
rel. pos. of max. flow reduction t_e mean	63.4%	38.0%	63.8%
rel. pos. of max. flow reduction t_e st. dev.	11.5%	12.2%	16.8%
rel. area of flow function A mean	56.0%	49.9%	59.1%
rel. area of flow function A st. dev.	3.5%	5.6%	5.0%

Table 2.4: Source signal properties of different voice types, measured with normal speakers (10 male), esophageal speakers (8 male and 2 female), and TE speakers (9 male and 3 female, [QW95, p. 545])

2.5.2   Objective Measures and Analysis

Robbins et al. used principal component analysis (PCA) on a set of duration measures in order to identify the least redundant subset that allows to classify recordings of a sustained vowel and recordings of a standard text into one of the groups "laryngeal", "esophageal" and "tracheo-esophageal" automatically. Mean intensity during reading, mean maximum phonation time and number of words per phrase were the three measures that differentiated all three groups ([Rob84], cf. Table 2.5, 2.6 and 2.7). However, duration measures cannot give information about the acoustic quality of the voice. For this purpose, frequency-based methods have to be applied. Usually, objective evaluation relies on sustained vowels only [PJ01]. This vowel is /a/ in most of the cases, spoken at normal communication intensity and recorded by a headset. For analysis, it is often selected due to its sensitivity for jitter [Hor80, PC89]. Some other examples are known where additionally the vowels /i/ and /u/ are examined [MPM+04, WP03, BP83]. Mendelsohn et al. measured latency and duration of the consonant /s/ in analysis of telephone speech [MMG93].

Fundamental frequency: The fundamental frequency F_0 (i.e. periodicity) is the most important feature in all acoustic voice category systems [GFV+05, LJR01]. Its variation is also very important for the task. Due to the high degree of aperiodicity, only few TE speakers can be analyzed by usual frequency-based methods [AHKA98]. Indeed, the binary voiced-unvoiced decision is sometimes more helpful than numerical F_0 values (see Chapter 7.3). Debruyne et al. state that it is easier to detect F_0 in TE than in esophageal voices, although the mechanism for voicing is, except for the different air supply, the same [DDWU94].

Jitter: Jitter, i.e. fluctuations of F_0, is a typical measure for irregularity. It is applied to acoustic or electroglottogram signals (EGG, [BKG+96, Kli91, Sat05]), or to signals describing the spatial vibrations of vocal folds [Döl02]. Many studies involve the "percent jitter". The time Δt_k between the maxima of two successive oscillations defines the duration of cycle k in milliseconds.

The jitter (in percent) for the number n of pharyngoesophageal cycles is then given as

$$J = \frac{\sum_{k=1}^{n} |\Delta t_{k+1} - \Delta t_k|}{\sum_{k=1}^{n} \Delta t_k} \cdot 100 \quad . \tag{2.4}$$

It represents the percentage of jitter which considers the dependence of absolute jitter on the F_0 level (jitter relative to average F_0). Like for F_0, it is often difficult to compute jitter in highly pathologic voices. Moerman et al. consider F_0 values within 25% of the mean over all voiced frames as "reliable" and thus suitable for the computation of jitter [MPM+04]. They performed speech/non-speech classification for 10 ms frames by computing the average energy of five surrounding frames and marking the frame as speech when for its energy E held $E > 1.25E_{min} + 0.05E_{max}$. For combined high-speed video and audio recordings of the PE segment of 9 TE speakers, Lohscheller reports percent jitter J_{PE} between 5.3% and 23.2%, obtained from the video sequence. The jitter from the corresponding audio signal J_{ac} ranged from 1.7% to 22.9%. The reasons for the differences in both measures are the different sample rate for audio and video channel and the fact that the PE vibrations are a 3-D movement while the audio signal is one-dimensional [Loh03, p. 53].

Shimmer: Analogous to jitter, shimmer describes the perturbations in intensity. Like percent jitter, shimmer S is often given as a percentage relative to the mean intensity in n samples which is computed from the intensity values I_k in all samples k:

$$S = \frac{\sum_{k=1}^{n} |I_{k+1} - I_k|}{\sum_{k=1}^{n} I_k} \cdot 100 \tag{2.5}$$

The time over which jitter and shimmer are computed varies across different studies. Moran et al., for instance, involve 3, 5 and 55 fundamental periods [MRCL06]. Robbins et al. examined jitter, shimmer and several measures derived from them in normal, esophageal and TE voices [RFBS84a, RFBS84b], confirming that the acoustic quality of TE voices is much closer to normal voices than esophageal voices. Results are summarized in Table 2.5, 2.6 and 2.7 (see also the parameters measured from airflow in Table 2.4).

Harmonics-to-Noise Ratio (HNR):

$$\mathrm{HNR} = 10 \cdot \log_{10} \frac{E_p}{E_{ap}} \tag{2.6}$$

is the harmonics-to-noise ratio computed from the energies E_p in the harmonic or periodic signal and E_{ap} in the aperiodic noise components. They are obtained from the quefrency domain of the cepstrum whose lower region corresponds to the vocal tract system; the region around the highest cepstral peak at the fundamental period expresses the harmonic part of the excitation, and the remaining region corresponds to the noise part of the excitation [LJW+04, YAD98, Kro93]. For details on the computation of the HNR, see e.g. [MRCL06, RML04, Kro93] or the overview in [Bud00]. HNR is often computed in several frequency bands. In the frequency area of the first formant, it was reported between 22 and 31 dB for normal laryngeal voices. TE speakers only reach about 1 to 9 dB [FBMP96]. HNR (or the signal-to-noise ratio SNR [Bud00]), jitter and shimmer in voiced speech are sufficient to discriminate between normal and pathologic

measure	laryngeal sp. #subj.	value	esophageal sp. #subj.	value	TE speakers #subj.	value	study
F_0 mean (/a/)	10 m	120 Hz	10 m	64 Hz	10 m	89 Hz	[Blo84]
F_0 mean (/a/)	15 m	103 Hz	15 m	65 Hz	15 m	83 Hz	[RFBS84a]
F_0 mean (/a/)	10 m	132 Hz	8 m/2 f	82 Hz	9 m/3 f	86 Hz	[QW95]
F_0 mean (/a/)	10 f	179 Hz	9 f	107 Hz	7 f	119 Hz	[BLG01]
F_0 st. dev. (/a/)	10 m	4 Hz	10 m	11 Hz	10 m	19 Hz	[Blo84]
F_0 st. dev. (/a/)	15 m	24 Hz	15 m	31 Hz	15 m	43 Hz	[RFBS84a]
F_0 st. dev. (/a/)	10 m	27 Hz	8 m/2 f	48 Hz	9 m/3 f	27 Hz	[QW95]
F_0 st. dev. (/a/)	10 f	17 Hz	9 f	54 Hz	7 f	37 Hz	[BLG01]
F_0 range (/a/)	10 m	20 Hz	10 m	40 Hz	10 m	61 Hz	[Blo84]
F_0 range (/a/)	15 m	6 Hz	15 m	74 Hz	15 m	40 Hz	[RFBS84a]
F_0 mean (reading)	10 m	121 Hz	10 m	65 Hz	10 m	88 Hz	[Blo84]
F_0 mean (reading)	12 m/3 f	128 Hz	4 m/1 f	84 Hz	4 m/1 f	108 Hz	[PC89]
F_0 mean (reading)	15 m	103 Hz	15 m	77 Hz	15 m	102 Hz	[RFBS84a]
F_0 mean (reading)	10 f	178 Hz	9 f	112 Hz	7 f	148 Hz	[BLG01]
F_0 mean (reading)	—	—	—	—	10 f	109 Hz	[TQ90]
F_0 st. dev. (reading)	10 m	6 Hz	10 m	15 Hz	10 m	20 Hz	[Blo84]
F_0 st. dev. (reading)	12 m/3 f	39 Hz	4 m/1 f	10 Hz	4 m/1 f	34 Hz	[PC89]
F_0 st. dev. (reading)	15 m	15 Hz	15 m	23 Hz	15 m	23 Hz	[RFBS84a]
F_0 st. dev. (reading)	10 f	21 Hz	9 f	34 Hz	7 f	49 Hz	[BLG01]
F_0 st. dev. (reading)	—	—	—	—	10 f	18 Hz	[TQ90]
F_0 range (reading)	10 m	16 Hz	10 m	44 Hz	10 m	61 Hz	[Blo84]
F_0 range (reading)	12 m/3 f	129 Hz	4 m/1 f	177 Hz	4 m/1 f	170 Hz	[PC89]
F_0 range (reading)	15 m	86 Hz	15 m	118 Hz	15 m	142 Hz	[RFBS84a]
F_0 range (reading)	—	—	—	—	10 f	70 Hz	[TQ90]
jitter mean (/a/)	15 m	0.1 Hz	15 m	4.1 Hz	15 m	0.7 Hz	[RFBS84a]
jitter mean (/a/)	—	—	—	—	10 f	1.8 Hz	[TQ90]
jitter st. dev. (/a/)	15 m	0.1 Hz	15 m	4.4 Hz	15 m	0.9 Hz	[RFBS84a]
jitter st. dev. (/a/)	—	—	—	—	10 f	0.6 Hz	[TQ90]

Table 2.5: Acoustic properties of different voice types (derived from F_0 and jitter); subjects are abbreviated as 'm' (male) or 'f' (female).

measure	laryngeal sp. #subj.	value	esophageal sp. #subj.	value	TE speakers #subj.	value	study
intensity mean (/a/)	10 m	84	10 m	73	10 m	80	[Blo84]
intensity mean (/a/)	15 m	77	15 m	74	15 m	88	[RFBS84a]
intensity st. dev. (/a/)	10 m	5.1	10 m	6.4	10 m	8.6	[Blo84]
intensity st. dev. (/a/)	15 m	0.8	15 m	3.5	15 m	1.2	[RFBS84a]
intensity mean (reading)	10 m	84	10 m	70	10 m	82	[Blo84]
intensity mean (reading)	15 m	70	15 m	59	15 m	79	[RFBS84a]
intensity mean (reading)	—	—	—	—	10 f	71	[TQ90]
intensity st. dev. (reading)	10 m	7.9	10 m	7.4	10 m	8.2	[Blo84]
intensity st. dev. (reading)	—	—	—	—	10 f	5.2	[TQ90]
intensity range (reading)	15 m	14	15 m	11	15 m	14	[RFBS84a]
shimmer mean (/a/)	15 m	0.3	15 m	1.9	15 m	0.8	[RFBS84a]
shimmer mean (/a/)	—	—	—	—	10 f	1.9	[TQ90]
shimmer st. dev. (/a/)	15 m	0.2	15 m	1.6	15 m	0.6	[RFBS84a]
shimmer st. dev. (/a/)	—	—	—	—	10 f	1.6	[TQ90]
SNR mean	10 f	14.9	9 f	−1.9	7 f	−2.2	[BLG01]
SNR st. dev.	10 f	2.4	9 f	2.5	7 f	2.2	[BLG01]
HNR mean	88 m+f	25.2	—	—	—	—	[MFS98]
HNR mean	—	—	—	—	12 m/12 f	−1.8	[PFKB89]
HNR mean	—	—	—	—	19 m/10 f	0.8	[BPH95]
HNR st. dev.	88 m+f	3.6	—	—	—	—	[MFS98]
HNR st. dev.	—	—	—	—	12 m/12 f	5.2	[PFKB89]
HNR st. dev.	—	—	—	—	19 m/10 f	1.5	[BPH95]

Table 2.6: Acoustic properties of different voice types (derived from intensity and shimmer); subjects are abbreviated as 'm' (male) or 'f' (female). The measures from [RFBS84a] are given in dB (A), i.e. perception characteristics of the human auditory system are considered; all other values are in dB (SPL) regarding the physical measure of sound energy only.

measure	laryngeal sp. #subj.	value	esophageal sp. #subj.	value	TE speakers #subj.	value	study
syllables/min	10 f	249	9 f	186	7 f	201	[BLG01]
syllable dur. mean (ms)	15 m	220	15 m	310	15 m	280	[RFBS84a]
syllable dur. st. dev. (ms)	15 m	30	15 m	56	15 m	43	[RFBS84a]
words/min	15 m	173	15 m	99	15 m	128	[RFBS84a]
words/min	12 m/3 f	159	4 m/1 f	94	4 m/1 f	152	[PC89]
words/min	—	—	—	—	10 f	138	[TQ90]
words/min st. dev.	15 m	23	15 m	25	15 m	21	[RFBS84a]
words/min st. dev.	12 m/3 f	24	4 m/1 f	23	4 m/1 f	16	[PC89]
words/min st. dev.	—	—	—	—	10 f	40	[TQ90]
words/phrase	15 m	9.8	15 m	3.0	15 m	7.2	[RFBS84a]
words/phrase	12 m/3 f	12.2	4 m/1 f	3.6	4 m/1 f	8.1	[PC89]
words/phrase st. dev.	15 m	2.6	15 m	0.9	15 m	1.4	[RFBS84a]
words/phrase st. dev.	12 m/3 f	1.4	4 m/1 f	0.7	4 m/1 f	1.0	[PC89]
pause time mean (ms)	15 m	625	15 m	650	15 m	890	[RFBS84a]
pause time mean (ms)	—	—	—	—	10 f	1300	[TQ90]
pause time st. dev. (ms)	15 m	195	15 m	135	15 m	215	[RFBS84a]
pause time st. dev. (ms)	—	—	—	—	10 f	1100	[TQ90]
% pause time	15 m	18	15 m	36	15 m	24	[RFBS84a]
% pause time	—	—	—	—	10 f	31	[TQ90]
% pause time st. dev.	15 m	6.0	15 m	6.7	15 m	5.6	[RFBS84a]
% pause time st. dev.	—	—	—	—	10 f	12.2	[TQ90]
% periodicity	15 m	80	15 m	42	15 m	78	[RFBS84a]
% periodicity st. dev.	15 m	8.0	15 m	11.0	15 m	15.5	[RFBS84a]
MPT mean (s)	15 m	22	15 m	2	15 m	12	[RFBS84a]
MPT mean (s)	12 m/3 f	25	4 m/1 f	2	4 m/1 f	16	[PC89]
MPT st. dev. (s)	15 m	9.1	15 m	0.7	15 m	5.2	[RFBS84a]
MPT st. dev. (s)	12 m/3 f	5.4	4 m/1 f	0.6	4 m/1 f	5.7	[PC89]

Table 2.7: Duration measures of different voice types; subjects are abbreviated as 'm' (male) or 'f' (female). "MPT" means "maximum phonation time".

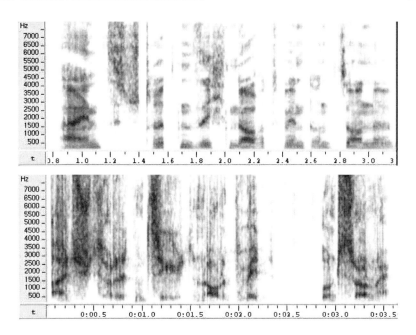

Figure 2.6: Spectrum of the first phrase ("Einst stritten sich Nordwind und Sonne") of the text "The North Wind and the Sun" (see Appendix A.1) from a normal and a TE speaker

speakers [MRCL06, MFS98, Kro95]. It was, however, not examined whether it is also possible to divide these two classes into further subgroups, like e.g. "good" and "bad" TE speakers. According to van Gogh et al., there are three categories of TE voices [GFV⁺05]:

1. good voices with low-frequency harmonics, and noise taking over at higher frequencies,

2. moderate voices consisting of repetitive bursts of sound energy with low repetition rate and a weak periodicity due to high levels of voice in all frequencies,

3. poor voices with no detectable or very weak F_0 or envelope periodicity.

Figure 2.6 contains the spectra of recordings of a normal and a TE speaker. The high noise level in the substitute voice is clearly visible. Only the voices from the first two categories could be reliably analyzed automatically and correlated well to perceptually evaluated voice quality parameters in van Gogh's study. HNR was found to be associated with "gurgling" sound, F_0 represented the voice criterion "deviancy". F_0, intensity, F_0 stability (jitter), HNR in low and mid-frequencies, and high frequency noise were the measures that were suitable for the automatic analysis, and also F_0 salience (in dB) which denotes the peak level in a spectrum region relative to the average level in a region around this peak. Van Gogh found that F_0 salience below 7 dB defined voices of category 3, between 7 and 11 dB of category 2 and above 11 dB of category 1.

Linear Prediction Coefficients (LPC):   Like HNR, the spectral slope is significantly smaller in severely pathologic noisy voices. It is obtained as follows: When a voice signal is analyzed by Linear Prediction (LP, [AS67]), and the logarithmic spectrum of the all-pole LP filter is available, the polynomial coefficients of a 1st-order linear function are computed. The function fits the discrete spectral data, its slope is the spectral slope which is independent of F_0 [LJW$^+$04]. Further objective measures based on Linear Prediction Coefficients were used by Gu et al. [GHSS05]. One of them is the Itakura-Saito Distortion Measure (IS; cf. [HP98]):

$$\text{IS}(\boldsymbol{a}_d, \boldsymbol{a}_\varPhi) = \left(\frac{\sigma_\varPhi^2}{\sigma_d^2}\right) \cdot \left(\frac{\boldsymbol{a}_d \boldsymbol{R}_\varPhi \boldsymbol{a}_d^T}{\boldsymbol{a}_\varPhi \boldsymbol{R}_\varPhi \boldsymbol{a}_\varPhi^T}\right) + \log\left(\frac{\sigma_\varPhi^2}{\sigma_d^2}\right) - 1 \qquad (2.7)$$

Here, $\sigma_\varPhi^2$ and σ_d^2 represent the all-pole gains for the average normal speaker and the average test patient, respectively. The LPC vectors for both speaker groups are $\boldsymbol{a}_\varPhi$ and $\boldsymbol{a}_d$. The normal speech is available as sequence of samples $x_\varPhi(k)$, its autocorrelation matrix is $\boldsymbol{R}_\varPhi$. The Log-Likelihood Ratio (LLR; see also [WH96, TY99]) is similar to the IS measure – without considering the variance terms, however:

$$\text{LLR}(\boldsymbol{a}_d, \boldsymbol{a}_\varPhi) = \log\left(\frac{\boldsymbol{a}_d \boldsymbol{R}_\varPhi \boldsymbol{a}_d^T}{\boldsymbol{a}_\varPhi \boldsymbol{R}_\varPhi \boldsymbol{a}_\varPhi^T}\right) \qquad (2.8)$$

In the study of Gu et al., these measures were compared to a 5-point rating scale of human listeners evaluating the dysarthric speech of 14 patients with Alzheimer's disease. Their correlation to the speech quality score was best for IS ($r = 0.76$) and remarkably worse for LLR ($r = 0.64$). The application of these measures on substitute voices might be interesting because there are similarities of the examined type of voices to substitute voices, like the possibly hoarse sound and the reduced ability of articulation. However, this holds for voices with a low degree of pathology only. In severe cases there will be problems due to the high aperiodicity. The autocorrelation function will not be very successful on these signals. Moreover, the described measures are only suitable for recordings of vowels again, so the approach was not further examined in this thesis.

Formant Analysis: Vowels are expected to have a harmonic structure with peak amplitudes close to the harmonics, i.e. the multiples of the F_0. The first two formants, together with vowel duration, are the most relevant parameters in human vowel perception [CMG01]. Formant frequencies, their bandwidths, and the FFT spectrum of amplitude measurements were used for objective voice evaluation by Wokurek et al. [WP03]. The formants were estimated as the pole frequencies of the LPC. The voice quality parameters open quotient (OQ), glottal opening (GO), skewness of glottal pulse (SK), rate of closure (RC), amplitude of voicing (AV), and completeness of closure (CC), identified in [SH95b, Slu95, CDJ$^+$98], could then be obtained. While all parameters except RC could distinguish between male normal speakers and male pathological speakers, only OQ and AV could do the same for female speakers. The reason for this might be the higher energy loss due to less complete glottal closure and a stronger spectral tilt in female speakers [HC99].

Approximate Entropy: An example for the use of the electroglottogram (EGG) for objective voice evaluation of male larynx cancer patients was given by Manickam et al. [MMW$^+$03]. Their test persons were no laryngectomees but patients after organ-preserving radiotherapy. Perturbations in the spectrum of the electroglottogram were determined by computation of the Approximate Entropy (ApEn, [Pin91]). This measure states the probability of a sequence of two patterns in the spectrum where the second one is not similar to the first one, i.e. the value of ApEn rises with the degree of irregularity. If a sequence s_n consists of n measured values and m denotes the length of a subsequence, i.e. a pattern, then $p_m(i)$ is the pattern of length m beginning at measurement i. Two patterns $\omega_m(i)$ and $\omega_m(j)$ are called similar when the difference between all corresponding pairs of measurements in them is smaller than a given similarity criterion r. P_m denotes the set of all patterns of length m within s_n, and $v_{im}(r)$ is the number of patterns in P_m that are similar to $\omega_m(i)$. With

$$\gamma_{im}(r) = \frac{v_{im}}{n - m + 1} \qquad (2.9)$$

and

$$\gamma_m(r) = \frac{1}{n} \sum_{i=1}^{n} \gamma_{im}(r) \quad , \qquad (2.10)$$

the ApEn is defined as

$$\text{ApEn}(s_n, m, r) = \ln \frac{\gamma_m(r)}{\gamma_{m+1}(r)} \quad . \qquad (2.11)$$

In the experiments described in Manickam's study, the quality enhancement one year after radiotherapy could be measured, and the correlation to the similarly raised subjective ratings was promising. However, the method has the big disadvantage that it does not use speech signals which can be recorded much easier than an electroglottogram.

Since acoustic parameters are very hard to obtain from severely pathologic voices, Li et al. proposed a two-step classification scheme. The severe cases should be eliminated from the evaluation first, then the second step should classify normal and less noisy voices [LJW$^+$04]. This means, however, in view of an automatic evaluation system, that there must be some objective features defining what a "severely pathologic" voice is. These again must be automatically computable which is, according to the assumption, not possible. Therefore, it might be a better way to process all test data equally and do some validity check on the results afterward.

As pointed out before, for the frame of this thesis measurements were required that do not only allow to classify a speaker into the classes "normal" or "pathologic"/"TE speaker", but the goal was to find features which are able to do an objective, quantitative description of voice or speech quality within the group of persons with substitute voice. Unfortunately, there is very few information on this particular topic in the literature. From the measures introduced in this section, the fundamental frequency F_0, jitter, shimmer and some other measures derived from these are used in the prosody module that will be described in Chapter 5.5. The final part of the current chapter will give a short summary of two products on objective voice evaluation that are in use for several years already.

2.5.3 The Dysphonia Severity Index (DSI)

The Dysphonia Severity Index (DSI, [WdM$^+$00]) is an objective and quantitative measure of voice quality. It was developed from a database with more than 1000 normal and pathologic voices. More than 45 voice characteristics and measurements were collected for each patient together with a voice quality evaluation according to the grade of hoarseness as described in the GRBAS scale (Chapter 2.4.2). A multivariate statistical analysis revealed 4 parameters that could differentiate between healthy and pathological voices: the maximum phonation time (MPT) in seconds, the highest frequency $F_{0,h}$ in Hertz, the lowest intensity I_l in decibels, and jitter J in percent. The DSI was then defined as:

$$\text{DSI} = 0.13 \cdot \text{MPT} + 0.0053 \cdot F_{0,h} - 0.26 \cdot I_l - 1.18 \cdot J + 12.4 \qquad (2.12)$$

The extremal values of the DSI are +5 for a normal voice and –5 for a severely bad voice. A voice with a DSI of more than 1.6 is considered to be normal. The DSI shows high correlation to the "Grade (G)" measure of the GRBAS scale (Chapter 2.4.2).

2.5.4   The Hoarseness Diagram

A commercial product for analyzing voices is the Hoarseness Diagram (*Göttinger Heiserkeits-diagramm*, [FMSK00, Mic00, MSK97]). It displays its result in a two-dimensional diagram with the axes "irregularity" and "noise" (see Figure 2.7). The basis of the computation is a sustained vowel recorded with a specific microphone provided with the program. The irregularity component representing hoarseness is computed from jitter, shimmer, and short-time cross-correlation of adjacent cyclic periods; on the ordinate the glottal-to-noise excitation (GNE, [MGS97]) describes the breathiness. The GNE is based upon correlations between the Hilbert envelopes of different frequency bands. It is independent from jitter and shimmer and expresses how the voicing is excited by glottal activity or turbulent noise. Thus it is a measure for breathiness. Further measures involved are F_0 mean and standard deviation, pitch perturbation quotient (PPQ) as a measure for jitter [Bud00, p. 140], amplitude perturbation quotient (APQ) as a measure for shimmer [Bud00, p. 158], HNR, furthermore voice turbulence index describing the ratio of high frequency noise energy to the harmonic energy of the signal, and also the short-time cross-correlation of two adjacent cyclic periods. The standard deviation of F_0 was described as valid acoustic parameter for the determination of phonatory stability [ZB92]. While normal voices show hoarseness values of 2.5 to 3 and breathiness of about 0.5 to 1.5, the coordinate values of pathologic voices in the diagram are, dependent on the degree of the disorder, much higher. In extreme cases they reach 9 and 5, respectively [KMZB97].

   The success of the program is undisputed, but it was neither made for substitute voices nor adapted to them. Therefore, especially the computation of the fundamental frequency F_0 is sometimes not successful in the respective test data [TBS+06]. In Chapter 7.3.3, the measures from this program will be compared to the corresponding measures obtained by the prosody module of the Chair of Pattern Recognition.

2.5.5   Summary

In this chapter, the concept of voice rehabilitation with substitute voice was introduced. Since about 1980, many patients whose larynx had to be removed were equipped with a shunt valve between the trachea and the esophagus which allows them to use the entire lung volume for voicing again. Many research studies examined the properties of substitute voices, but often with subjective methods only. For voice therapy, it would be a big advantage if this evaluation could be done automatically because it would be less expensive with respect to time and personnel. The main advantage of automatic methods is their objectivity. Different therapists might evaluate a given voice differently according to their experience (inter-rater discrepancy), and also one single rater might have a different opinion if he or she listens to a voice recording some time

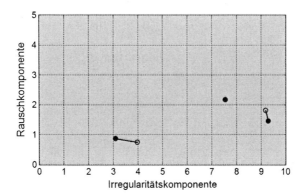

Figure 2.7: Visualization of the vowel /a/ in the Hoarseness Diagram by a normal, an average and a severely pathologic TE speaker (from left to right); the irregularity (abscissa) and the noise component (ordinate) during phonation are depicted. For the samples longer than 500 ms, a second position was computed.

later again (intra-rater discrepancy). Automatic methods are deterministic, their result will not change on the same data, and they can serve as a reference independent from a particular human expert's career. Established methods for objective evaluation, however, analyze only recordings of sustained vowels in order to find irregularities in the voice. This does not reflect a real communication situation. In these approaches, only the voice is examined. For the patient, speech is more important in daily life. Since the automatic processing of completely free speech is very difficult, for this thesis the test persons read a given standard text. This text was then analyzed by methods of automatic speech recognition. The fundamental frequency F_0, jitter and shimmer that were explained in detail in this chapter serve as the basis for prosodic features that combine the evaluation of voice and speech. They will be discussed in Chapter 5.5.

When an automatic method has to be tested on data that were only processed by humans before, then the human evaluation is the only reference that is available. In order to get a representative reference, several raters have to be taken into account. The degree of their agreement and the agreement to the automatically computed results have to be determined by some mathematical method. The following chapter will introduce such approaches.

Chapter 3

Agreement Measures

In the previous chapter, basic measures for automatic voice evaluation have been introduced. When automatic processing of data is supposed to be done, the question arises how to find a reliable reference for the evaluation when all former methods were subjective. For this thesis, the speech data were rated by a group of human experts (see also Chapter 4.4.3) whose average scores were defined to be the reference. For the comparison of the human results among different raters and for the comparison of human and automatic results, appropriate agreement measures have to be applied. This chapter introduces those which were used during the experiments summarized in Chapter 7.

3.1 Correlation Coefficients

3.1.1 Pearson's Product-Moment Correlation Coefficient r

A common way of describing the correlation between two series of real-valued measurements is *Pearson's product-moment correlation coefficient* [Pea01], also denoted as "sample correlation coefficient" and abbreviated as r. Very often it is used as a synonym for the term "correlation". It can be determined for two random variables $X = \{x_1, ..., x_n\}$ and $Y = \{y_1, ..., y_n\}$. They should be normally distributed, otherwise r may not be reliable. The correlation coefficient is then given as

$$r_{xy} = \frac{n \sum_{i=1}^{n} x_i y_i - \sum_{i=1}^{n} x_i \sum_{i=1}^{n} y_i}{\sqrt{n \sum_{i=1}^{n} x_i^2 - (\sum_{i=1}^{n} x_i)^2} \sqrt{n \sum_{i=1}^{n} y_i^2 - (\sum_{i=1}^{n} y_i)^2}} \tag{3.1}$$

or shortly, with use of the mean values μ and the standard deviations σ:

$$r_{xy} = \frac{\sum_{i=1}^{n} [x_i - \mu(x)][y_i - \mu(y)]}{(n-1) \cdot \sigma(x)\sigma(y)} \tag{3.2}$$

For a positive linear relationship between both random variables, r will be positive with a maximum of 1 in the case of perfect correlation. If there is a negative linear relationship, then the coefficient is also negative with a possible minimum of –1. The closer r is to 0, the smaller is the correlation.

It is dependent on the context and the purpose of the particular experiment whether the cor-

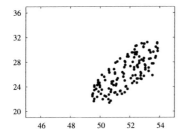 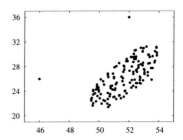

Figure 3.1: Effects of outliers on the correlation coefficients by Pearson (r) and Spearman (ρ):
Left: Data without outliers ($r = 0.76$, $\rho = 0.76$); *Right:* Data with outliers ($r = 0.69$, $\rho = 0.75$).

relation is "good". Nevertheless, Cohen suggested to interprete $|r| \geq 0.50$ as "large" correlation
and $0.30 \leq |r| < 0.50$ as "medium" [Coh88]. For this thesis, Pearson's r serves as a measure for
the correlation between the human evaluation of substitute voices and automatically computed
measures.

3.1.2   Spearman's Rank-Order Correlation Coefficient ρ

By Spearman's correlation coefficient ρ (see e.g. [Spe04] or [Alt91, pp. 285–288]), not the exact
values of the input data are represented but their respective ranks within the ordered values.
The rank of the largest element is set to 1, and the rank of the smallest element is set to n.
Then (3.1) is applied using these ranks instead of the actual data. In this way it describes to which
degree the numerical order in one random variable is kept in the corresponding values of another
variable. In medical and social studies, Spearman's ρ is often used with ordinal data because it
is much less sensitive against outliers in the data than Pearson's r (see Figure 3.1). This is also
valid when, as for the purpose of this thesis, the correlation between ratings by two experts is
computed. A problem arises, however, when a rater has to be compared to a measure which is
not ordinally scaled as it is the case for the word accuracy of an automatic speech recognizer,
for instance (see Chapter 7). The same situation occurs when the ordinal-scaled data of more
than one human rater are averaged. Clinical studies often compare the "average rater" to other
measures which should therefore not be evaluated by Spearman's method. Furthermore, if some
of the input values of one data series are equal, then they get the same rank, too. In this case,
the rank correlation does not make sense. Because of these reasons, Pearson's r will be used
throughout this thesis instead. For selected experiments, however, also ρ will be given where
applicable. For approximately normally distributed data, both correlation coefficients show very
similar values.

For the comparison of a human rater to another one, i.e. measuring the agreement in scores of
the same range, the coefficient r should actually not be applied since it standardizes the scores.
This means that two experts who perfectly agree get $r = 1$, and two coders who always differ by
the same value will also reach $r = 1$. This is one of the reasons why there is a wide variety of
further measures for inter-rater agreement. Some of them are described below.

3.2 Cohen's κ and its Extensions

3.2.1 Chance vs. Competence

When human beings have to evaluate any kind of data using pre-defined categories, then the rater's decision is dependent on many factors that might influence the scoring. In the case of pathologic speech data, the evaluation is done by listening. If a rater caught a cold, for instance, then his or her hearing ability will be reduced which can lead to different results than under normal circumstances. The rater might have also listened to several similar recordings or patients immediately before which can cause a kind of training effect or affect the decision by unknowingly comparing the current patient to the ones before. Because of these facts it is highly recommended to do multiple evaluations of the same data. In clinical research, this is mostly done by different therapists who do their examinations independently of each other.

After the evaluations have been done, it is necessary to find out in what way or to which degree the raters agreed. Two sources of agreement have to be differentiated. The first one is the agreement that occurs by competence, i.e. the agreement that arises from the experience of the raters with the patients and their (speech) data. This is the kind of agreement that is actually interesting for the respective study. It can, however, not simply be extracted from the given data; this is only possible for the *observed agreement* [Kru99] where it is inherent. The other portion is a certain amount of equal ratings possible already by chance which is called *expected agreement*. Therefore, a measure is needed which allows to see the proportion of agreement by competence alone, and a kind of "chance correction" has to be done. Generally, such a measure will look like

$$\kappa = \frac{o - e}{1 - e} \quad (0 \le o \le 1 \, ; \, 0 \le e < 1) \tag{3.3}$$

where o is the observed agreement and e is the portion of matches expected by coincidence. The maximum of κ is 1 when there is perfect agreement between the raters; κ is 0 when the observed agreement is only as high as the portion e that was expected by chance. Note that κ can also be smaller than 0 when the raters show less consensus than expected by chance. One of the first and most widespread measures of the mentioned kind is Cohen's κ [Coh60] which was originally designed for the comparison of two independently generated binary findings. For the experiments described in this thesis, an agreement measure is needed which can handle

- an arbitrary number of raters,

- an arbitrary number of rating categories,

- and a weighting for the cases where raters disagree.

Since the introduction of the κ measure, a lot of extensions have been proposed that fulfill some or even all of these requirements (see overview e.g. in [LK75, Fei85, Dun92] or Chapter 13 of [Fle81]). One of those measures was used for this thesis and will be introduced in Chapter 3.2.4. The mathematical background is described in the following sections.

3.2.2 A Model for Agreement Measuring

The following model for an agreement measure was described by Krummenauer (see [Kru99]). The number $n \in \mathbb{N}$ will always denote the size of a set of data elements which are classified into exactly one of $c \in \mathbb{N}$ categories by $k \in \mathbb{N}$ raters (see also the example in Table 3.1). Such a chance experiment can be described by the indicators

$$X_{ax} = \begin{cases} 1 & \text{``rater } a \text{ chose category } x\text{''} \\ 0 & \text{else} \end{cases} \quad (1 \le a \le k; 1 \le x \le c) \qquad (3.4)$$

and the entire data set by the random variables $X_{ax}^{[1]}, ..., X_{ax}^{[n]}$ with

$$X_{ax}^{[j]} = \begin{cases} 1 & \text{``rater } a \text{ chose cat. } x \text{ for element } j\text{''} \\ 0 & \text{else} \end{cases} \quad (1 \le a \le k; 1 \le x \le c; 1 \le j \le n) \ . \qquad (3.5)$$

Their common distribution is given by the k-variate probabilities

$$\pi_{x_1,...,x_k} = \mathrm{P}(X_{1,x_1} = 1, ..., X_{k,x_k} = 1; \text{ all other indicators} = 0) \qquad (3.6)$$

with $1 \le x_1, ..., x_k \le c$. For pairwise rater comparison, the bivariate marginal distributions

$$\pi_{xy}^{(a,b)} = \mathrm{P}(X_{a,x} = 1, X_{b,y} = 1) \quad (1 \le x, y \le c; 1 \le a < b \le k) \qquad (3.7)$$

are useful. $\pi_{xy}^{(a,b)}$ denotes the probability that an element of the data set is classified to category x by rater a and to category y by rater b. Let finally be

$$\pi_x^{(a)} = \mathrm{P}(X_{a,x} = 1) \quad (1 \le x \le c; a = 1, ..., k) \quad . \qquad (3.8)$$

The measure for observed agreement would then be the diagonal sum concordance

$$o^{(a,b)} = \sum_{x=1}^{c} \pi_{xx}^{(a,b)} \qquad (3.9)$$

which sums up the occurrences of all cases where the results x of two raters a and b match exactly. The agreement between the raters expected by coincidence is given by

$$e^{(a,b)} = \sum_{x=1}^{c} \sum_{y=1}^{c} \pi_x^{(a)} \pi_y^{(b)} \quad . \qquad (3.10)$$

The original work by Cohen [Coh60] proposed a chance-corrected measure as introduced in (3.3) only for the case of two raters and two categories ($k = 2$, $c = 2$). However, many ordinal classification scales used in sociology or medicine offer more than two possibilities to choose from, i.e. $c > 2$ (see Chapter 2.4). In the following section, an appropriate extension of Cohen's κ will be described.

3.2.3 Weighted κ Measures

If two raters do not agree, then not only the fact that they disagree should be taken into consideration but also the degree of disagreement. If one expert rates voice quality with '2' and a second rater with '3', for instance, then there is obviously some more agreement than if the second rater voted for a '5'. Therefore, Fleiss et al. [FCE69] introduced a normalized weighting function $w : \{1, ..., c\}^2 \rightarrow [0, 1]$ with weights $w_{xy} \in [0, 1]$. Then instead of $o^{(a,b)}$, a weighted concordance probability $o^{(a,b)}(w)$ can be applied:

$$o^{(a,b)}(w) = \sum_{x=1}^{c} \sum_{y=1}^{c} \pi_{xy}^{(a,b)} \cdot w_{xy} \tag{3.11}$$

The weights can be chosen as proposed by Cicchetti [Cic76] with

$$w_{xy} = 1 - \left| \frac{x - y}{c - 1} \right| \tag{3.12}$$

or

$$w_{xy} = 1 - \left(\frac{x - y}{c - 1} \right)^2 \quad . \tag{3.13}$$

The original non-weighted version of κ can be expressed by the special cases $w_{xy} := 1$ for $x = y$, and $w_{xy} := 0$ otherwise. The agreement between the raters expected by coincidence is given by

$$e^{(a,b)}(w) = \sum_{x=1}^{c} \sum_{y=1}^{c} \pi_x^{(a)} \pi_y^{(b)} \cdot w_{xy} \quad , \tag{3.14}$$

and the "weighted κ" is defined as

$$\kappa^{(a,b)}(w) = \frac{o^{(a,b)}(w) - e^{(a,b)}(w)}{1 - e^{(a,b)}} \quad . \tag{3.15}$$

Since the true probability values for a given application are usually not available, κ is estimated from the data collection with

$$\hat{\pi}_{xy}^{(a,b)} = \frac{n_{xy}}{n} \quad (1 \le x, y \le c) \quad , \tag{3.16}$$

i.e. the proportion of all cases where rater a decided for category x and rater b decided for category y. With $\hat{\pi}_{xy}^{(a,b)}$, $\hat{\pi}_x^{(a)}$, and $\hat{\pi}_y^{(b)}$ obtained in this way and used in (3.11) and (3.14), the weighted κ measure for raters a and b is then given by

$$\hat{\kappa}^{(a,b)}(w) = \frac{\hat{o}^{(a,b)}(w) - \hat{e}^{(a,b)}(w)}{1 - \hat{e}^{(a,b)}(w)} \quad . \tag{3.17}$$

It has asymptotically Gaussian distribution for a sufficiently large number of ratings n [FCE69].

3.2.4 Multi-Rater Agreement with κ Measures

As mentioned before, Cohen's original κ only gives the agreement between two raters. If a measure for a multi-rater agreement is needed, like it is necessary for the inter-rater correlation of an entire rater group, an extension of this measure is required. Fleiss introduced the first κ measure for the simultaneous comparison of more than two judgments for each patient or, in general, data element [Fle71]. It is valid for the case that the sources of these $k \in \mathbb{N}$ findings for each person are not distinguishable, i.e. it does not require that there is a fixed number of raters but only a fixed number k of ratings for each test person. The derivation and definition of this variant will not be given here. In the experiments for this thesis, the κ measure by Davies and Fleiss was applied which is valid for the situation that each one of $n \in \mathbb{N}$ data elements is rated by $k \in \mathbb{N}$ identifiable raters and put into one of $c \in \mathbb{N}$ categories. All elements have to be rated by the same raters [DF82, Kru99].

The estimation for the $\hat{\kappa}_{\mathrm{DF}}(w)$ value by Davies and Fleiss is based on a linear combination of the observations of the pairwise rater comparison introduced in Chapter 3.2.3. Therefore,

$$\hat{\kappa}_{\mathrm{DF}}(w) = \frac{\sum\limits_{a=1}^{k} \sum\limits_{\substack{b=1 \\ b \neq a}}^{k} [1 - \hat{e}^{(a,b)}(w)] \cdot \hat{\kappa}^{(a,b)}(w)}{\sum\limits_{a=1}^{k} \sum\limits_{\substack{b=1 \\ b \neq a}}^{k} [1 - \hat{e}^{(a,b)}(w)]} \tag{3.18}$$

can be divided into the pairwise expectation values $\hat{e}^{(a,b)}(w)$ with the nominal weighting function w and the weighted $\hat{\kappa}^{(a,b)}(w)$ for the comparison of the two raters a and b ($1 \leq a \leq b \leq k$). The terms containing $\hat{e}^{(a,b)}(w)$ occur due to the prerequisite that the raters are identifiable so that the degree of expected agreement can be computed for rater pairs.

3.2.5   Restrictions of the κ Measure

Cohen's κ and its extensions are still widely used measures for inter-rater agreement especially in medical and sociological applications. However, for special input data they show unexpectable behavior [Gwe02]. The κ value may be low even if the level of agreement is high because κ depends on assumptions about the decision-making of raters [Ueb87, FC90, CF90]. Therefore, the often mentioned intervals of a "moderate" agreement for $0.4 \leq \kappa \leq 0.75$ and a "good" agreement for $\kappa > 0.75$ are actually obsolete [Fle81, Kru99]. For the reliable computation of κ, it is required that every rater chooses each one of the possible categories at least once. One solution if this is not the case was proposed by Crewson where unused categories were filled with "dummy" observations, and in a second table a control variable contained the positions of these dummy values [Cre01]. This method, however, was especially developed for a commercial statistics software. A more severe problem is when one rater does not give a judgment at all for some of the test data. This violates the definition and computation rules which means that κ cannot be computed for the respective data. A measure which is able to cope with both of these commonly occurring problems is Krippendorff's α. It will be introduced in the next section.

3.3   Krippendorff's α

3.3.1   Introduction

Krippendorff's α [Kri03, Kri02] is a generalization of Scott's π [Sco55] which is a statistic very similar to Cohen's κ except for the way chance is calculated. Many researchers use *Cronbach's α* for the computation of inter-rater reliability instead [Cro51]. It measures, however, only covariation after standardizing the means and variances of data from different raters and might thus be inappropriate for the task [HG90]. Krippendorff's α does not change the mean values. For this reason, it was preferred for the experiments in this thesis. According to [Kri02], the α measure applies to

- any number of raters, not just two (like the multi-rater κ in Chapter 3.2.3);

- any number of categories, scale values, or measures;

- any metric or level of measurement (see below);

- incomplete or missing data (as opposed to κ);

- large and small sample sizes alike, not requiring a minimum.

The last two items may be an advantage for clinical evaluations when it is difficult to obtain enough data. A further appropriate measure of (inter-rater) consistency in the case of multi-valued scales is Kendall's τ [Stu83] which will not be presented in detail here.

3.3.2 Computation

While for computation of κ in (3.3) the agreement o between two raters was the basic component, α uses the disagreement D. The general formula of the measure is

$$\alpha = 1 - \frac{D_o}{D_e} \tag{3.19}$$

with the observed disagreement D_o and the expected disagreement D_e that would be a product of chance. The observed disagreement D_o is obtained by the number of cases n_{xy} where one rater decided for category (number) x and the other one for category y. For the case $D_o = D_e$, α will be 0 which means that the agreement observed was just a product of chance, not of the raters' competence. If the raters agree perfectly and $D_o = 0$, α reaches its maximum at 1.

For the case that a rating is made by multiple observers using a nominal scale, α would be computed like this: For all raters and all rated data elements, e.g. speech files, a *reliability data matrix* M is computed where the element $m_{a\chi}$ of the column vector m_χ contains the score that was assigned to data element χ by rater a. The total number of available ratings for data element χ is denoted by μ_χ.

The reliability matrix contains v different values for all the $m_{a\chi}$. These define the size of the *coincidence matrix* N, i.e. the dimension of this matrix is $v \times v$. For each column vector m_χ of the matrix M it is counted how often the category pair (x, y) occurs in it, i.e. how often one rater decided for x and another other one for y when evaluating a certain data element:

$$n_{xy} = \sum_\chi \frac{\tau \cdot \#(x, y) \text{ in } m_\chi}{\mu_\chi - 1} \quad \text{with} \quad \begin{cases} \tau = 2 & \text{for } x = y \\ \tau = 1 & \text{for } x \neq y \end{cases} \tag{3.20}$$

The matrix N is symmetric because every occurrence of (x, y) is also an occurrence of (y, x). This is why for the case $x = y$ the number is doubled by τ. The column or the row sums of N

$$n_x = \sum_x n_{xy} = \sum_y n_{xy} \tag{3.21}$$

which are also equal are summed up to the total number of ratings:

$$n = \sum_x \sum_y n_x n_y \qquad (3.22)$$

The rating categories do not necessarily have to be numerical when an appropriate metric weighting the "distance" between two categories x and y is defined. In the case of numerical scales, like the integer scores for voice evaluation, the distance metric is chosen of the interval metric type, i.e. the values differ algebraically:

$$_{\text{interval}}\delta^2_{xy} = (x - y)^2 \qquad (3.23)$$

With this metric, the observed disagreement is given by

$$D_o = \frac{1}{n} \sum_x \sum_{y>x} n_{xy}\,_{\text{interval}}\delta^2_{xy} \qquad . \qquad (3.24)$$

Similarly, the expected disagreement is computed as

$$D_e = \frac{1}{n(n-1)} \sum_x \sum_{y>x} n_x n_y\,_{\text{interval}}\delta^2_{xy} \qquad , \qquad (3.25)$$

and the final result of α is

$$_{\text{interval}}\alpha = 1 - \frac{D_o}{D_e} = 1 - (n-1) \frac{\sum_x \sum_{y>x} n_{xy}\,_{\text{interval}}\delta^2_{xy}}{\sum_x \sum_{y>x} n_x n_y\,_{\text{interval}}\delta^2_{xy}} \qquad . \qquad (3.26)$$

This computation is possible even when there is data missing, e.g. when a rater accidentally forgot to make a decision on a criterion during a listening experiment. The inter-rater reliability is usually regarded as being sufficient if α is greater than approximately 0.70 ([Kri03], see the example in Table 3.1).

In this chapter, statistic methods for rater agreement have been introduced. They are necessary when the agreement between human raters has to be judged and also when human and automatic evaluation results have to be compared (see Chapter 4.4 and 7). The next chapter will describe the speech data that are the basis for the evaluation task, i.e. recordings of TE speakers. There will also be a look at the way the human experts analyzed these data. But also other speech corpora have to be considered. They serve as the training and test sets for the automatic recognition system and thus define the kind of "experience" that the system has with voice analysis, similar to the listening experience of a human being. The agreement between the results of the automatic processing of the speech signals and the human ratings is done by means of the agreement measures that were described in the previous sections.

		rater B			
		1	2	3	4	5
	1	40	10	5	3	2
	2	5	35	15	10	5
rater A	3	5	10	40	10	5
	4	2	3	10	10	10
	5	2	3	10	20	30

		rater B			
		1	2	3	4	5
	1	0	10	25	10	5
	2	0	25	35	15	5
rater A	3	0	10	25	30	5
	4	0	2	8	10	15
	5	0	0	5	20	40

Pearson's r	0.63
Spearman's ρ	0.63
Cohen's κ	0.39
weighted $\kappa_{DF}(w)$	0.53
Krippendorff's α	0.63

Pearson's r	0.54
Spearman's ρ	0.53
Cohen's κ	0.16
weighted $\kappa_{DF}(w)$	0.33
Krippendorff's α	0.42

Table 3.1: Example for agreement measures; each of the upper tables represents ratings for $n = 300$ items by $k = 2$ raters using integer scores from 1 to 5 ($c = 5$). The numbers in the upper tables show on how many items the raters agree and disagree. In the table on the right side, rater B never gives a score of 1. For this reason, the κ-based values may be unreliable.

Chapter 4

Speech Corpora

In this chapter, the speech data for the experiments in this thesis are introduced. The EMBASSI corpus (Chapter 4.1) was used for preliminary tests on the recognition of reverberated signals. Verification of selected results on this corpus was done using the Fatigue corpus (Chapter 4.2) and the VERBMOBIL corpus (Chapter 4.3) which was also the recognizer training base for the analysis of substitute voices (Chapter 7). The test data for these experiments were recordings of TE speakers (Chapter 4.4) and normal speakers as control groups (Chapter 4.5). Speech recognition in reverberated environment is important for a free communication situation, i.e. it should be possible to record patients in a way that doesn't give them a feeling of being watched or controlled. One step towards this goal is recording by distant-talking microphones. However, with rising distance the degree of reverberation in the signals grows which makes it necessary to adapt the speech recognition in an appropriate way. In the frame of this thesis, no distant-talking recordings of laryngectomees were available. Collecting such data would have been too exhausting for the patients because they already had to read a standard text once while wearing a headset and once again on the telephone where they also read their PLTT sheet (see Chapter 7.4). For this reason, the speech recognition in noisy environment was performed with normal speech (EMBASSI and Fatigue corpus). The findings on these data were verified on artificially reverberated TE speech (see Chapter 7.5).

4.1 The EMBASSI Corpus

One of the goals of the EMBASSI[1] project was the creation of a speech interface for home entertainment devices. The microphones recording the user's utterances in such a scenario will most probably be integrated in the devices themselves or distributed within the room. However, on the long way from the speaker to the microphone(s), many different kinds of distortions may influence the signal. One of them is reverberation.

4.1.1 Influence of Reverberation on Human Perception

Reverberation is caused by sound that is reflected by any kind of surface. In contrast to the *direct sound*, it does not take the shortest way from the sound source to the listener or microphone. Different "copies" of the original signal reach the recipient at different times and influence the

---

[1]http://www.embassi.de

perceptive impression of the sound or the quality of the recording, respectively. Dependent on the signal itself, the positions of source and receptor, and the material and arrangement of the surfaces in the room, a characteristic reflection pattern can be measured which is usually done by sending a very short signal, ideally a Dirac pulse, and measuring the "answer" of the room with a microphone. This pattern is called *room impulse response*. It consists of a first pulse, a set of early reflections (up to about 50 ms), and a reverberation tail [OSM98]. The spectrum appears smeared (see Figure 4.4). Reverberation is often described by means of the early-to-late energy ratio C and the reverberation time T_{60}. These values can be computed as follows [Sab64]: T_{60} is the time interval in which reverberation decreases by 60 dB after the sound source was switched off. Given the values for the size s_w of the wall surface in the room, the room volume V, the speed of sound c, and the mean wall absorption coefficient $\bar{\alpha}_w$, it is determined as

$$T_{60} = \frac{\ln 10^6 \cdot 4V}{c \cdot \bar{\alpha}_w \cdot s_w} \approx \frac{0.161 V}{\bar{\alpha}_w \cdot s_w} \tag{4.1}$$

where the approximation is valid for metric values and $c = 343.24$ m/s. With the help of a directivity factor d and the source-microphone distance r, the early-to-late energy ratio is defined:

$$C = 10 \log_{10} \left(-\frac{s_w \cdot d \cdot \ln(1 - \bar{\alpha}_w)}{16\pi \cdot (1 - \bar{\alpha}_w) \cdot r^2} \right) \tag{4.2}$$

It represents the steady-state ratio between the direct and reverberated sound energies. These formulae are valid for the diffuse sound field assumption only, i.e. an acoustic environment with multiple reflections where a listener could not determine exactly where a sound comes from. The early-to-late energy ratio (in dB) can also be defined as the relation of the energy of early reflections to the energy of reflections after a selected "critical delay time" t_e:

$$C_{t_e} = 10 \log_{10} \left(\int_0^{t_e} p^2(t) \, \mathrm{d}t \, \Big/ \int_{t_e}^{\infty} p^2(t) \, \mathrm{d}t \right) \tag{4.3}$$

In this equation, $p(t)$ denotes the room impulse response. Surprisingly, early reflections can improve human speech and music perception where the critical delay time t_e is about 50 ms for speech and 80 ms for music [DIN00]. This is because of the temporal integration inherent in the human auditory system. Early reflections are thus combined with the original signal and not perceived separately. This causes a change in the magnitude impression of formants [Pet27]. Noise in general mainly affects the perception of place, stop and frication information followed by nasality and voicing [GS79]. The confusion under reverberation is highest among /p/, /t/, /k/ and /m/, /n/, /N/ in final position. However, these show the highest error rates in quiet condition as well. Utterance-initial consonants are less affected because there are no reflections from earlier events. Higher levels of reverberation in smaller rooms cause more uniform masking noise than in a large room and are thus more difficult to handle [NR78]. Reverberation strongly affects the phase of a speech signal which is, however, irrelevant for phone discrimination [Ste05, p. 51].

4.1.2 EMBASSI Corpus Overview

In order to obtain realistic data with respect to environmental noise, a German speech corpus was recorded by the Chair of Pattern Recognition and the Chair of Multimedia Communica-

	number	μ	σ	min.	max.
male	10	24-4	3-2	19-4	29-10
female	10	24-3	3-4	20-4	28-8
total	20	24-3	3-3	19-4	29-10

Table 4.1: Age statistics for the EMBASSI test speakers; average, standard deviation, minimum and maximum values are given in years and months.

tions and Signal Processing in Erlangen. The data were collected in a room which was in its acoustic properties equal to a living-room. The size of this room was approx. 35 square meters (see Figure 4.1). All walls of the room were equipped with a curtain which resulted in a reduced reverberation time of $T_{60} = 150$ milliseconds. In this room, recordings of 20 speakers were made (10 male, 10 female) who were between 19 and 29 years old (see Table 4.1). A close-talking microphone (headset) and an array of 11 microphones were used for synchronous recording (see Figure 4.2). Experiments in an early phase of the EMBASSI project had shown how people would talk to a TV set or a video cassette recorder if speech input were supported. Taking these into account, sentence templates were modeled, and an automatic text generator produced the sentences to be read by the speakers. Examples of such commands are "I'd like to see 'Tatort' please." or "What is running at one o'clock on RTL?" The recordings contain different scenarios involving noise and a disturbing speaker. In two sessions (number 5 and 10), however, the readers were not disturbed by any noise. These data were used for the experiments described later on. The distance to the microphone array was 1 meter in session 5 and 2.5 meters in session 10. One session lasted between approx. 150 and 180 seconds. During this time, the speaker was alone in the room, sitting on a chair and reading 60 sentences without a break.

The 20 persons read a total of 15360 commands. Many sentences occurred more often than once; the number of different commands was 6816. The texts differed among speakers as well as among sessions. Only speakers 19 and 20 read the same texts as speakers 1 and 2, respectively. The total duration of the corpus is about 11 1/2 hours. The data were recorded in digital audio tape (DAT) quality, i.e. with 48 kHz sampling frequency and quantized with 16 bit. The data were also downsampled to 16 kHz. These signals were used for the experiments in Chapter 6. The EMBASSI corpus is described more in detail in [HN03] and [HSN03].

4.1.3   Training Data for the EMBASSI Baseline Recognizer *EMB-base*

In order to cope with reverberation during speech recognition, different speech features with many different parameters were examined (Chapter 5.2). For each parameter value changed in the feature extraction process, a complete recognizer training had to be performed in order to evaluate the effects of the change. For the pilot experiments, a small training set was chosen in order to accelerate the procedure. The training data for the baseline recognizer *EMB-base* were the close-talking recordings of the EMBASSI corpus where the speakers were not disturbed by any noise (session 5 and 10). In order to enhance the training, these files were semi-automatically cut into sections containing one sentence each. The corresponding reverberated signals from the central array microphone (#6) were then cut at the same timestamps. The training data consisted of the recordings of speaker 1 to 12 (6 men, 6 women); speaker 13 (male) and 14 (female) were the validation set (see Table 4.2). The test group consisted of the remaining 3 men and

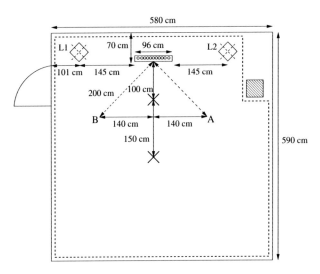

Figure 4.1: The EMBASSI recording room; the two crosses mark the speaker positions. 'A' and 'B' are the "disturber" positions; 'L1' and 'L2' denote the loudspeakers in the room. The curtain at the walls is symbolized by the dashed line. The height of the room was 3.10 meters.

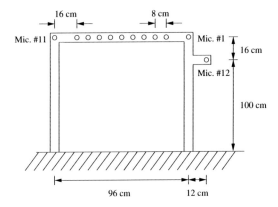

Figure 4.2: The microphone array for the EMBASSI recordings; microphone #12 was reserved for speaker localization methods (not used in this thesis).

	session	mic. dist.	speakers	duration	words	vocab.
EMB-base						
training	5, 10	close-talk	1–12 (6 m, 6 f)	60 min	8325	455
validation	5, 10	close-talk	13–14 (1 m, 1 f)	10 min	1439	261
EMB-rev						
training	5	1 m	1–12 (6 m, 6 f)	30 min	4126	455
	10	2.5 m	1–12 (6 m, 6 f)	30 min	4199	
validation	5	1 m	13–14 (1 m, 1 f)	5 min	727	261
	10	2.5 m	13–14 (1 m, 1 f)	5 min	712	
EMB-12						
training	5, 10	close-talk (artif. reverberated)	1–12 (6 m, 6 f)	12*60 min = 720 min	99780	455
validation	5, 10	close-talk (artif. reverberated)	13–14 (1 m, 1 f)	12*10 min = 120 min	17268	261
EMB-2						
training	5, 10	close-talk	1–12 (6 m, 6 f)	60 min	8325	455
	5, 10	close-talk (art. rev.)	1–12 (6 m, 6 f)	60 min	8325	
validation	5, 10	close-talk	13–14 (1 m, 1 f)	10 min	1439	261
	5, 10	close-talk (art. rev.)	13–14 (1 m, 1 f)	10 min	1439	

Table 4.2: Training and validation sets for the EMBASSI recognizers (acoustic modeling)

session	mic. dist.	speakers	duration	words	vocabulary
5, 10	close-talk	15–20 (3 m, 3 f)	30 min	4184	377
5	1 m	15–20 (3 m, 3 f)	15 min	2094	300
10	2.5 m	15–20 (3 m, 3 f)	15 min	2090	307

Table 4.3: Test sets for the EMBASSI recognizers

3 women (see Table 4.3). Their close-talking recordings of sessions 5 and 10 were the first subset of the test data. The synchronously recorded distant-talking signals from microphone #6 were the second (session 5, 1 m distance) and third (session 10, 2.5 m distance) subset.

The language model for all EMBASSI-based recognizers was trained with 700,000 and validated with 100,000 sentences created in the same way as the sentences for the test speakers.

4.1.4 Training with Distant-Talking EMBASSI Data

In order to get a reference for later experiments in speech recognition on signals with reverberation, a speech recognizer was created where the training data were reverberated. The signals from microphone #6 from the middle of the microphone array served as training data because these recordings were synchronously recorded with the close-talking training data. As two sessions were involved (number 5 and 10), half of the data was recorded at a distance of 1 m and the other half at 2.5 m distance (see Table 4.2). The situation for the validation data was analogous. Only the test data were exactly the same as before, i.e. three sets from three microphone distances (see Table 4.3). The language model training data stayed the same as well. The new system will be referred to as *EMB-rev.*

4.1.5   Artificial Reverberation of Speech Data

Reverberation may not only have positive effects on human perception (cf. Chapter 4.1.1), but also automatic speech recognition can get benefits from the early portions of reverberation. Gölzer et al. convolved close-talking speech with different sections of room impulse responses in order to examine their influence on the recognition task. The initial parts of room impulse responses between the first 25 ms and 50 ms served best for this purpose [GK03] which held for both RASTA-PLP [HM94] features with their long-term filtering and MFCC [DM80]. In general, for acoustic environments that are present in the training data, the recognition results can be enhanced. If the goal is a recognizer which works sufficiently in many environments, the training data should provide recordings that were made in a lot of different places. This, however, would mean bringing a lot of technical equipment to many rooms with different impulse responses and placing the microphone(s) in different angles and distances from the speaker. By reverberating close-talking speech artificially with the help of pre-defined room impulse responses, this problem can be avoided. Couvreur et al. proposed the use of artificially reverberated training data to improve performance of speech recognition in reverberant rooms [CC00, CCR00]. In order to represent the acoustic properties in the target environment as good as possible, they used room impulse responses matching the corresponding early-to-late energy ratio C and the reverberation time T_{60} (see Chapter 4.1.1). Their method outperformed systems trained on clean speech with integrated normalization methods like Cepstral Mean Subtraction (CMS, [Fur81]) or RASTA algorithms [HM94, KM97], i.e. with robust feature extraction from the distorted signals. The reason is that the duration of the room impulse response is longer than the window size of these frame-based preprocessing methods. Couvreur et al. used a hybrid HMM/MLP recognizer in which the multi-layer perceptron (MLP) estimated the acoustic modeling.

Stahl et al. added noise to clean speech and filtered it with room impulse responses in order to match the speech quality of the training material and the test data from a distant-talking microphone. They found out that the room impulse response of the target environment is obviously less important for the recognition task than additive noise in the signals [SFB01]. The difference of most other studies to the work described in this thesis is that other approaches assume a known target environment. If it is unknown, however, a very "general" system has to be designed that should be able to handle any kind of reverberation in the test data. In the next sections, the setup of such a system will be described.

4.1.6   Selecting Room Impulse Responses

For multiplying the amount of available training data, 12 room impulse responses were used. The close-talking training data of the EMBASSI and VERBMOBIL baseline recognizers (see also Chapter 5) were convolved with each one of them separately, and thus 12 differently reverberated versions of the original data sets were created. The convolution was done by a Matlab® script which was also used for the experiments described in [Her05]. The room impulse responses were measured in the room where also the EMBASSI corpus was recorded (Figure 4.1). However, the reverberation time was changed from $T_{60} = 150$ ms to $T_{60} = 250$ ms and to $T_{60} = 400$ ms, respectively, by removing sound-absorbing carpets and sound-absorbing curtains from the room.

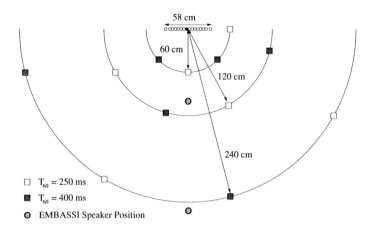

Figure 4.3: Recording setup for room impulse responses; the measuring positions (squares) start at angle 0° at the right-hand side of the microphone array and end at 165°. The used microphone #8 is marked black. The circles mark the real EMBASSI speaker positions.

The impulse responses were measured for loudspeaker positions on three semi-circles in front of the microphone array at distances 60 cm, 120 cm, and 240 cm. The speaker positions started at an angle of 0 degrees on the innermost circle and continued in 15-degree steps while alternating through the semi-circles. The microphone array contained 16 microphones, but only the signals from microphone #8 (closest to the middle) were used. An overview about the impulse responses is given in Table 4.4. Figure 4.3 shows the recording setup graphically. Figure 4.4 gives an overview about the spectra taken from a short section of a speech signal in different acoustic environments. In comparison to the close-talking recording, the spectra of the distant-talking recording and the artificially reverberated recording appear to be strongly smeared which seems, however, to be by far stronger in the artificial signal as its intensity level was not reduced by microphone distance but stayed the same as in the close-talking recording.

4.1.7 Artificially Reverberated Training Data in EMBASSI Recognizers

The close-talking training data of the baseline recognizer *EMB-base* were convolved with each one of the impulse responses separately, i.e. 12 hours of reverberated data resulted from one hour of close-talking speech. The recognizer trained with these data is named *EMB-12* (see Table 4.2).

Since the test sets contain also close-talking signals and a "general" speech recognizer should also be able to handle undistorted speech, a third training set was combined from clear and reverberated data. One part of the training set was the entire training set of the *EMB-base* recognizer (see Table 4.2). The other part consisted of one twelfth of the artificially reverberated training files used for the *EMB-12* approach, i.e. the new training set was twice as big as for the baseline system *EMB-base*. For this reason, it is denoted as *EMB-2* (see Table 4.2). The reverberated data were selected like this: In every reading session, 60 sentences were read by each

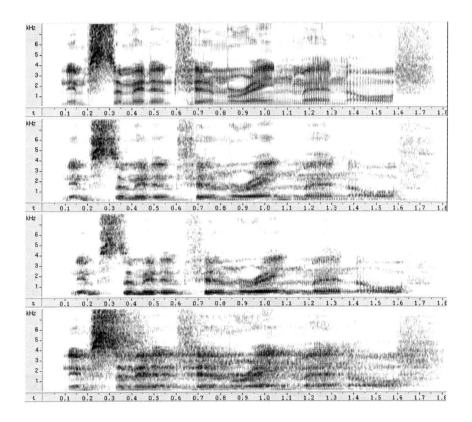

Figure 4.4: Spectra of a short section (1.8 s) of a speech signal; the uppermost image shows the original close-talking recording, below it is the synchronously recorded signal with 2.5 m microphone distance. The next picture shows the signal beamformed from 11 array microphones (see also Chapter 6.3); the last one is the artifically reverberated close-talking recording (T_{60} = 400 ms, angle: 165°). The text spoken was "Nimmst du mir den Film 'Rain Man' auf?" ("Will you record the film 'Rain Man' for me?"; EMBASSI speaker 15, male, session 10, sentence 3)

impulse response	T_{60} (ms)	dist. (cm)	angle (°)	sentences
none (close-talk)	—	≈3–5	90	1–60
h411000	250	60	0	1–5
h422015	400	120	15	6–10
h413030	250	240	30	11–15
h421045	400	60	45	16–20
h412060	250	120	60	21–25
h423075	400	240	75	26–30
h411090	250	60	90	31–35
h422105	400	120	105	36–40
h413120	250	240	120	41–45
h421135	400	60	135	46–50
h412150	250	120	150	51–55
h423165	400	240	165	56–60

Table 4.4: Impulse responses for artificially reverberating the close-talking training data; the rightmost column gives the numbers of the respective sentences within one session for the training data of the EMBASSI recognizer *EMB-2*.

speaker. The baseline training data consisted of all sentences from session 5 and 10 from the readers 1 to 12 (i.e. 12×120 sentences). For each of the 12 corresponding artificially reverberated versions, 10 of the 120 sentences from each speaker were selected, namely 5 sentences from session 5 and 5 sentences from session 10 (cf. Table 4.4). The validation set was composed analogous; the test sets stayed the same as before (Table 4.3). For the experiments with the EMBASSI-based recognizers, see Chapter 6. The next sections will introduce further corpora that were used for the verification of the results obtained with the EMBASSI data.

4.2 The Fatigue Corpus

Like the EMBASSI corpus, the Fatigue corpus was recorded at the Chair of Multimedia Communications and Signal Processing in Erlangen. The Chair of Pattern Recognition was responsible for the acquisition of the test persons and the reading material. The speech data were obtained from a fatigue experiment, i.e. six persons were kept awake a whole night and had to read texts, play computer games etc. The test persons were medically supervised; blood pressure, pulse rate and reaction times were measured. For the experiments described here, however, only the speech signals from the reading sessions were used. All persons (characterized in Table 4.5) were native German speakers, all texts were also in German. The very first and very last text read by the test persons was the German version of the text "The North Wind and the Sun" (see also Chapter 4.4.1). Between those two sessions, 12 other reading sessions, referred to as "reading session" 1 to 12, took place. The texts were transliterations of dialogues from the SMARTKOM[2] project (sessions 1 to 5, 11, 12) and VERBMOBIL recordings (sessions 6 to 10, cf. Chapter 4.3) which were reread by the test persons. Since the relevant experiments were made with a VERB-

---

[2]http://www.smartkom.org

speaker	sex	age (yy-mm)	size (cm)	weight (kg)
1	m	24-9	192	93
2	m	32-4	174	65
3	f	48-9	153	63
4	f	29-3	164	66
5	f	36-9	168	57
6	m	42-6	184	87

Table 4.5: Speakers in the Fatigue experiment

MOBIL recognizer, only the texts from that database were used as test set. For the texts and further details, see [Had02]. By a mistake of the organizers, not the text reference was read but the word-based VERBMOBIL transliterations which contained broken words, corrections and filled pauses the original speakers had produced, and so those were sometimes repeated by the test speakers. However, the rate of such errors is negligible, and the corpus could still be used for the planned experiments. Since the texts of session 6 to 10 were transliterations of VERB-MOBIL dialogues, the Fatigue vocabulary is a subset of the VERBMOBIL vocabulary. For this reason, it was possible to use this part of the Fatigue corpus as test data for a VERBMOBIL-based recognizer. For more information about the particular test set, see Chapter 4.3.2.

The corpus was recorded in an office with a reverberation time T_{60} of 300 ms. A close-talking microphone on a headset and an array of 15 further microphones (Figure 4.5) recorded the speakers synchronously. The array stood in a distance of approx. 70 cm in front of the speaker's mouth (Figure 4.6). The distance from the array to the back of the chair the speaker was sitting on was exactly 1 meter. The data were recorded in DAT quality (48 kHz sampling frequency, quantized at 16 bit). For the speech recognition experiments, however, they were resampled using a frequency of 16 kHz and 16 bit resolution.

4.3   The VERBMOBIL Corpus

The German part of the VERBMOBIL corpus served as training data for the recognizers both for the experiments with the distant-talking test data (Chapter 6) and the substitute voices (Chapter 7). The subject of the first phase (1993–1996) of the VERBMOBIL project [Wah00] was the automatic translation between the language pairs German/English and German/Japanese. In the second phase (1997–2000), the dialogue system was extended to other domains, like hotel reservation, and the system could work as a server that was accessible by telephone. The speech data recorded during the project is distributed by the Bavarian Archive for Speech Signals [BAS]. The VERBMOBIL-*German* corpus contains native German speakers. For all dialogues, the spoken word sequence was transliterated following the rules in [KLP+94]. More information on the VERBMOBIL corpus in general is summarized in [Ste05, pp.38–42]. A subset of the corpus was used for this thesis. It consists of about 29 hours of speech signals (cf. [Had02, Gal02, Ste05]). In [Had02] and [Ste05], it was denoted as "VERBMOBIL small", but throughout this thesis the term "VERBMOBIL" will be used. This subset of the VERBMOBIL CDs 1 to 5, 7 and C contains 12030 files[3]. The total duration of these files, neglecting the pauses at beginning and end of each

---

[3][Gal02]: 12033 files (recordings 3G201A:BLA045, 3G203A:BLA012, and 5M050N:SAW019 were removed)

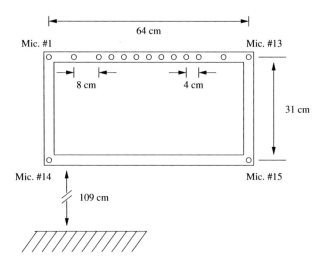

Figure 4.5: The microphone array used during the Fatigue experiment

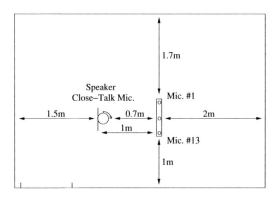

Figure 4.6: Location of speaker and microphone array in the office during the Fatigue experiment; the reverberation time T_{60} was 300 ms. Rows of windows were in the walls which are at the top and right side in the graphics. The height of the room was 3.20 m.

file, is 27.7 hours. For further details, see [Had02].

4.3.1   Training Data for the VERBMOBIL-based Recognizers

The training and validation data for the baseline VERBMOBIL recognizer (*VM-base*) was the same set as used in [Ste05]. For the recognizers derived from this one, the original close-talking signals were entirely or partially replaced by their artificially reverberated versions as it was done for the EMBASSI recognizers in Chapter 4.1.7. The important difference, however, is that the size of training and validation set was kept the same for all recognizers, so the changes in the results are only dependent on the degree of reverberation in the data because the acoustic model of a specific phone gets the same amount of training data in all the training processes, and only the signal quality differs. Even when differently reverberated signals and, if needed, also close-talking files are combined to form a new training list, each one of the original utterances was used exactly once in one specific quality. Concerning the training set, three different recognizers were set up comparable to those from the EMBASSI signals in Chapter 4.1 (see also Table 4.6):

- **VM-base:** This is the baseline VERBMOBIL recognizer as described in [Had02, Ste05]. It was trained with close-talking recordings only.

- **VM-12:** All close-talking recordings were replaced by reverberated versions. The used impulse responses (Chapter 4.1.6) were iterated with each utterance in order to prevent the case that all signals from one speaker are convolved with the same acoustic properties. In the end, each impulse response was used on 1002 or 1003 files, respectively. The total amount of data for this recognizer is the same as for the baseline version.

- **VM-2**: Like in the *EMB-2* training set (Chapter 4.1.7), half of the training set consisted of close-talking signals and the other half of reverberated files. The training list was created as follows: 12 utterances were taken from the close-talking list, the next 12 from the reverberated versions, then again 12 from the original files and so on. In this way it was ensured that each utterance from the original data set was represented in the new list, too, and the 12 room impulse responses were equally distributed among the reverberated half of the training set. The validation list was built in a similar way.

The fact that only 48 utterances were in the original VERBMOBIL validation set was inconvenient for the test series as each one of the 12 room impulse responses was represented in it by only 4 files. Nevertheless, the file list was not changed in order to get comparable results with earlier experiments [Had02, Gal02, Ste05]. The language model for the recognizers was created using the same file lists for training, validation and test as for the acoustic training.

4.3.2   Test Sets for the VERBMOBIL-based Recognizers

The recognizers introduced in the previous section were evaluated on 4 data sets (see Table 4.7 and 4.8):

- The original VERBMOBIL test set (268 close-talking recordings) as defined in [Gal02].

- The artificially reverberated VERBMOBIL test set: The original data were convolved with the 12 room impulse responses that were also used for the corresponding training data. The 268 files were homogeneously distributed to these responses.

	mic. dist.	speakers	duration	words	vocabulary
		VM-base			
training	close-talk	578 (304 m, 274 f)	27 h	257,810	6390
validation	close-talk	30 (14 m, 16 f)	7 min	1042	367
		VM-12			
training	close-talk (artif. reverberated)	578 (304 m, 274 f)	27 h	257,810	6390
validation	close-talk (artif. reverberated)	30 (14 m, 16 f)	7 min	1042	367
		VM-2			
training	close-talk close-talk (art. rev.)	578 (304 m, 274 f)	13.5 h 13.5 h	257,810	6390
validation	close-talk close-talk (art. rev.)	30 (14 m, 16 f)	3.5 min 3.5 min	1042	367

Table 4.6: Training and validation sets for the VERBMOBIL recognizers (acoustic modeling)

- The Fatigue close-talking set: As summarized in Chapter 4.2, this data collection consists of close-talking recordings where six speakers read sections of the VERBMOBIL transliteration again. The signals were segmented automatically; the segment boundaries were mostly set so that one file contained one entire utterance of one speaker each. In several cases the utterances were also split to smaller units. The average file duration on the 1445 files is 6.4 seconds whereas the VERBMOBIL sentences show an average length of 8.7 seconds which is also much longer than for the EMBASSI data (2.3 seconds, see Table 4.8).

- The Fatigue distant recordings: They are synchronous with the close-talking data and were recorded by one of the array microphones (#7, Figure 4.5) 70 cm away from the speaker.

The acoustic properties of the recording rooms are arranged in Table 4.9. An important addition has to be made to the description of the Fatigue test sets: As the texts read by the speakers were transliterations from VERBMOBIL CD 1 and 2, all utterances were in the training data of the language model. Hence, better results than for the VERBMOBIL sets were expected when the usual 4-gram language model was enabled during recognition. The results for the pure acoustic recognition, however, were expected to be lower than their VERBMOBIL counterparts (cf. Chapter 6). The "language model" was in this case just represented by assigning uniform probabilities to all words in the vocabulary ("0-gram language model").

The *VM-base* recognizer was not only used for the experiments on reverberated speech data, it served also as the basis for the recognizer variants for the evaluation of substitute speech. The test data for the latter will be introduced in the following sections.

4.4 Recordings of Laryngectomized Speakers

A wide variety of large speech databases for normal, laryngeal speech existed already in the 1990s (see e.g. an overview in [HTW+97]). Data collections of specific speech disabilities, however, are mostly not commercially available. For the purpose of this thesis, the speech data

	mic. dist.	speakers	duration	words	vocabulary
VM close-talk	close-talk	16 (2 m, 4 f; 10 n/a)	30 min	4781	752
VM artif. reverb.	artif. rev.	16 (2 m, 4 f; 10 n/a)	30 min	4781	752
Fatigue close-talk	close-talk	6 (3 m, 3 f)	150 min	24738	865
Fatigue distant	1 m	6 (3 m, 3 f)	150 min	24738	865

Table 4.7: Test sets for all VERBMOBIL recognizers; gender information was not available for all VERBMOBIL test speakers

corpus subset of corpus	EMBASSI session 5, 10	VERBMOBIL ("small")	Fatigue session 6–10
files	2400	12030	1445
total duration	60 min	27.7 h	150 min
avg. duration	2.3 s	8.7 s	6.4 s
st. dev. duration	0.8 s	7.4 s	4.5 s
min. duration	0.3 s	0.1 s	0.7 s
max. duration	8.4 s	85.1 s	45.3 s
empty files	0	16 (0.13%)	2 (0.14%)
files $\leq$ 0.5 s	2 (0.08%)	62 (0.52%)	0
files $\geq$ 20 s	0	927 (7.71%)	16 (1.11%)
words (total)	13948	263,633	24738
size of vocabulary	473	6445	865

Table 4.8: File statistics for the used speech corpora; the time information refers to the close-talking recordings or to the recordings of one single microphone, respectively. Files with silence only ("empty") were not removed in order to keep the same data sets as in earlier experiments.

of the laryngectomees and the elderly reference speakers were recorded at the Department of Phoniatrics and Pedaudiology in Erlangen.

4.4.1   The Text "The North Wind and the Sun"

Each test person read out the standard text "Nordwind und Sonne", a fable by Aesop which is known as "The North Wind and the Sun" in the Anglo-American language area. It is also used for speech evaluation in other languages [IPA99, NN06]. The German version is a phonetically rich text and includes all possible phonemes of the German language. It consists of 108 words (71 disjunctive) and 172 syllables and is used in speech therapy in German-speaking countries. For "normal" speakers it takes approx. 43 seconds on average to read the text loudly, i.e. at 4 syllables per second [SHN+06]. The full text can be found in Appendix A.1.

The basis for objective voice or speech evaluation (Chapter 2.5.2) in English-speaking countries is often the Rainbow Passage ([Fai44] or [Fai60, p. 127]) which is also used with TE speakers, e.g. in [Blo84, RFBS84a, BPH95]. It consists of 330 words; therefore often only the first paragraph (6 sentences with 98 words) or even less is read [SHC89, TQ90]. The term "Rainbow Passage" is obviously not used consistently in the literature. Sometimes, it refers to the first

	EMBASSI	Fatigue	IR measuring
reverb. time T_{60}	150 ms	300 ms	250/400 ms
room size	5.8 m × 5.9 m	4.5 m × 4.3 m	5.8 m × 5.9 m
room height	3.1 m	3.2 m	3.1 m
mic. distance	1 m/2.5 m	1 m	0.6/1.2/2.4 m

Table 4.9: Acoustic properties of the recording rooms for the EMBASSI and Fatigue corpus, and for measuring the room impulse responses (IR) for artificial reverberation

paragraph only. Often, only the second sentence of the Rainbow Passage is used for F_0 detection in fluent speech, because the mean F_0 of this sentence correlates highly with that of the entire paragraph [Hor79].

4.4.2 Speaker Groups *laryng41* and *laryng18*

The group denoted as *laryng41* consists of 41 TE speakers with an average age of 62 years. The youngest person was 44 years and 7 months at the time of recording, the oldest was 84 years and 11 months old. Two of the speakers are women. Detailed information on the age of each single speaker can be obtained from Table 4.10. All speakers were provided with a Provox® shunt valve (see Chapter 2.2.5). Unfortunately, no information was available about how many patients used the first and second generation of the valve and whether they used an additional stoma filter or stoma valve (Chapter 2.2.6). All patients were native German speakers using local Franconian dialect. Informed consent had been obtained by all participants prior to the examination. The test data were recorded with a "dnt Call 4U Comfort" headset[4] at a sampling frequency of 16 kHz and quantized with 16 bit linear. All recordings were made in a small room in the Department of Phoniatrics and Pedaudiology in Erlangen. For the first 33 files, a self-developed recording software was applied under Linux which was replaced by a new program for Microsoft® Windows® XP® (file names beginning with "00" in Table 4.10). Table 4.11 contains a comparison of the recorded speaker groups concerning articulation rate, spoken vocabulary and similar measures. It has to be noted that the transliteration of all groups was made at different times within a two-year interval. This might have caused varieties in the handling of words outside the regular vocabulary of "The North Wind and the Sun". Therefore, all values based upon the number of words and syllables uttered may not be fully comparable. In the very first experiments with the *laryng18* group (see below) that were published e.g. in [HSN⁺04, HNS⁺05, HSNS05], a preliminary, more detailed version of the transliteration was applied which lead to a number of out-of-vocabulary (OOV) words of 32. For the *kom18* group (Chapter 4.5), the number of words in the text reference plus the number of OOV words is larger than the total number of uttered words. This can be explained by the fact that some speakers left out a few words they should have read.

Some of the preliminary tests were made with the data set *laryng18*, an initially recorded subset of the *laryng41* group. It was obtained from 18 male TE speakers who were on average 64.2 years old. For age information of the single speakers, see Table 4.10. 14 of the patients had undergone total laryngectomy because of laryngeal cancer and 4 because of hypopharyngeal

---

[4]DNT GmbH, 63128 Dietzenbach, Germany

file	sex	age
m000011s01*	m	54-2
m000012s01*	m	58-2
m000013s01	m	61-10
m000014s01*	m	60-1
m000017s01	m	58-1
m000018s01*	m	84-11
m000019s01	m	54-9
m000052s01	m	48-6
m000054s01	m	69-2
m000055s01	m	44-7
m000057s01*	m	67-5
m000058s01*	m	63-0
m000059s01*	m	76-4
m000060s01	m	60-0
m000061s01	m	58-5
m000062s01*	m	61-2
m000063s01	m	53-9
m000064s01	m	66-0
m000067s01	m	61-2
m000069s01	m	60-5
m000073s01	m	66-9
m000074s01	m	64-3

file	sex	age
m000304s01*	m	66-2
m000305s01*	m	70-2
m000306s01*	m	49-6
m000307s01*	m	59-0
m000329s01*	m	62-1
m000437s01*	m	68-0
m000467s01*	m	56-5
m000500s01	m	64-4
m000504s01*	m	62-9
m000506s01*	m	68-4
m000507s01*	m	58-6
001257.nw-nah.01	m	68-1
001264.nw-nah.02	m	70-1
001265.nw-nah.01	m	55-4
001266.nw-nah.02	m	64-6
001274.nw-nah.01	f	54-5
001275.nw-nah.01	m	67-10
001279.nw-nah.01	f	70-10
001280.nw-nah.02	m	52-10

Table 4.10: The *laryng41* tracheoesophageal speaker group; files marked with an asterisk form the subgroup *laryng18*. The age of the persons is given in years and months.

speaker group	*laryng41*	*laryng18*	*kom18*	*bas16*
speakers (male/female)	41 (39/2)	18 (18/0)	18 (18/0)	16 (9/7)
average age (years)	62.0 ± 7.7	64.2 ± 8.3	65.4 ± 7.6	n/a (≈ 25)
total duration (min)	46.0	21.2	15.6	12.5
avg. duration (s)	67 ± 20	71 ± 23	52 ± 8	47 ± 6
words (total, reference text)	4428	1944	1944	1728
words (total, uttered)	4445	1980	1964	1728
words/speaker	108.4	110.0	109.1	108.0
size of vocabulary	84	82	93	71
OOV words (distinct)	13	11	22	0
articulation rate (syllables/s)	2.9 ± 0.7	2.8 ± 0.8	3.5 ± 0.6	4.2 ± 0.5

Table 4.11: Time statistics on "The North Wind and the Sun" recordings of the TE speaker groups and the normal-speaking control groups

cancer at least one year prior to the investigation. At the time of recording, the patients had used the Provox® device for between 5 and 136 months (63.2 ± 35.7 months).

4.4.3 Evaluation by Human Experts

For the automation of the clinical voice evaluation methods, a human evaluation reference had to be defined. For this reason, a set of five raters (four men and one woman) working in the Department of Phoniatrics and Pedaudiology at the University of Erlangen-Nuremberg listened to the recordings of the *laryng18* group in an evaluation session in December 2003. 26 months later, in January 2006, another session with the same raters was held in the same room where the experts evaluated the entire *laryng41* group. Note that for all experiments with the *laryng18* group the first rating was used; for all experiments with the *laryng41* data – including the *laryng18* subset – the second evaluation was applied. The raters (in the following named K, L, R, S, and U) were familiar with substitute voices as each one of them had several years of practical experience in speech therapy. The raters received written instructions before the listening experiment. Firstly, three example recordings were played in order to allow the raters to prepare for the test. The listeners were then asked to rate the voices heard during the session and judge according to their previous experience with substitute voices. It was explicitly stated that the TE voices should not be compared to laryngeal voices but only to other TE voices.

The evaluation sheet (Table 4.12) had also been designed at the Department of Phoniatrics and Pedaudiology[5]. The abbreviations for the criteria names that will be used in this thesis are also given in that table. The criteria were rated on a 5-point Likert scale ([Lik32], cf. Chapter 2.4.1), i.e. one out of 5 (quality criterion: 4) named alternatives had to be chosen. For the purpose of automatic analysis, the scores had to be converted to integer numbers. These were not printed on the evaluation sheet. The overall quality score was not Likert-based: A gray bar with a width of 10 cm was printed on the sheet. The label at the left end said "very good", the label at the right end was "very bad". The raters were asked to mark their impression of the overall voice quality by a vertical line on this visual analog scale (VAS, cf. Chapter 2.4.1) without regarding their results for the single criteria before. The distance in centimeters of the drawn line from the left boundary was measured by hand with a precision of 0.1 cm and used as the value of the overall quality score, i.e. possible values for this criterion were between 0.0 and 10.0.

4.4.4 Intra-Rater and Inter-Rater Correlation

The evaluation criteria were chosen with respect to their use in speech therapy (see Chapter 2.4.1). Some of them, however, are highly correlated with each other. The correlation between the ratings for the different criteria on the *laryng41* group is shown in Table 4.13. One of the highest correlations is between the intelligibility and the overall quality (+0.96). This indicates the importance of the intelligibility for the overall perceptive impression of TE speech. Vocal tone (+0.96) and ability for prosody (+0.88) seem to be further important aspects for human listeners.

Before comparing automatic and human evaluation results, it has to be determined how homogeneous the expert group rated the test data. For the example of the intelligibility criterion,

---

[5]The "voice penetration" criterion was defined by Pahn et al. as the voice capacity to penetrate background noise [PDP01]. Since no background noise was present at the time the raters listened to the *laryng41* recordings, the respective scores are obsolete.

(1)	(2)	(3)	(4)	(5)
quality of the substitute voice *(quality)*				
very good	rather good	rather bad	bad	—
hoarseness *(hoarse)*				
very high	high	moderate	low	none
speech effort *(effort)*				
very high	high	moderate	low	none
voice penetration *(penetr)*				
very high	high	moderate	bad	extremely bad
prosody *(proso)*				
very good	good	moderate	low	none
match of breath and sense units *(brsense)*				
very good	good	moderate	low	none
distortions by insufficient occlusion of tracheostoma *(noise)*				
very high	high	moderate	low	none
vocal tone *(tone)*				
very high	high	moderate	low	none
change of voice quality during reading *(change)*				
very high	high	moderate	low	none
overall intelligibility *(intell)*				
very high	high	moderate	low	none
overall quality score *(overall)*				
very good				very bad

Table 4.12: Schematic diagram of the TE speech evaluation sheet; the Likert scales for the rating criteria were transformed to integer numbers (first line, not printed on the original sheet). The overall quality score was marked graphically in a box of width 10 cm and then measured by hand. The abbreviations of the criteria (in italics) were also not visible for the raters.

	hoarse	effort	penetr	proso	brsense	noise	tone	change	intell	overall
quality	−0.85	−0.83	+0.73	+0.88	+0.81	−0.50	+0.94	−0.43	+0.93	+0.97
hoarse		+0.65	−0.46	−0.79	−0.70	+0.38	−0.89	+0.35	−0.79	−0.82
effort			−0.60	−0.79	−0.86	+0.54	−0.82	+0.57	−0.77	−0.82
penetr				+0.66	+0.56	−0.47	+0.61	−0.20	+0.74	+0.73
proso					+0.91	−0.46	+0.86	−0.40	+0.83	+0.88
brsense						−0.45	+0.82	−0.48	+0.80	+0.83
noise							−0.50	+0.36	−0.63	−0.55
tone								−0.52	+0.92	+0.96
change									−0.49	−0.53
intell										+0.96

Table 4.13: Correlation r between rating criteria (average of the 5 experts) on the *laryng41* data

raters	r	ρ	κ	$\kappa(w)$	α
K vs. L	+0.79	+0.80	+0.44	+0.62	+0.79
K vs. R	+0.72	+0.72	+0.25	+0.49	+0.70
K vs. S	+0.72	+0.73	+0.16	+0.41	+0.63
K vs. U	+0.69	+0.69	+0.16	+0.36	+0.52
L vs. R	+0.73	+0.68	+0.20	+0.47	+0.70
L vs. S	+0.82	+0.81	+0.33	+0.57	+0.75
L vs. U	+0.65	+0.62	+0.27	+0.41	+0.54
R vs. S	+0.74	+0.68	+0.07	+0.40	+0.63
R vs. U	+0.72	+0.72	−0.04	+0.28	+0.50
S vs. U	+0.79	+0.76	+0.29	+0.54	+0.74

Table 4.14: Inter-rater agreement for the criterion „intelligibility" between rater pairs evaluating the *laryng41* data; given are Pearson's r, Spearman's ρ, Cohen's κ, the weighted $\kappa(w)$ after Cicchetti and Krippendorff's α (using interval metric).

rater	K	L	R	S	U
r	+0.81	+0.84	+0.80	+0.87	+0.80

Table 4.15: Inter-rater agreement for the criterion „intelligibility" between one rater and the average of the others evaluating the *laryng41* data

the inter-rater agreement between all rater pairs is given in Table 4.14 according to the agreement measures that were introduced in Chapter 3. In comparison to Cohen's κ, the weighted version of κ shows by far higher values. This reveals the fact that it is closer to an intuitive agreement measure where small differences between ratings of two experts would be assigned a smaller "error" value than large differences. The correlation of each single rater's intelligibility score to the average scores across the other four persons can be found in Table 4.15. Remember that κ and α cannot be computed for this case because of the occurring non-integer values. For the entire group of the 5 raters as a whole, these measures are defined again. The unweighted multi-rater κ_{DF} is 0.21 only while the weighted κ_{DF} reaches a value of 0.45; Krippendorff's α is 0.66. Both values represent "moderate" agreement (cf. Chapter 3) which demonstrates that also human experts often disagree. For the corresponding values on the *laryng18* group, see [SNH+05, SHN+06].

4.5 Normal-Speaking Control Groups

Two corpora of non-pathologic, laryngeal speech served as control groups for some experiments with the TE speakers. The first speaker group ("control group men", *kom18*) consisted of 18 normal-speaking men forming an age-matched group with respect to the 18 tracheoesophageal speakers of the *laryng18* set (Chapter 4.4.2). Their average age was 65.4 years. The data were recorded in the same environment using the same technical equipment as for the *laryng18* speakers. The second group, denoted as *bas16*, consisted of 9 men and 7 women and was taken

kom18				bas16	
file	sex	age		file	sex
m000474s01	m	66		erld4580	f
m000537s01	m	52		esnd4580	f
m000563s01	m	62		hdbd4580	m
m000570s01	m	69		heid4580	m
m000571s01	m	70		hord4580	m
m000572s01	m	69		hsbd4580	m
m000576s01	m	65		jand4580	m
m000582s01	m	73		jehd4580	m
m000583s01	m	67		lind4580	m
m000590s01	m	64		mxbd4580	f
m000702s01	m	69		obld4580	m
m000711s01	m	68		ptzd4580	f
m000722s01	m	58		spid4580	m
m000723s01	m	58		wagd4580	f
m000741s01	m	82		weld4580	f
m000743s01	m	59		wind4580	f
m000751s01	m	53			
m000771s01	m	74			

Table 4.16: The normal-speaking *kom18* and *bas16* speaker groups; the age information for *kom18* was provided in years only, for the *bas16* group it was not available at all.

from the "BAS Strange Corpus 1 (,Accents')" from the Bavarian Archive for Speech Signals at the University of Munich [BAS]. These data were chosen in order to get an approximately age-matched set with respect to the training speakers of the speech recognizer (Chapter 4.3). However, no exact age information was provided with the corpus. Since all persons were university students, their average age was assumed to be about 25 years. All subjects were native German speakers, they were recorded with a Sennheiser microphone (MKH 20 P48) on digital audio tape (DAT) at 48 kHz sampling frequency and 16 bit resolution. The data were then downsampled to 16 kHz. More information on the BAS Strange Corpus 1 is summarized in [Ste05, pp. 38–41]. Each speaker of the control groups read the text "The North Wind and the Sun" (Chapter 4.4.1) where the BAS version showed some minor differences (see Appendix A.1). For details on both data sets, see Table 4.11. The speaker overview is given in Table 4.16.

For the experiments, it was necessary to provide a word-based transliteration of the recordings. These were prepared for the first 33 signals of the *laryng41* group, the *bas16* and the *kom18* group by a computer scientist experienced in speech recognition. The transliteration of the remaining *laryng41* recordings were done by a student of computational linguistics. The guidelines for the transliteration follow those defined in [KLP+94] which had been designed for the VERB-MOBIL project.

In this chapter, the speech databases were defined that are necessary to do the automatic evaluation of TE speech and the evaluation of reverberated speech signals. The next chapter will describe the corresponding speech analysis methods.

Chapter 5

Automatic Speech Analysis

Automatic speech recognition is the key technology for deterministic evaluation of speech quality. This chapter introduces the recognition system that was used for the experiments in Chapter 6 and 7. It will also describe how speech disorders can be displayed graphically so that medical personnel can easily compare a patient's individual disability with other affected persons.

5.1 The Recognition System

5.1.1 Introduction

The speech recognition system was developed at the Chair of Pattern Recognition since 1978, shortly after the introduction of Hidden Markov Models (HMMs) in speech recognition [JBM75, Bak75]. It was continuously extended and revised in order to provide an automatic speech understanding system which requires very few acoustical, lexical, and grammatical restrictions on the speech input. One of the working fields at the institute is *speech recognition* which tries to capture the spoken word or phone sequence correctly, e.g. by adaptation to the respective speaker group [SHSN03, Gal02, GNNW02, AHG+98]. An important part of this is *grammar modeling* which provides linguistic models of language and thus avoids the recognition of word sequences that do not make sense [Haa01, Bor01, BHW+98]. The latest version of the system is described in [Ste05]; for more details on the aspects mentioned in the following sections, cf. [SN93].

The system was also the basis for dialogue systems where research was done on *semantic analysis*. It obtains the meaning of the spoken word sequence [GAB+98, NHW+99] and passes it to the *dialogue manager* which asks the user for further information if this is necessary and provides the desired or alternative information [Eck96]. The system EVAR for train timetable information was the first commercial, conversational dialogue system in the world that was connected to the public telephone line [GAB+98].

5.1.2 Acoustic Models

Training of the acoustic models was performed using the speaker-independent system called ISADORA ("Integrated System for Automatic Decoding of Observation Sequences of Real-valued Arrays", [Sch95, SNE+92, SNE+93]). It represents structural knowledge by a constituent network whose nodes correspond to speech concepts, like phonetic units, morphemes, words, syntactical constituents, sentences, vocabularies, finite-state grammars and so on. Each node is

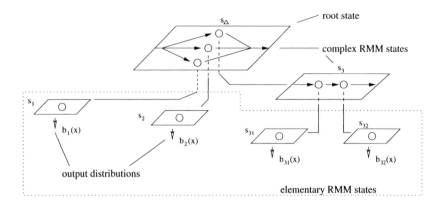

Figure 5.1: Recursive Markov Model (RMM, [Sch95, p. 274])

acoustically represented by a *Recursive Markov Model (RMM)*. A state of an RMM can contain a whole RMM or an elementary state like a standard HMM (Figure 5.1). The Markov models for the atomic acoustic nodes are given explicitly as left-to-right HMMs with a varying number of states, each state being connected to itself and its immediate successor. The models for the other node types can be recursively constructed from the acoustic models of their successor nodes. Phonetic modeling in ISADORA is done by so-called *polyphones* [SNE+93]. Those are phone-like units which generalize the well-known concept of triphone units. Whereas triphones are restricted to a context of one phone symbol to the left and to the right, the context of a polyphone may be arbitrarily large. The context items may also include suprasegmental markers, like syllable, morpheme, or word boundaries. In *generalized polyphones*, introduced in [Gal02], this is extended by phone categories, like "vowel", "fricative", etc. The concept allows to organize the models of the subword units in a tree hierarchy which has the most general units (monophones) at its top and the most specific units (polyphones) with an arbitrary context length at the leaves (Figure 5.2).

For the training of the acoustic models, the propagation-based APIS algorithm is used. It is a modification of the Baum-Welch training [BPSW70] to utilize the generalization/specification relation between the subword units that is defined by the tree structure. Each subword unit which occurs often enough (e.g. more than 50 times) in the training data is represented by a linear HMM with one to four states. Semi-continuous HMMs with full-covariance Gaussian densities in the codebook are used. Four steps are performed during each reestimation:

1. *Accumulation* of HMM statistics using the Baum-Welch algorithm; sufficient statistics for the most specific HMMs in the tree are computed from the training data.

2. *Propagation* of statistics through the generalization tree from the bottom to the top; each state passes forward its current statistics to the unique predecessor.

3. *Interpolation* to increase the robustness of the parameter estimation; the probability density function of a Markov state is averaged with the respective function of its predecessor.

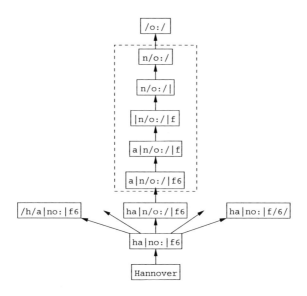

Figure 5.2: Polyphone structure for the word "Hannover" (after [SN93])

4. *Smoothing* of the state parameters with their values of the previous training iteration; the convergence is slowed down which avoids overadaptation to the training data.

5.1.3 Feature Extraction

The feature extraction module was developed by Rieck [Rie95]; for newer implementations see [Ste05, Hac01]. Short-time analysis uses a Hamming window with a length of 16 ms which is, at a sample rate of 16 kHz, equivalent to 256 samples (see Figure 5.3). The frame shift rate is 10 ms. The Fast Hartley Transform (FHT, [Bra84]) computes the short-time spectrum from which the Mel spectrum is obtained by employing an auditory-based filterbank. The filters are uniformly spaced on the Mel scale and overlap each other. For the EMBASSI-based recognizers, the filterbank consists of 18 trapezoid filters as introduced in [Rie95]. For the later experiments with VERBMOBIL-based recognizers, a filterbank of 25 triangle filters was used based on the findings by Stemmer [Ste05]. The lower bound of the first filter is 62.5 Hz, the upper bound is 6250 Hz in the former and 6000 Hz in the latter case, respectively. The Mel spectrum coefficients are normalized to values between 10^{-6} and 1. After this step, usually the logarithm of the values is further processed. However, this operation has disadvantages which will be discussed in Chapter 5.2. The Discrete Cosine Transform (DCT) leads to the cepstrum domain [OS68, OS75]. The first of the 12 Mel-Frequency Cepstrum Coefficients (MFCCs, [DM80]) is replaced by the smoothed short-time energy. After Dynamic Adaptive Cepstral Subtraction (DACS) and smoothing with the respective values of the preceeding and succeeding frame, the static part of the feature vector is complete. The vectors also contain dynamic features as introduced

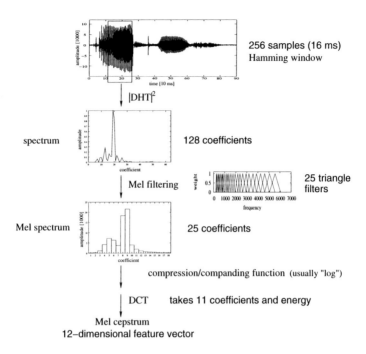

Figure 5.3: Feature extraction (static features) in the VERBMOBIL-based speech recognizers; in the EMBASSI-based recognizers, a filterbank with 18 trapezoid filters was used.

in [Fur86]. The first-order derivative of all 12 static features is approximated by the slope of a linear regression line over 5 consecutive frames (56 ms) as proposed in [Ste05]. For the EMBASSI-based recognizers, 9 frames (96 ms) were used based on the previous feature extraction method ([Rie95]; cf. the discussion in [Ste05, pp. 105–106]). Hence, for each 16 ms frame, a 24-dimensional feature vector is computed.

5.1.4   Language Model and Decoding

For decoding, a separate decoder is used [Kuh95, GSN96] due to suboptimal performance of the ISADORA system on this task. The recognition process is done in two steps. First, a beam search is applied which generates a word graph. The beam search uses a category-based bigram language model. In the second phase, the best-matching word sequence is determined from the word graph by an A^* search which rescores the graph with a second language model. For the experiments with reverberated speech data, this was a 4-gram model. For the evaluation of substitute voices, however, only a unigram model was used because the number of recognition errors was supposed to be a measure for intelligibility (see Chapter 7). A higher-level language model would have removed many errors and hence made this measure inapplicable. The models of non-verbal sounds and non-speech phenomena, like pauses or noise, have fixed language model probabilities determined during earlier stages of the recognition system [Zei01, SZNN01]. The A* search was completely reimplemented in [War03] allowing now to generate word graphs which have been used to compute confidence measures [Ste01, SSN+02].

5.1.5 Recognizer Training Procedure

The training procedure for the semi-continuous acoustic models is derived from the *bootstrap-training method* [Kuh95, pp. 174–178] with some modifications [Ste05, p. 85]. A set of training utterances which are transliterated on the word level serves for the estimation of the HMM parameters. For their initialization, a frame-wise transcription of the data on a sub-phonetic level is needed. The training procedure repeatedly generates such a transcription and simultaneously improves the acoustic models. Firstly, an initial codebook is built by the k-means algorithm [Mac67]. Secondly, all other HMM parameters, i.e. initial state probabilities, transition and emission probabilities, are initialized uniformly. Next, the training procedure iteratively repeats three steps: In the *labeling step*, a sub-phonetic label for each feature vector is created by forced alignment of the training data. During the *initialization step*, the HMM parameters are initialized using these labels while the codebook is not changed. In the *reestimation step*, the APIS training algorithm is iterated 10 times; the codebook is also reestimated. The three steps are repeated as long as the negative log-likelihood of the validation data decreases. For the theoretical background of the described methods, see e.g. [Nie03, Sch95, Nie90].

5.1.6 Speech Recognizers for the Evaluation of TE Speech

The baseline recognizer for the experiments with tracheoesophageal speakers was in principle the same as the *VM-base* recognizer (Chapter 4.3). Only the recognition vocabulary was changed to the 71 words of the text "The North Wind and the Sun" (Chapter 4.4.1). Like the VERBMOBIL-based recognizers, this recognizer is polyphone-based (see Chapter 5.1.2) and will therefore be denoted as *NW-base-poly*. Another important difference to *VM-base* is that *NW-base-poly* applies a unigram language model for the A* search only so that the recognition results are mainly dependent on the acoustic models. Both recognizers use a codebook with 500 classes.

Many TE voices show a very low quality. The highly specialized polyphone models may be a drawback in these cases. For this reason, *NW-base-poly* was also converted to a corresponding monophone-based recognizer called *NW-base-mono*. Here, no differentiation is made between different phone contexts for one core phone. There is one single model for all occurrences of the same phone which makes this phone model more robust against distortions. An aspect that had also to be considered is the difference in the age of training and test speakers. The *laryng41* test speakers (Chapter 4.4.2) were elderly persons with an average age of 62 years while the VERBMOBIL training speakers show a completely different age distribution. Personal data like date of birth and place of residence, however, were only available from 336 of the 578 speakers. 79.2% of these speakers were between 20 and 29 years old, 7.4% were between 40 and 63 which was the highest age occurring in the data. The age distribution of all 578 speakers can be assumed to be close to that depicted in Figure 5.4.

Tissue tension, lung pressure and peak airflow are reduced in elderly speakers [HCK01]. Shape, size and periodicity of the glottal pulses change with increasing age; the harmonics-to-noise ratio (HNR) becomes lower [Fer02, Jun00]. The recognition error rate for speakers is significantly higher [ALB+99]. Wilpon et al., however, stated that the age relevant for significant

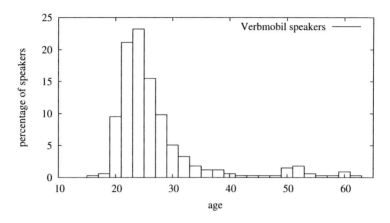

Figure 5.4: Age distribution of the VERBMOBIL speakers; age information was available for 336 of the 578 speakers only.

changes in automatic speech recognition does not start until about 70 [WJ96]. For these reasons, the *kom18* and *bas16* control groups were recorded. They are age-matching with respect to the age of the test and training speaker groups, respectively (Chapter 4.5). Their evaluation results give information about the influence of age on speech recognition. For more information about the voice and speech of elderly people, cf. [Ste05, pp. 17–20].

The reason why all recognizers were trained with young, normal-speaking persons was that there were not enough training data from elderly or laryngectomized speakers. On the other hand, it was important for the TE speech evaluation that the system simulates a naïve listener, i.e. a human being that has never heard TE speech before because this is the situation that the patients face in their daily life. However, there are situations where a high recognition rate is required also for distorted speech. For this reason, the next sections will give some examples how to improve the processing of speech signals where distortions are caused by the environment (reverberation) and by the anatomy of the speaker (substitute voice).

The special output symbols representing pauses and non-verbal phenomena in the recognizers are shown in Table 5.1. There is no "pure" version of the symbol [-"ah-] without enclosing silence because in earlier projects with the same recognition system there were too many misinterpretations of regular German 'e' or 'ä' (/E/, /e:/) phones by this kind of filled pause.

5.2   Modified Features for Reverberated Environment

If there is an acoustic mismatch between training and test data of a speech recognizer, then there are many ways to reduce the influence of this discrepancy. It is beyond the scope of this thesis to describe them all in detail; only some examples will be given in the following.

symbol	meaning
[-], [--], [---]	pauses of different duration
[Atmung] / [-Atmung-]	breath (alone or enclosed in silence period)
[NV] / [-NV-]	non-verbal sound (dto.)
["ahm] / [-"ahm-]	"erm" (dto.)
[-"ah-]	"...er...", enclosed in silence period

Table 5.1: Types of silences and non-verbals in the recognizers used for voice and speech analysis

5.2.1 Handling Acoustic Mismatch between Training and Test Data

One possibility for noise-robust speech recognition is the adaptation of an HMM-based speech recognizer to the test data which can be achieved by model adaptation techniques, like e.g. the maximum a posteriori (MAP or Bayesian) learning [GL94] or the maximum likelihood linear regression (MLLR; [LW94]). For more adaptation techniques, cf. [Jun00, pp. 51–66] or [GM98]; studies on adaptation to reverberated speech are summarized in [OSM98, p. 88].

Much effort is spent in the literature on the identification of noise-robust features. Many approaches concern the duration of the sections in a signal from which features are obtained. In MFCC-based recognition, dynamic features are used which are invariant to slowly varying linear (convolutive) distortions [BHM96]. In the case of the recognizers for this thesis, the window for the computation of these features is 56 or 96 ms long, respectively (Chapter 5.1.3). Much longer windows for the computation of dynamic features were proposed for noisy speech [Fur81, AH91]. In the presence of additive noise, the cepstral dynamic features alone were reported to be more robust than the static features alone [HA90]. In addition, Yang et al. proposed the introduction of different exponential weights for the log-likelihood of static and dynamic features during decoding to make this advantage more efficient [YSL05, Her97]. Long-term log spectral subtraction (LTLSS) was also shown to improve recognition performance [ATH97]. Combined with short-term noise filtering, the word error rate on a digit recognition task could be reduced from 26.3% to 7.2% [GM02]. For the log-spectral subtraction, the signal spectrum is split into phase and magnitude components. From the latter, the mean value of a certain number of frames is subtracted and then recombined with the original phase spectrum. The incorporation of long-term temporal information into the acoustic model is also one of the principles of the TRAPs features that are commonly used for speech recognition in noise [AHE04, CZM04, HS98].

Often, artificial neural networks (ANN) and especially multi-layer perceptrons (MLP) are used for noise-robust speech recognition. Kirchhoff et al. [Kir98] combined HMM-based and ANN-based recognizers using modulation spectrum features which are very robust in noisy and reverberant conditions [GK97]. This has also been confirmed for a hybrid HMM/MLP recognizer with syllable-based recognition [WKMG98]. Modulation spectrum features are derived from normalized amplitude envelopes computed for each channel of a filterbank; they are based on the spectral energy of modulations in low frequencies (2–16 Hz).

In the case of reverberation, the time-variant room impulse response (Chapter 4.1.1) can be modeled as a stochastic process which is integrated into the decoding phase [SZK06, Zel06]. Thus, not only the signal but also the filter, i.e. the impulse response, is processed frame-wise. This, however, requires also a revision of the Viterbi algorithm [Vit67, For73], and the computational costs of this method are very high.

Although many of the mentioned methods are more or less successful, Guinness et al. object that several signal processing schemes that improve recognition in mismatched conditions fail when the conditions during training and test are similar [GRS+05]. They applied noise-masking by separating the input signals into 64 channels and let the channels with the higher energy dominate. This reduced error during recognition. However, their test data were created by artificially distorting a portion of the training data and were hence not independent from the training set.

Noise can also be removed from the signal before the speech recognition phase by preprocessing algorithms. For reverberation this will be described in Chapter 6.3. The next two sections will introduce two feature types that were examined for their ability to cope with convolutive noise. A closer look at speech recognition in noisy environments in general is taken e.g. in [Jun00, Gon95, Hun99].

5.2.2   The Root Cepstrum

Feature extraction methods are very often based on a model of the speech production process, e.g. the Linear Prediction (LP, [AS67]), the Perceptual Linear Prediction (PLP, [Her90]), the cepstrum [OS68, OS75], or the Mel-frequency cepstrum [DM80].

The feature extraction of Mel-Frequency Cepstrum Coefficients (MFCC) which were used in the baseline recognizers was described in detail earlier in this chapter (see also Figure 5.3). For the experiments relevant for the recognition under the influence of reverberation, the focus was on one special property of the MFCC features. The problem with the logarithmic compression of the filterbank coefficients is that it is most sensitive to spectral parts with the lowest power, i.e. where the signal-to-noise ratio (SNR) is usually worst. Furthermore, low feature or coefficient values smaller than 1 might not be exactly represented due to the limitations of the float number range of the computer. Replacing $\log(x)$ by $\log(x + c)$ may solve this problem where c is a small constant or a minimum threshold to which critical values will be set. On the other hand, it is possible not to use the pure logarithm at all and apply functions with more suitable companding characteristics (see also Chapter 5.2.3). The root cepstrum, introduced in [Lim79], simply replaces the logarithm by a root function $\sqrt[n]{x}$. Bourlard et al. assume that root-spectral compression improves modeling spectral envelope zeros which occur in nasalized and fricative sounds and thus is beneficial for recognition [BHM96].

In addition to the MFCC features of the baseline recognizers (Chapter 4.1 and 4.3), the coefficients of the root cepstrum were used as feature set. Initial tests were made with a root cepstrum parameter of $n = 3$ which is reported in the literature as the optimal value for low signal-to-noise ratio (SNR, [Hun99]). However, results on the EMBASSI test data were so much worse than with MFCC features that only values between 4 and 9 were further examined (see Chapter 6.2.1).

5.2.3 μ-Law Features

The logarithm for compressing the Mel-filtered spectrum coefficients was also replaced by another function that is usually used for data compression in telecommunications in order to achieve histogram equalization and a better signal-to-noise ratio. The μ-law (often written as "mu-law" or "μ-law") coding has the formula

$$f(x) = \text{sign } x \cdot \frac{\log(1 + \mu|x|/x_{\max})}{\log(1 + \mu)} \quad \text{where } \text{sign } x = \begin{cases} +1 & \text{for } x > 0, \\ 0 & \text{for } x = 0, \\ -1 & \text{for } x < 0. \end{cases} \quad (5.1)$$

In the feature extraction described in Chapter 5.1.3, $x_{\max}$ is equal to 1 because before the companding step an energy normalization is made. While low feature or coefficient values below 1 are always set to a minimum threshold when using logarithmic compression, the μ-law coding attenuates this problem. It "compands" the input, i.e. it raises low values and compresses high values; the compression is even stronger than by a logarithmic function. A similar idea has also been used within the RASTA methodology when in J-RASTA the logarithm before the filtering was replaced by $\log(1 + \vartheta x)$ in each frequency band where ϑ is a user-defined factor [KMH⁺94, MH92] just like μ in (5.1). Using the μ-law function during feature extraction, different values for μ were analyzed (see results in Chapter 6.2.2).

The methods described up to now are suitable for data distorted by some kind of noise. In the case of a substitute voice, the distortion is in the voice itself which means that the recorded signal cannot be separated easily into "signal" and "noise". The next section will describe a method to adapt the acoustic models of a speech recognizer to a small test set in order to improve recognition results. It can also be applied to speech data from voices with "in-built" noise.

5.3 Recognizer Adaptation to TE Voices

5.3.1 Basic Principles

The HMM interpolation technique was originally used for the sparse data problem. When a speech recognizer has to be built for a domain with a small amount of training data, then its acoustic models can be made more robust by interpolation with models from another recognizer. Stemmer describes an interpolation method which was used to adapt a recognition system to non-native speech without using a second recognizer [Ste05, pp. 139–145]. It is based upon an algorithm introduced in [SSH⁺03] which allows to select not only one but a variable number of interpolation partners for each HMM. The same approach was applied now to adapt the baseline speech recognizer to substitute voices.

First, the polyphone-based recognizer *NW-base-poly* (cf. Chapter 5.1.6) was converted into the monophone-based recognizer *NW-base-mono*. The polyphone models of *NW-base-poly* became the candidates for the adaptation of the monophone models to TE speech. This was done unsupervised as follows: In contrast to [SSH⁺03], the adaptation was not done with the help of a validation set on which the recognition results were optimized. Instead, the *laryng18* data set (Chapter 4.4.2) was processed by the original recognizer, i.e. the best word sequence was computed, and the result was assumed to be correct. Then the monophones underlying the best word sequence were interpolated.

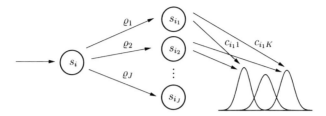

Figure 5.5: Interpretation of the linear interpolation problem (5.2) as a semi-continuous HMM [SSH$^+$03]; the arrows denote state transitions.

5.3.2   Linear Interpolation of Hidden Markov Models

The description of the interpolation algorithm in the next sections for the general case of J interpolation partners follows [SSH$^+$03]. All J hidden Markov models are assumed to have the same number of states. Another condition is that the recognizer is based on semi-continuous HMMs, i.e. all HMMs share one common codebook consisting of K Gaussian densities. The K output mixture weights c_{ik} of one HMM state s_i are interpolated with the mixture weights c_{i_jk} of the interpolation partners s_{i_2}, ..., s_{i_J}, where $s_{i_1} = s_i$ and $c_{i_1k} = c_{ik}$, as follows:

$$\forall k: \quad \hat{c}_{i_k} = \varrho_1 \cdot c_{i_1 k} + \ldots + \varrho_J \cdot c_{i_J k} \quad \text{with} \sum_{j=1}^{J} \varrho_j = 1 \tag{5.2}$$

Afterward, the transition probabilities of state s_i are interpolated with the same interpolation weights ϱ_j.

5.3.3   Estimation of the Interpolation Weights

The interpolation is done using the EM algorithm [JM80]. The overall number of parameters to be estimated is very large because each HMM state that has to be interpolated has its own set of interpolation weights ϱ_j. Instead of a validation set, the recognition result of the *laryng18* data set on the polyphone-based recognizer *NW-base-poly* was defined as a reference, i.e. the underlying polyphone HMM sequence was assumed to be correct and therefore suitable as interpolation partners for the monophone models of *NW-base-mono*. Since this is equivalent to the approach that uses a second recognizer and a validation data set for the interpolation, in the following just the term "validation set" will be used. The estimation formulae for the interpolation weights are based on [Sch95, p. 305].

The EM algorithm can be used to estimate the weights ϱ_j iteratively when the problem (5.2) is interpreted as a semi-continuous HMM (see Figure 5.5). The estimates of the parameter values serve as the basis for the further interpolation. Again, the interpolation partners of state $s_i = s_{i_1}$ are the states s_{i_2} to s_{i_J}. The interpolation weights ϱ_j represent the transition probabilities from state s_i to the states s_{i_j}. The mixture weights c_{i_jk} correspond to the output probabilities of the HMM. For a given set of estimates ϱ, the probability of being in state s_{i_j} if the output is codeword k can be calculated as

$$P(s_{i_j} \mid k, s_i, \boldsymbol{\varrho}) = \frac{P(s_{i_j}, k \mid s_i, \boldsymbol{\varrho})}{P(k \mid s_i, \boldsymbol{\varrho})} = \frac{\varrho_j \cdot c_{i_j k}}{\sum_{j=1}^{J} \varrho_j \cdot c_{i_j k}} \tag{5.3}$$

which can be used to obtain transition probabilities ϱ_j:

$$\varrho_j = P(s_{i_j} \mid s_i, \boldsymbol{\varrho}) = \sum_{k=1}^{K} P(k \mid s_i, \boldsymbol{\varrho}) \cdot P(s_{i_j} \mid k, s_i, \boldsymbol{\varrho}) \tag{5.4}$$

In order to get new estimates of the transition probabilities, the term $P(k \mid s_i, \boldsymbol{\varrho})$ in (5.4) is replaced by the probability $\zeta(i, k) = P(s_i \mid \boldsymbol{X}, \boldsymbol{\lambda})$ where $\boldsymbol{X}$ is the sequence of observations and $\boldsymbol{\lambda}$ is the HMM sequence. This is calculated on the validation set.

$$\tilde{\varrho}_j = \sum_{k=1}^{K} \zeta(i, k) \cdot \frac{\varrho_j \cdot c_{i_j k}}{\sum_{j=1}^{J} \varrho_j \cdot c_{i_j k}} \tag{5.5}$$

The new estimates of the transition probabilities have to be normalized afterward in order to fulfill the condition $\sum_{j=1}^{J} \varrho_j = 1$ again:

$$\hat{\varrho}_j = \frac{\tilde{\varrho}_j}{\sum_{j=1}^{J} \tilde{\varrho}_j} \tag{5.6}$$

The algorithm stops when the $\hat{\varrho}_j$ do not change any more. The success of the HMM interpolation can be evaluated without recomputing the likelihood $P(\boldsymbol{X} \mid \boldsymbol{\lambda})$ of the validation set by a quality measure defined in [Sch95, p. 305]:

$$\ell(\varrho_1, \ldots, \varrho_J) = \log \prod_{k=1}^{K} \left(\sum_{j=1}^{J} \varrho_j \cdot c_{j k} \right)^{\zeta(i,k)} = \sum_{k=1}^{K} \zeta(i, k) \log \left(\sum_{j=1}^{J} \varrho_j \cdot c_{j k} \right) \tag{5.7}$$

5.3.4   Determination of the Interpolation Partners

For each HMM that is supposed to be interpolated, a set of good interpolation partners has to be selected. For this purpose, each HMM of one speech recognizer (here: *NW-base-mono*) is interpolated with all models of the other recognizer (here: *NW-base-poly*) individually, and n possible partners are selected with the help of the quality function (5.7). Regarding the relative improvement of the quality function, however, it is not useful simply to choose the n-best list. It was determined that HMMs which represent polyphones (Chapter 5.1.2) with the same core phone and similar left and right context often show similar improvement alone, but in combination there is no further improvement any more. New interpolation partners should have a distance above a certain threshold to the already selected set. For this purpose, the Kullback-Leibler divergence between corresponding HMM states is used as distance measure:

$$d(s_i, s_j) = \sum_{k=1}^{K} c_{ik} \cdot \log \frac{c_{ik}}{c_{jk}} \tag{5.8}$$

For the experiments with tracheoesophageal voices, first one single interpolation partner was chosen for each HMM. Then, in a second step, the number of partners was set to 40 because this number had achieved the best results in [SSH+03]. The results of the experiments on substitute voices will be summarized in Chapter 7.2.

HMM adaptation can not only serve for enhancing recognition results but also for the graphical representation of a person's voice or speech properties and even speech pathology. How this can be achieved will be presented in the next section.

5.4   Visualization of Recognizer Adaptation

5.4.1   Introduction

For speech therapists, it might be very helpful to get some automated and objective support for the evaluation and classification of pathologic voices or speech. However, the results of such an automatic evaluation are often sequences of numbers or multi-dimensional measures. For a human user, it is much more convenient to get a graphical visualization of these data. This means that the high-dimensional data representing a person's voice or speech properties have to be reduced to one single pair (2-D graphics) or triple (3-D graphics) of coordinates by an adequate reduction of dimension. Additionally, this method should allow to compare a new speaker's properties to an existing database of previously processed persons.

The basis of the distance measure between different speakers are the HMM parameters of a speech recognition system that are changed when the recognizer is adapted to the current test speaker. This is very similar to the procedure that was introduced in Chapter 5.3. Here, the interest does not focus on recognition or accuracy purposes in the first place but to gain insight into individual voice disorders. The results of the recognizer adaptation are presented graphically. A mapping technique, the so-called *Sammon* mapping [Sam69], allows the graphical representation of abstract data unveiling underlying structures and configurations. This method of mapping data is not new, but it has not been applied to this concrete problem before (see also [HZS+06, HZN+06]). The features computed to express the differences between speakers are obtained from the adaptation of a speech recognizer to the current test speaker. With the interpolation method from [SSH+03, SSHN04] (cf. Chapter 5.3) for recognizers based on semi-continuous Hidden Markov Models (SCHMMs), the output weights of an existing *NW-base-mono* recognizer (Chapter 5.1.6) are adapted to individual speaker characteristics. Like in the previous section, this is done with a small amount of adaption data, i.e. the standard text "The North Wind and the Sun" (Chapter 4.4.1) uttered by the respective speaker. For a given group of speakers, in this way a set of speaker-adapted recognizers is achieved. The output weights of each recognizer are used for the mapping procedure.

5.4.2   A Distance Metric for Semi-Continuous HMMs

The Sammon mapping (Chapter 5.4.3) is a non-linear transformation preserving data topology. This topology is represented within a matrix of respective "utterance distances". The quality and information quantity of a Sammon map is fully determined by this metric and not by the mapping itself. Thus, it is extremely important to have a suitable distance metric. On the other hand, the distance metric can be chosen without any mathematical restrictions, like linearity, etc.

The great advantage of the Sammon Transform against some other dimension reduction operations, like the Principal Component Analysis (PCA), is that the transform is not linear and therefore loses less information. For the purpose of this thesis, a good distance calculus for speaker-adapted SCHMMs is needed in order to get the distance between a pathologic voice and the normal voices represented by the baseline recognizer, or between two pathologic voices. A measure computed from the distances of the respective elementary SCHMMs of different speaker-dependent speech recognizers fulfills this requirement. The arithmetic mean of these model distances serves as the final result. The basic problem is the definition of the distance between the states of two SCHMMs. Distance calculation has to use the interpolation weights but still take into consideration the densities from the recognizer codebook containing the Gaussian output densities. This is due to the varying information load which can be considered higher for densities with low variance and vice versa. If a simple Euclidean distance of the weight vectors were used, this information would get lost and the quality of the distance metric would diminish. The codebook itself is static and common to all speakers.

The distance metric for HMM states is based upon the Mahalanobis distance [Mah36] of corresponding codebook densities of two recognizers. In the adapted recognizers, for each state s_i of a Markov model p the mean vector $\boldsymbol{m}_{ik}(p)$ of each codebook density k is scaled with the corresponding output weight $c_{ik}(p)$:

$$\hat{\boldsymbol{m}}_{ik}(p) = c_{ik}(p) \cdot \boldsymbol{m}_{ik}(p) \tag{5.9}$$

Given two HMMs p and q, the Mahalanobis distance for such a pair of weighted mean vectors is

$$d_{ik}(p,q) = \sqrt{(\hat{\boldsymbol{m}}_{ik}(p) - \hat{\boldsymbol{m}}_{ik}(q))^{\mathrm{T}} \cdot S_i(p,q)^{-1} \cdot (\hat{\boldsymbol{m}}_{ik}(p) - \hat{\boldsymbol{m}}_{ik}(q))} \tag{5.10}$$

where the estimate S_i for the global covariance of two HMM states is computed from the weighted covariances of the K single densities:

$$S_i(p,q) = \frac{1}{2} \sum_{k=1}^{K} (c_{ik}(p) + c_{ik}(q)) \cdot \mathrm{cov}(k) \tag{5.11}$$

In the end, the resulting set of K density distances $d_{ik}(p,q)$ is summed up to provide a single state distance between the corresponding states s_i of models p and q. The overall HMM distance δ_{pq} between p and q is the sum of all N state distances:

$$\delta_{pq} = \sum_{i=1}^{N} \sum_{k=1}^{K} d_{ik}(p,q) \tag{5.12}$$

The HMM distance in (5.12) is computed for each pair of elementary HMMs. It fills up a matrix holding the speaker distances. This matrix is symmetric, so for n utterances $\frac{n^2-n}{2}$ distances have to be calculated.

5.4.3 Sammon Mapping

The Sammon mapping performs a topology-preserving reduction of data dimension. It minimizes a "stress function" between the topology of the low-dimensional Sammon map and the high-dimensional original data. The latter topology is defined by the distances between utterances or speakers, as defined in Chapter 5.4.2. The low-dimensional Sammon map is usually visualized as 2-D or 3-D image. With respect to [SN04], a Sammon map is called a *cosmos* while a mapped utterance inside a cosmos is called a *star*.

The heart of Sammon's method is its special error function E which yields a stress factor between the actual configuration of stars in T-dimensional target domain and the original data in R-dimensional space ($T < R$):

$$E = \frac{1}{\sum_{p=1}^{n-1} \sum_{q=p+1}^{n} \delta_{pq}} \sum_{p=1}^{n-1} \sum_{q=p+1}^{n} \frac{(\delta_{pq} - \nu_{pq})^2}{\delta_{pq}} \tag{5.13}$$

δ_{pq} denotes the distance between HMMs with number p and q, as in (5.12), ν_{pq} is the distance between $star(p)$ and $star(q)$ in the cosmos map. E is within $[0, 1]$ where $E = 0$ means a lossless projection from R- to T-dimensional space. Due to (5.13), utterances forming clusters in original space will tend to cluster also in destination space. The same holds for utterances being far apart from each other. In order to achieve the final map, standard steepest descent is applied to (5.13). For more details, see [Zor06] or [HZS$^+$06].

5.4.4   Mappings of Voice Disorders

An example for the application of the previously described methods is depicted in Figure 5.6. It is clearly visible that different speaker groups were almost completely separated into different areas. In addition, the genders of the hoarse and young reference speakers were separated. The degree of voice pathology is growing from right to left with the hoarse speakers located between the laryngectomees and the normal speakers. Pitch is growing from the top to the bottom of the cosmos. However, which voice properties are arranged in which direction by the Sammon Transform, is dependent on the data and not known in advance. This phenomenon was already reported in [SN04] where a cosmos map was suggested to have an unlimited number of axes. Most of them represent complex properties of the data and are thus difficult to describe.

With a slightly modified mapping method, it is possible to project an unknown speaker into an existing cosmos of well-known and previously evaluated cases of pathologic voices [Zor06]. The pre-computed cosmos serves as a reference, and the new speaker's degree or even the type of pathology can be determined by the position where the recording is projected into the map. For experiments on the visualization of substitute voices, see Chapter 7.6.

The Sammon Transform can be applied to various problems; it is not at all restricted to the analysis of speech signals. Another example is the visualization and graphical separation of classes of written digits [NW79]. A newer approach for data clustering which is even suitable for data that are not represented in a vector space was introduced by Roth et al. [RLKB03]. It can handle data units for which a pairwise proximity is defined, e.g. between the items of psychometric tests. For the combination of automatic voice analysis and human evaluation (see Chapter 2.4), this might be an interesting alternative.

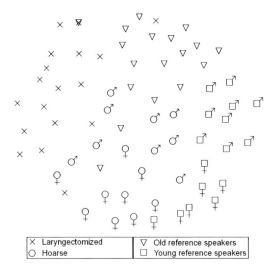

Figure 5.6: Cosmos of four speaker groups and their arrangement by the Sammon Transform [Zor06]; the laryngectomized speakers were the *laryng18* group (see Chapter 4.4.2). Symbols without additional gender specification denote male speakers.

5.5 Prosodic Analysis

5.5.1 Overview

One of the voice criteria that the human experts had to evaluate was the use of prosody in the test data (see Table 4.12) because this is an important aspect of natural speech. Older listeners rely on prosodic elements during speech perception more than younger people do [Bau03, WWS92]. The main reason might be their reduced hearing ability. The communication partners of laryngectomees are often persons of the same age, i.e. elderly people, so it is even more relevant that the ability for producing prosodic elements is tested during speech therapy. As the goal of this thesis is to provide methods for speech analysis and not only for voice evaluation, the prosodic analysis of the TE speech test data was an important part of the task. This means that it is not sufficient to take into account a sustained vowel only like other approaches for measuring voice quality [GFV$^+$05, RML04, WP03]. On a spoken text, it is possible to evaluate the patient's voice and speech together. A similar approach was introduced by Moerman et al. [MPM$^+$04], but the text consisted of only 18 words there. Correlations to human ratings are only given for the "overall impression" of the substitute voice, and they do not exceed $r = 0.49$.

Gandour and Weinberg state that TE speakers can produce simple intonational contrast (like e.g. rise vs. fall) as good as normal speakers [GW83]. They used test sentences like "*Bev* loves Bob." vs. "*Bev* loves Bob?" and "Bev loves *Bob*." vs. "Bev loves *Bob*?" that were read out by the patients. 40 listeners unfamiliar with substitute voices evaluated the recordings. Indeed, some alaryngeal speakers were able to produce prosodic patterns which means that they can control and regulate the fundamental frequency in speech. In a study with 9 esophageal and 10 TE speakers by Rossum et al., all speakers were able to convey word accent. When they were not able to control F_0, they used alternative strategies [RKNQ02]. For this thesis, the analysis of intonation was not of high priority since the patients read a standard text without any questions, exclamations, etc. Further prosodic properties in pathologic speech have been examined (see also Chapter 2): Ainsworth and Singh reported that the rhythm of a sentence is judged to be normal if the intervals between stressed syllables are fairly equal [AS92]. In a study with German speakers, the voice quality correlated with the word stress [CDJ+98].

The analysis of prosodic features from acoustic measures, even though done by hand, was already described by Robbins et al. in 1984 [RFBS84a]. This study involved pause durations, the number of pauses, percentage of total reading time and more, like it is done automatically by the prosody module described in the next section.

5.5.2   The Prosody Module

The Chair of Pattern Recognition has a profound experience in the analysis of prosody in speech, e.g. published in [BFH+03, Hub02, GNNW02, NBK+00, Kom97, Nöt91, NK88], which lead to the development of the *Prosody Module* during the VERBMOBIL [Wah00] and the SMARTKOM project [Wah06]. The major role of prosody in human-human communication is segmentation and disambiguation. Prosodic information is attached to speech segments which are larger than a phoneme, i.e. syllables, words, phrases, and whole turns of a speaker. To these segments, perceived properties like pitch, loudness, speaking rate, voice quality, duration, pause, rhythm, etc., can be attributed. In human-human communication, the listener extracts information out of the perceived phenomena. The prosodic functions which are generally considered to be the most important ones are the marking of boundaries, accents, sentence mood, and emotional state of the user [NBK+00]. The task of the automatic prosodic evaluation is to identify features which highly correlate with these perceived properties, e.g. the acoustic feature fundamental frequency (F_0) which correlates to *pitch*, and the short time signal energy correlating to *loudness*. For the analysis of substitute voices, features have to be identified that correlate with the human rating criteria defined in Chapter 4.4.3.

Basic prosodic features are extracted from the pure speech signal without any explicit segmentation into prosodic units. Examples are the frame-based extraction of F_0 and energy. Structured prosodic features are computed over larger speech units (syllable, syllable nucleus, word, turn). Some of them are based on the basic prosodic features, e.g. features describing the shape of the F_0 or the energy contour. Others are based on segmental information that can be provided from the output of a word recognizer, e.g. features which describe durational properties of phonemes, pauses, or other speech units. For this reason, the prosody module processes two means of input. The first one is the speech signal itself, the second one is a word hypotheses graph (WHG) which is the output of the word recognition module on this signal. A WHG is a directed acyclic graph [ON93] where each edge corresponds to a word hypothesis which has attached to it its acoustic probability, its first and last time frame, and a time alignment of the underlying phoneme sequence. In this way, the time alignment and the information about the underlying phoneme classes (e.g. "long vowel") can be used by the prosody module.

Since it is not clear in advance which prosodic features are relevant for different classification problems and how the different features are interrelated [NBK+00], a highly redundant feature set is used. In earlier projects, like VERBMOBIL and SMARTKOM, a neural net classifier was supposed to find the relevant features and their optimal weighting. Experiments on the use of prosodic information for linguistic analysis showed that it was always the best to use all features if there are enough training data available [BBH+99]. However, the effort needed to find the optimal set usually does not pay off in terms of classification performance [BBH+01]. In this thesis, the correlation between the prosodic feature values and human ratings (see Chapter 4.4.3) was used to decide which features are the most suitable. The features proved to be effective for linguistic and emotion analysis [BFH+03], so they were expected to be sufficient for the analysis of the rating criteria used in this thesis.

Local prosodic features are computed for every word, syllable or other speech unit defined by the user. For the experiments on substitute voices, only word-based features were used. The word is a well-defined unit in word recognition which can be provided by any standard recognizer. A fixed reference point from which all positions are measured is chosen at the end of the currently processed word. The features are obtained by analyzing silent and filled pauses, the signal energy, word and syllable durations, and the fundamental frequency F_0. Usually the basic prosodic features cannot be directly used for prosodic classification because they contain speaker-dependent properties, like the specific articulation rate or F_0. For this reason, many of the features are normalized with respect to their mean values across the whole utterance or even the entire training database. The local features are (with their name components in parentheses):

- **Duration features (Dur)**: absolute duration (Abs) of the speech unit, normalized duration (Norm) with respect to the entire utterance; the normalization is done using the global value DurTauLoc which is determined from a global table containing the durations of words or subword units, respectively. For details see [BBN+00]. AbsSyl is the absolute duration divided by the number of syllables and represents another sort of normalization.

- **Energy features (En)**: regression coefficient within the speech unit (RegCoeff) and mean square error (MseReg) of the energy curve with respect to the regression curve; mean energy (Mean), maximum energy (Max) with its position on the time axis (MaxPos), absolute (Abs) and normalized (Norm) energy values; for the normalization with the global value EnTauLoc which represents the relative average sentence energy, see [BBN+00].

- **F_0 features (F0)**: regression coefficient (RegCoeff) and mean square error (MseReg) of the F_0 curve with respect to the regression curve; mean (Mean), maximum (Max), minimum (Min), onset (On), and offset (Off) values as well as the positions of Max (MaxPos), Min (MinPos), On (OnPos), and Off (OffPos) on the time axis. All F_0 values are not stored as absolute values but transformed into semitone values and normalized with respect to the utterance-specific mean value F0MeanG.

- **Length of pauses (Pause)**: duration of the silent pause before (Pause–before) and after (Pause–after), and filled pause before (PauseFill–before) and after (PauseFill–after) the respective word in context.

The speech unit which is the basis for the computation is appended to the feature name; for this thesis, this marker is "Word".

For each reference point, 95 local prosodic features over word intervals of different sizes are extracted (see Table 5.2): The current word, i.e. after which the reference point is set, gets the number 0. The interval containing only this word is denoted by "0,0". The interval containing the two words before word 0 and the pause between them is called "-2,-1" because it begins at word -2 and ends at the end of word -1 (Figure 5.8). In the same way, words after the reference point get positive numbers. The interval code is added to the feature name. For instance, the feature EnMaxWord1,2 denotes the maximum energy value in the two words after the reference point, and F0MeanWord-1,0 contains the mean F_0 of the interval including the current word and the previous one. The high degree of redundancy is obvious; for instance, there is a strong correlation between the normalized word duration DurNormWord for the contexts 0,0 and -1,0. For a detailed description of all features, see [Hub02].

In addition to the local features, 15 global features for the entire file are computed regarding jitter, shimmer, and voiced/unvoiced decision. These features are explained in Table 5.3. The names are used according to [BFH$^+$00].

Figure 5.7 shows how some prosodic features, like the F_0 at voice onset and offset or the F_0 minimum and F_0 maximum, are determined for a single word. The positions of these features are negative for the current word and all words before because they are situated before the reference point. If no voiced frame is found in the word, then all F_0 values are set to 0, and all F_0 positions are set to -1.

The linear regression coefficients of F_0 contour and energy contour are computed over 6 different word intervals (see Table 5.2). An important difference to the prosodic analysis by other research groups is that the F_0 contour is not "stylized", i.e. no hard decisions are made, and no contour labels, like "hat contour", "rise", "rise fall", "high tone", etc., are assigned, because in this way information gets lost. The features of the prosody module describe the F_0 and the energy contour implicitly: High values at the beginning of a word and low values at the end of the word can be combined to a "fall" label when it is required, but the values themselves can also be used directly for classification and leave the decision about the appropriate label to the classifier.

For the detection of disfluencies in pathologic speech, Liu et al. [LSS03] proposed the coupling of word-based and part-of-speech-based methods. Another suggestion of them is to define possible interruption points in the language model. Part-of-speech features can also be obtained by the prosody module, and interruption points can be integrated into the acoustic-phonetic network of the ISADORA system (Chapter 5.1; see also [NNH$^+$00]). However, due to the low number of disfluency phenomena in the test data, only the word-based prosodic analysis was applied, and the ISADORA network was not changed.

The particular experiments with the prosody module will be described in Chapter 7.3. In the next chapter, experimental results on the problem of distant-talking speech will be addressed.

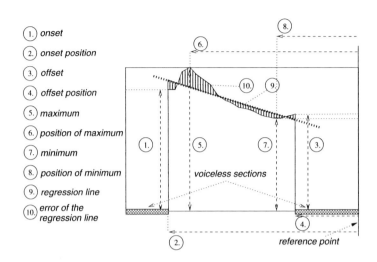

Figure 5.7: Computation of prosodic features within one word [War03, p. 68]; depicted is the F_0 trajectory over time where in the beginning and end no F_0 is detectable (voiceless sections).

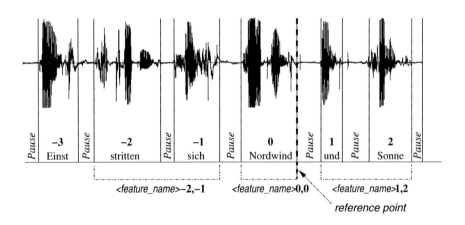

Figure 5.8: Examples for computation intervals for prosodic features on the first phrase of the text "The North Wind and the Sun"

features	context size -2	-1	0	1	2
DurTauLoc; EnTauLoc; F0MeanG			•		
Dur: Abs, Norm, AbsSyl		•	•	•	
En: RegCoeff, MseReg, Mean,		•	•	•	
Max, MaxPos, Abs, Norm		•	•	•	
F0: RegCoeff, MseReg, Mean,		•	•	•	
Max, MaxPos, Min, MinPos		•	•	•	
Pause–before, PauseFill–before		•	•		
F0: Off, OffPos		•	•		
Pause–after, PauseFill–after			•	•	
F0: On, OnPos			•	•	
Dur: Abs, Norm, AbsSyl	•			•	
En: RegCoeff, MseReg, Mean,	•			•	
Abs, Norm	•			•	
F0: RegCoeff, MseReg	•			•	
Dur: Norm		•			
En: RegCoeff, MseReg		•			
F0: RegCoeff, MseReg		•			

Table 5.2: 95 local prosodic features and their computation intervals ("context", [BBN$^+$00])

feature	description
StandDevF0	standard deviation of F_0 for entire file
MeanJitter	mean jitter in all voiced sections
StandDevJitter	standard deviation of jitter in all voiced sections
MeanShimmer	mean shimmer in all voiced sections
StandDevShimmer	standard deviation of shimmer in all voiced sections
#+Voiced	number of voiced sections in file
#–Voiced	number of unvoiced sections in file
Dur+Voiced	duration of voiced sections in file (in frames)
Dur–Voiced	duration of unvoiced sections in file (in frames)
DurMax+Voiced	maximum duration of voiced section
DurMax–Voiced	maximum duration of unvoiced section
RelNum+/–Voiced	ratio of number of voiced and unvoiced sections
RelDur+/–Voiced	ratio of duration of voiced and unvoiced sections
RelDur+Voiced/Sig	ratio of duration of voiced sections and duration of signal
RelDur–Voiced/Sig	ratio of duration of unvoiced sections and duration of signal

Table 5.3: 15 global prosodic features computed by the prosody module for each file

Chapter 6

Speech Recognition in Reverberated Environment

This chapter contains the experiments for the enhancement of speech recognition in reverberated environment. Three different approaches were examined. The first one concerns the training data. Artificially reverberated speech signals were used in order to cover many possible test environments (see Chapter 6.1). The second kind of modifications of the baseline recognizer involved the feature extraction (Chapter 6.2). Finally, a preprocessing step was taken into consideration. Recordings from multiple microphones were combined by beamforming in order to create a single, less distorted test signal (Chapter 6.3). The speech recognizers used in this chapter are the EMBASSI- and VERBMOBIL-based recognizers introduced in Chapter 4.

6.1 Experimental Results on Reverberated Training Data

6.1.1 Experiments with the EMBASSI Baseline System *EMB-base*

The word accuracy (WA) which is based upon the Levenshtein distance [Lev66] between the recognized and the reference word sequence was used as the basic measure for the evaluation of a recognition system. If the number of words in the reference is denoted by n_{all} and the number of substituted (n_{sub}), inserted (n_{ins}), deleted (n_{del}) and correctly recognized words (n_{corr}) are also known, then the word accuracy in percent is computed as

$$\text{WA} = 100 \cdot \left(1 - \frac{n_{sub} + n_{del} + n_{ins}}{n_{all}} \right) \quad . \tag{6.1}$$

A prototype of the *EMB-base* recognizer was trained with a 4-gram language model and a pre-trained codebook from [Ste05]. It achieved a word accuracy of 94.0% on the EMBASSI close-talking test data (Chapter 4.1.3). With a 0-gram model, however, the word accuracy was only 54.7%. In order to attenuate this effect of the purely acoustic-based recognition, the word penalty parameter which has an influence on the length of the recognized words was altered. Figure 6.1 shows how the word accuracy depends on the word penalty. Due to these findings, the parameter was set to 10^{-6} for all 0-gram experiments, and it was left at 0.1 throughout this thesis when a 4-gram model was applied. The latter value was a result of earlier experiments in the working group.

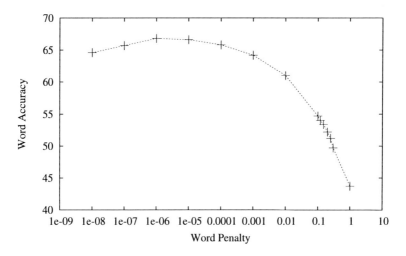

Figure 6.1: Word accuracy for different word penalty values on a prototype version of the *EMB-base* recognizer (EMBASSI close-talking test set; 0-gram language model)

On the baseline system *EMB-base* with close-talking training data and a 4-gram language model, the word accuracy for the close-talking test data was 94.3%. For the distant-talking recordings, 90.2% were reached for 1 m microphone distance and 84.1% for 2.5 m distance. With 0-gram language model and with the optimal value of 10^{-6} for the word penalty, 70.0% for close-talking data, 52.4% for the 1 m distance, and 37.5% for the 2.5 m distance are the baseline results (see also Table 6.1). The error correction effect of the more complex language model is clearly visible especially for the distant-talking data.

The training of an *EMB-base* recognizer on an AMD Athlon® XP 2800+ machine with 2.08 GHz clock frequency and 1 GB of main memory took about 3 to 4 hours, depending on the number of codebook reestimation iterations (cf. Chapter 5.1).

6.1.2   The *EMB-rev* Recognizer with Distant-Talking Training Data

The reference for the recognition in reverberated environment is a recognizer whose training data were recorded under the same acoustic properties as the reverberated test data. The recognizer *EMB-rev* (Chapter 4.1.4) was trained with the signals from a distant-talking microphone that recorded synchronously with the close-talking microphone. One half of the training data for *EMB-rev* were recorded at a distance of 1 m and the other half at 2.5 m distance (see also Table 4.2). The validation data were composed in the same way. Only the test data were exactly the same as for *EMB-base*. Table 6.1 shows that much better results were achieved on the reverberated test data. Both microphone distances which were represented in the training data show word accuracies of far beyond 90% when the 4-gram language model is used. Compared to the baseline system, the signals from 1 m distance reach 94.1% which is almost 5 percent points more than on *EMB-base*. With a 0-gram language model, the WA is 66.3%; it had been

mic. dist.	lang. model	EMB-base	EMB-rev	EMB-12	EMB-2
close-talk	4-gram	94.3	87.5	91.7	**95.5**
close-talk	0-gram	70.0	40.0	57.7	**71.4**
1 m	4-gram	90.2	*94.1*	*94.0*	***94.4***
1 m	0-gram	52.4	***66.3***	*61.9*	*63.0*
2.5 m	4-gram	84.1	***93.1***	*88.4*	*89.6*
2.5 m	0-gram	37.5	***63.2***	*52.4*	*55.3*

Table 6.1: Word accuracy for EMBASSI-based recognizers (MFCC features) on test data with different microphone distances; results in italics are significantly better ($p \leq 0.01$) than on *EMB-base*. The best results in each line are printed in boldface.

only 52.4% on the baseline system. The recordings at 2.5 m distance almost catch up to the 1 m signals with 93.1% where the baseline value was 84.1%. Even with only the 0-gram model, the WA is now 63.2% in contrast to poor 37.5% before. The disadvantage in this approach is with the high-quality close-talking signals. Already with the 4-gram language model, the loss is severe (87.5% vs. 94.3% on *EMB-base*), and with the 0-gram model only 40.0% WA are achieved which is 30 percent points below the baseline result. Training a recognition system with reverberated speech is a rather easy way to improve the results on test data recorded with a certain distance from speaker to microphone, but the goal is to train a recognizer in one single surrounding with its specific acoustic properties and then apply it successfully in any other room. In the described experiment with the *EMB-rev* recognizer, the acoustic properties of the training data are the same as in the distant-talking test data. Further examinations have been made with artificially reverberated data. These will be described in the next section.

6.1.3   Artificially Reverberated Training Data in EMBASSI Recognizers

The *EMB-12* recognizer was trained with approx. 12 hours of artificially reverberated training data which was basically the one hour of *EMB-base* training data in 12 different acoustic qualities (see also Chapter 4.1.7). The results for the recognition experiments are summarized in Table 6.1. Especially interesting are the results of the test data recorded with a distant-talking microphone. As expected, the recognition rates of the close-talking test data are lower than for the baseline system, and the reverberated data were recognized better. Training a speech recognizer in different acoustic environments can obviously enhance the recognition also on signals from an environment that was not included in the training material. However, recognition on the close-talking training data lost some accuracy, yet not so much as with the *EMB-rev* approach. With 4-gram language model, still 91.7% instead of 94.3% as on the baseline system are reached. The results for the close-talking test data, however, get worse when only a 0-gram model is used (57.7% vs. 70.0% on *EMB-base*).

A mixture of reverberated and clear training data was tested for its ability to keep the recognition rates for the near and distant microphones on their high level. One part of the training set were the entire training data of the *EMB-base* recognizer. The other part consisted of one twelfth of the artificially reverberated training files for *EMB-12*, i.e. the final training set was twice as big as for the baseline system (see Table 4.2). For this reason, it is denoted as *EMB-2* (see details in Chapter 4.1.7). The results for this approach (Table 6.1) show that the recognition could be enhanced for all three test sets, even for the close-talking recordings. Although this was very pleasing at first sight, the question arose whether the reason for this improvement was only an effect of the reverberation of the training files. The baseline recognizer *EMB-base* had a very small training set of only about one hour of speech data because it was used for time-efficient testing of different features. The vocabulary size was 473, and the number of training speakers was 12, so the training set might have been simply too small for a robust estimation of all the phone models. When the same utterances are added to the data set again in another speech quality (*EMB-2*), it is very likely that the parameter estimation becomes more reliable by the larger amount of data, and hence the recognition performance could have been improved. If the same sentences are used 12 times, convolved with 12 room impulse responses (*EMB-12*), this effect is intensified even more.

Another aspect in the EMBASSI experiments was that the training and the test set were recorded in the same room (see Chapter 4.1). Even the impulse responses for the artificial reverberation of the close-talking signals were measured in the same room. This does not reflect a real application situation where the target environment is unknown before. These problems were solved by employing different speech databases. The respective experiments are subsumed in the next section.

6.1.4   Experiments on VERBMOBIL and Fatigue Data

Because of the different sizes in training data for the EMBASSI-based recognizers, further tests involving a bigger baseline set with constant size among all experiments were performed. This excluded under- or overadaptation, because always the same amount of training data was available for each phone model. The new training data were a part of the VERBMOBIL German corpus; the recognizers created with these data are named *VM-base*, *VM-12*, and *VM-2* (see also Chapter 4.3). In addition to the VERBMOBIL test sets, a subset of the Fatigue corpus was used as test data (Chapter 4.2). Similar experiments were also published in [HNH⁺05] where in the training phase always 10 iterations for the codebook reestimation were performed. In the frame of this thesis, however, the codebook was reestimated as long as the negative log-likelihood of the validation data decreased (cf. Chapter 5.1.5). Training of a VERBMOBIL-based recognizer takes about 6 days on a 2.08 GHz machine (AMD Athlon® XP 2800+) with 1 GB RAM when 10 codebook reestimation iterations are made. The numbers of respective iterations for the different recognizers are summarized in Table 6.5. Table 6.2 gives some information about the recognition performance of the *VM-base* recognizer. The real-time factor on the close-talking test data is about 2.5 and rises to about 4 on reverberated test data. The positive influence of the 4-gram language model not only for the recognition rates but also for the performance is impressively clear when looking at the corresponding factors for the 0-gram experiments. For distant-talking recordings from the Fatigue experiment, the factor is as high as 36.5. The reason is that, especially for the reverberated test sets, the search trees during the recognition phase were very complex.

Table 6.3 and 6.4 show the recognition results. The word accuracy for the Fatigue close-talking test set is highest for the *VM-base* recognizer (86.5% word accuracy when using a 4-gram language model) and lowest for *VM-12* (80.9%) where only reverberated files were in the training data. *VM-2* (85.1%) almost reaches the baseline result. Regarding the Fatigue data recorded at 1 m distance in a room with $T_{60} = 300$ ms, the close-talking recognizer *VM-base* shows least

test set	#files	lang. model	time	time/file	RTF
VERBMOBIL close-talk	268	4-gram	1.2 h	17 s	2.4
VERBMOBIL close-talk	268	0-gram	8.8 h	135 s	16.9
VERBMOBIL artif. reverb.	268	4-gram	1.9 h	26 s	3.7
VERBMOBIL artif. reverb.	268	0-gram	12.8 h	197 s	24.5
Fatigue close-talk	1445	4-gram	6.4 h	18 s	2.5
Fatigue close-talk	1445	0-gram	47.1 h	117 s	18.3
Fatigue reverberated	1445	4-gram	10.7 h	31 s	4.2
Fatigue reverberated	1445	0-gram	93.7 h	233 s	36.5

Table 6.2: Performance of full recognition phase on the *VM-base* recognizer (MFCC features) on a 2.08 GHz machine (AMD Athlon® XP 2800+) with 1 GB RAM; total recognition time and time per file are given for two language models. "RTF" denotes the real-time factor.

accuracy as expected (47.8%) and *VM-12* the highest one (69.8%). *VM-2* with 68.5% nearly reaches the same value. Taking the average of the results on Fatigue close-talking data and distant-talking data, the baseline word accuracy of 68.2% can be improved to 76.8% on *VM-2* which means a relative reduction of word error rate of 27.0% (Table 6.4). The texts read by the Fatigue test speakers were part of the training data of the language model (see Chapter 4.3.2). This is visible in the 4-gram results of the Fatigue test sets which are almost in all cases better than for the VERBMOBIL test data. The results for the 0-gram language model, however, are mostly lower than their VERBMOBIL counterparts which is most likely a consequence of the acoustic mismatch between training and test data.

The results show that artificially reverberated training data can help to improve the robustness of speech recognition in reverberant acoustic environments, even if there is a mismatch between the room impulse responses used for training and those inherent in the test files. The average values confirm the results from the EMBASSI recognizers (Table 6.1). They show that across different acoustic properties in the test signals, the *VM-2* recognizer is the best choice. In the next section, the combination of differently reverberated training data and different feature extraction methods will be examined.

6.2 Experimental Results on Modified Features

6.2.1 Root Cepstrum Features

All speech recognizers that were applied compute 24 features per 16 ms frame. For the *EMB-base* recognizer, the features were the signal energy, the 2nd to 12th MFCC, and the first derivatives of those 12 static features (see also Chapter 5.1.3). The problem with the logarithmic compression of the filterbank coefficients in the usual MFCC feature extraction (Figure 5.3) is that it is most sensitive to spectral parts with the lowest power, i.e. where the signal-to-noise ratio (SNR) is usually worst. Furthermore, the float number range of the computer may not be sufficient for feature values below 1. As an alternative to MFCC, the root cepstrum coefficients (RCC, [Lim79]) were applied. The root cepstrum replaces the logarithm by a root function $\sqrt[\gamma]{x}$. Experiments were made on the EMBASSI-based recognizers *EMB-base*, *EMB-12*, and *EMB-2* following the same

test set	lang. model	VM-base (MFCC)	VM-12 (MFCC)	VM-2 (MFCC)
VERBMOBIL close-talk	4-gram	**79.7**	69.0	76.6
VERBMOBIL close-talk	0-gram	**51.7**	36.7	46.7
VERBMOBIL artif. reverb.	4-gram	60.4	*65.2*	*64.9*
VERBMOBIL artif. reverb.	0-gram	28.9	*38.1*	*36.9*
Fatigue close-talk	4-gram	**86.5**	80.9	85.1
Fatigue close-talk	0-gram	**49.5**	37.3	45.4
Fatigue reverberated	4-gram	47.8	*69.8*	*68.5*
Fatigue reverberated	0-gram	12.4	*30.8*	*28.1*

Table 6.3: Word accuracy for VERBMOBIL-based recognizers (MFCC features); results in italics are significantly better ($p \leq 0.01$) than on *VM-base*. The best results in each line are printed in boldface.

test set	lang. model	VM-base (MFCC)	VM-12 (MFCC)	VM-2 (MFCC)
VERBMOBIL close-talk / artif. reverb.	4-gram	70.1	67.1	**70.8**
VERBMOBIL close-talk / artif. reverb.	0-gram	40.3	37.4	**41.8**
Fatigue close-talk / reverberated	4-gram	68.2	*75.4*	**76.8**
Fatigue close-talk / reverberated	0-gram	31.0	*34.1*	**36.8**

Table 6.4: Average word accuracy for VERBMOBIL-based recognizers (MFCC features) across different acoustic situations; results in italics are significantly better ($p \leq 0.01$) than on *VM-base*. The best results in each line are printed in boldface.

recognizer	VM-base (MFCC)	VM-12 (MFCC)	VM-2 (MFCC)	VM-base ($\mu = 10^5$)	VM-12 ($\mu = 10^5$)	VM-2 ($\mu = 10^5$)
iterations	7	4	6	6	9	10

Table 6.5: Number of codebook reestimation iterations for the VERBMOBIL-based recognizers; if the stop condition was not fulfilled after the 10th iteration, then the process was stopped.

scheme as in Chapter 6.1. Preliminary tests had shown that the word accuracy for $n = 10$ gets worse rapidly in comparison to the MFCC features. The same holds for $n \leq 3$. Therefore, the experiments described below are restricted to a range of $n \in [4; 9]$. Since the *fex4* feature extraction program expects the root parameter as $1/n$, the reciprocal values of n were given with the precision of 4 decimal places for the training procedure, e.g. 0.1428 for $n = 7$.

All results are summarized in Table 6.6 for the recognizers with the *EMB-base* training set, in Table 6.7 for the *EMB-12* training set, and in Table 6.8 for the *EMB-2* data. Concerning the number of cases where the MFCC word accuracies were reached or exceeded, the best results were achieved for $n = 7$. However, this happened only on a few test sets, and the improvement was not significant. The remaining test sets on the respective recognizer showed significantly worse results than with MFCC features. The reason for this is not clear. Taking into account the experiments altogether, the root cepstrum was not convincing in reverberated environment. For *EMB-base* the results are also displayed graphically in Figure 6.2 and Figure 6.3 in order to give an impression of the best interval for the root parameter n.

6.2.2 μ-Law Features in the EMBASSI Baseline System *EMB-base*

In the μ-law features, the logarithm that is usually applied to the Mel spectrum coefficients is replaced by a companding formula (see Chapter 5.2.3). Features with different powers of 10 for the user-defined factor μ were analyzed in order to find alternatives for MFCC features in reverberated environment. Preliminary experiments with $\mu = 10^2$ and $\mu = 10^3$ achieved bad results, above $\mu = 10^9$ the word accuracies declined as well. For this reason, the remaining experiments were restricted to integer exponents for μ between 4 and 9.

The recognition results are summarized in Table 6.9. In order to give an impression about the relation of MFCC and μ-law features, the results for these experiments are also presented graphically in Figure 6.4 and 6.5. With the *EMB-base* training set, improvement of the recognition results could be achieved for all test sets, i.e. for all three microphone distances and for 4-gram and 0-gram language model. With $\mu = 10^5$ and 4-gram language model, the close-talking signals reached a word accuracy of 95.0% (MFCC: 94.3%). The improvement for the recordings with 1 m microphone distance (92.3% vs. 90.2%) and the 2.5 m distance recordings (87.0% vs. 84.1%) was even more clearly and significant on a 0.01 level. The same holds also for the recognition with 0-gram language model. In contrast to the findings in [HSN03] where erroneously different initialization vectors for the features were used, there was no indication for the former assumption that the best value for μ is dependent on the degree of reverberation in the test data.

It was reported for Root Cepstrum Coefficients that – at least for Linear Frequency Cepstral Coefficients (LFCC) without a Mel-like filterbank – different root functions for training and test set can improve performance when noisy signals are tested on a recognizer trained with clear speech [AL93, LA94]. In order to find out whether this might also be valid for μ-law features, the data from 2.5 m microphone distance were tested on the *EMB-base* recognizer ($\mu = 10^9$) with some μ values smaller than the one for training. But in contrast to the baseline MFCC result of 84.1%, the word accuracy reached only about 75% for several steps between $\mu = 9 \cdot 10^8$ and $\mu = 10^9$, so this approach was not further examined.

EMB-base, root cepstrum features								
mic. dist.	lang. model	$n=4$	$n=5$	$n=6$	$n=7$	$n=8$	$n=9$	MFCC
close-talk	4-gram	90.6	93.6	94.0	**94.6**	94.4	94.2	94.3
close-talk	0-gram	47.0	59.2	63.8	69.2	66.7	66.3	**70.0**
1 m	4-gram	77.8	87.2	88.0	**91.1**	90.7	88.1	90.2
1 m	0-gram	27.3	42.4	48.3	48.6	47.9	46.6	**52.4**
2.5 m	4-gram	66.7	77.3	82.1	82.0	80.5	81.0	**84.1**
2.5 m	0-gram	20.2	29.0	32.2	34.5	33.8	34.5	**37.5**

Table 6.6: Word accuracy for *EMB-base* recognizers (root cepstrum features) with different root parameters n on test data with different microphone distances; the best results in each line are printed in boldface.

EMB-12, root cepstrum features								
mic. dist.	lang. model	$n=4$	$n=5$	$n=6$	$n=7$	$n=8$	$n=9$	MFCC
close-talk	4-gram	81.6	89.9	91.8	**92.6**	92.4	91.2	91.7
close-talk	0-gram	34.5	48.5	53.6	55.7	57.0	57.4	**57.7**
1 m	4-gram	78.4	89.3	93.3	92.7	92.3	91.7	**94.0**
1 m	0-gram	34.3	47.7	54.8	60.0	60.8	57.9	**61.9**
2.5 m	4-gram	69.6	84.8	87.6	**89.6**	89.0	89.0	88.4
2.5 m	0-gram	26.3	39.7	44.6	51.4	**52.9**	52.1	52.4

Table 6.7: Word accuracy for *EMB-12* recognizers (root cepstrum features) with different root parameters n on test data with different microphone distances; the best results in each line are printed in boldface.

EMB-2, root cepstrum features								
mic. dist.	lang. model	$n=4$	$n=5$	$n=6$	$n=7$	$n=8$	$n=9$	MFCC
close-talk	4-gram	91.6	94.2	94.7	95.0	94.8	93.8	**95.5**
close-talk	0-gram	50.6	62.1	66.6	69.4	69.2	67.1	**71.4**
1 m	4-gram	82.2	92.1	93.8	94.2	94.3	92.4	**94.4**
1 m	0-gram	36.5	52.4	58.0	61.5	61.1	59.3	**63.0**
2.5 m	4-gram	72.0	83.9	88.5	88.1	89.3	**89.7**	89.6
2.5 m	0-gram	25.7	40.3	46.6	47.9	49.9	51.2	**55.3**

Table 6.8: Word accuracy for *EMB-2* recognizers (root cepstrum features) with different root parameters n on test data with different microphone distances; the best results in each line are printed in boldface.

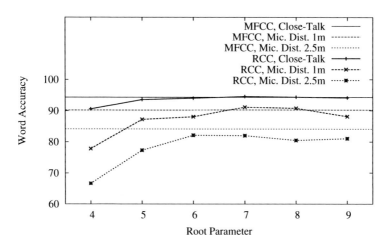

Figure 6.2: Word accuracy for *EMB-base* recognizers with root cepstrum features and a 4-gram language model; the horizontal lines represent the results for *EMB-base* with MFCC.

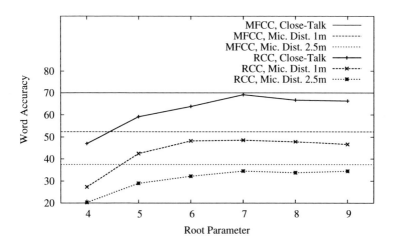

Figure 6.3: Word accuracy for *EMB-base* recognizers with root cepstrum features and a 0-gram language model; the horizontal lines represent the results for *EMB-base* with MFCC.

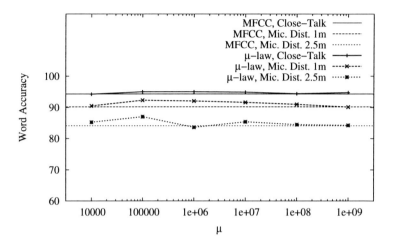

Figure 6.4: Word accuracy for *EMB-base* recognizers with μ-law features and a 4-gram language model; the horizontal lines represent the results for *EMB-base* with MFCC.

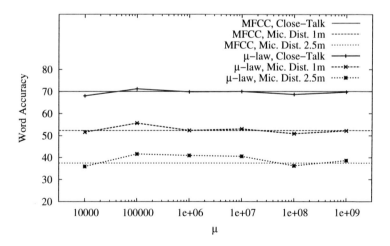

Figure 6.5: Word accuracy for *EMB-base* recognizers with μ-law features and a 0-gram language model; the horizontal lines represent the results for *EMB-base* with MFCC.

6.2.3 μ-Law Features and Artificially Reverberated EMBASSI Data

As pointed out in the previous section, the μ-law companding function shows advantages in speech recognition for undistorted and reverberated test environments on the *EMB-base* recognizer that was trained on clear speech. It was further examined whether this also holds for artifically reverberated training data on the *EMB-12* and *EMB-2* recognizer (Chapter 4.1.7). Again, powers of 10 were used as values for μ. The results are summarized in Table 6.10 for the bigger *EMB-12* training set and in Table 6.11 for *EMB-2*. In contrast to the *EMB-base* recognizer (Table 6.9), here the μ-law features show positive effects mainly on the reverberated test data only. There is also not only one single value for μ that could be identified as the best one. These values rather came from the entire range between 10^4 and 10^9. None of them reached a significance level of $p \leq 0.01$, however.

Again, the *EMB-2* recognizer with the training set consisting of close-talking speech and artificially reverberated recordings is the best compromise for all different test environments. For the close-talking test, however, MFCC are better than μ-law features. In Chapter 6.1.3, the problems arising from the different sizes of the EMBASSI training sets and their partial match of training and test environment were discussed. Because of these reasons, the EMBASSI experiments can only be seen as preliminary tests where the short training time helped to accelerate the search for better feature parameters. Selected experiments from this section were repeated on VERBMOBIL and Fatigue data. For the details, see the next section.

6.2.4 μ-Law Features and Artificially Reverberated VERBMOBIL Data

Since the training of a VERBMOBIL recognizer and the recognition experiments are very time-consuming (see Table 6.2), only the features and parameters were chosen that performed best on the EMBASSI approach. This means that the Root Cepstrum Coefficients (Chapter 6.2.1) were not taken into account any more as they mostly could not even reach the baseline results. Only the μ-law features with the value of $\mu = 10^5$ were examined and compared to the respective MFCC results.

Table 6.12 summarizes the results on the VERBMOBIL-based recognizers with μ-law features. It clearly shows the same tendency as for MFCC (cf. Table 6.3), i.e. that on average the recognizer *VM-2* with the combination of clean and artificially reverberated training speech is most suitable for the recognition in different acoustic environments (Table 6.13). This confirms the EMBASSI results from the previous section once more.

The results best representing a real-world experiment of a recognizer that does not have any information about the test environment are those from the Fatigue test data as their reverberated version does not match any of the room acoustics seen in the training data. Taking into account the recognition with a 4-gram language model, the average word accuracy on close-talking and reverberated Fatigue data could be improved from 68.2% on the *VM-base* recognizer with MFCC to 76.8% on the *VM-2* recognizer with MFCC and finally to 77.2% with μ-law features where the last step is unfortunately not a significant enhancement. Nevertheless, Table 6.12 shows that μ-law features perform better in all of the tested *VM-12* and *VM-2* cases, regardless whether the test signals were from a close-talking signal, artificially reverberated or recorded by a distant-talking microphone. One exception has to be noted: In contrast to the *VM-2* recognizer with MFCC, the word accuracy of the VERBMOBIL close-talking test set drops from 76.6% to 75.8%. The reason for this could not be identified; the corresponding recognition results with the 0-gram

EMB-base, μ-law features								
mic. dist.	lang. model	$\mu = 10^4$	$\mu = 10^5$	$\mu = 10^6$	$\mu = 10^7$	$\mu = 10^8$	$\mu = 10^9$	MFCC
close-talk	4-gram	94.3	**95.0**	**95.0**	94.9	94.4	94.8	94.3
close-talk	0-gram	68.1	**71.2**	69.9	70.0	68.7	69.7	70.0
1 m	4-gram	90.5	*92.3*	92.1	91.6	91.0	90.2	90.2
1 m	0-gram	51.7	*55.7*	52.4	53.1	50.9	52.2	52.4
2.5 m	4-gram	85.3	*87.0*	83.6	85.4	84.5	84.3	84.1
2.5 m	0-gram	35.9	*41.6*	41.0	40.6	36.3	38.6	37.5

Table 6.9: Word accuracy for *EMB-base* recognizers (μ-law features) with different values for μ on test data with different microphone distances; results in italics are significantly better ($p \leq 0.01$) than on *EMB-base* with MFCC. The best results in each line are printed in boldface.

.

EMB-12, μ-law features								
mic. dist.	lang. model	$\mu = 10^4$	$\mu = 10^5$	$\mu = 10^6$	$\mu = 10^7$	$\mu = 10^8$	$\mu = 10^9$	MFCC
close-talk	4-gram	92.3	91.9	91.8	**92.4**	92.3	92.0	91.7
close-talk	0-gram	57.2	56.2	57.7	56.3	56.6	57.1	**57.7**
1 m	4-gram	93.7	94.5	94.6	95.4	94.1	**95.0**	94.0
1 m	0-gram	62.9	62.8	62.6	62.9	61.8	**63.5**	61.9
2.5 m	4-gram	89.2	88.9	**90.0**	89.1	89.0	89.1	88.4
2.5 m	0-gram	54.6	**54.8**	54.6	54.3	53.5	53.9	52.4

Table 6.10: Word accuracy for *EMB-12* recognizers (μ-law features) with different values for μ on test data with different microphone distances; the best results in each line are printed in boldface.

EMB-2, μ-law features								
mic. dist.	lang. model	$\mu = 10^4$	$\mu = 10^5$	$\mu = 10^6$	$\mu = 10^7$	$\mu = 10^8$	$\mu = 10^9$	MFCC
close-talk	4-gram	95.4	95.3	95.3	94.8	95.0	95.2	**95.5**
close-talk	0-gram	70.8	69.4	70.0	68.6	70.3	70.5	**71.4**
1 m	4-gram	**94.7**	94.1	94.4	93.8	94.3	94.3	94.4
1 m	0-gram	64.2	63.2	63.2	64.6	**65.3**	63.6	63.0
2.5 m	4-gram	89.5	**90.7**	89.0	89.9	88.7	89.3	89.6
2.5 m	0-gram	53.9	52.1	**55.5**	54.7	54.2	54.9	55.3

Table 6.11: Word accuracy for *EMB-2* recognizers (μ-law features) with different values for μ on test data with different microphone distances; the best results in each line are printed in boldface.

test set	lang. model	VM-base $(\mu = 10^5)$	VM-12 $(\mu = 10^5)$	VM-2 $(\mu = 10^5)$
VERBMOBIL close-talk	4-gram	**79.9** (+0.2)	73.4 (*+4.4*)	75.8 (–0.8)
VERBMOBIL close-talk	0-gram	**50.2** (–1.5)	39.7 (*+3.0*)	49.1 (+2.4)
VERBMOBIL artif. reverb.	4-gram	57.3 (–3.1)	***68.1*** (*+2.9*)	*66.9* (+2.0)
VERBMOBIL artif. reverb.	0-gram	26.0 (–2.9)	***39.7*** (+1.6)	*38.4* (+1.5)
Fatigue close-talk	4-gram	**86.6** (+0.1)	82.1 (*+1.2*)	85.5 (+0.4)
Fatigue close-talk	0-gram	**48.2** (–1.3)	39.6 (*+2.3*)	46.6 (*+1.2*)
Fatigue reverberated	4-gram	44.4 (–3.4)	***71.1*** (*+1.3*)	68.7 (+0.2)
Fatigue reverberated	0-gram	11.1 (–1.3)	***31.7*** (+0.9)	*28.8* (+0.7)

Table 6.12: Word accuracy for VERBMOBIL-based recognizers (μ-law features); the values in parentheses are the difference to the corresponding result with MFCC (see Table 6.3). Results in italics are significantly better ($p \leq 0.01$) than on VM-base ($\mu = 10^5$) or on the corresponding recognizer with MFCC (in parentheses), respectively. The best results in each line are printed in boldface.

test set	lang. model	VM-base $(\mu = 10^5)$	VM-12 $(\mu = 10^5)$	VM-2 $(\mu = 10^5)$
VERBMOBIL close-talk / artif. reverb.	4-gram	68.7 (–1.4)	*70.8* (*+3.7*)	**71.4** (+0.6)
VERBMOBIL close-talk / artif. reverb.	0-gram	38.1 (–2.2)	*39.7* (*+2.3*)	**43.8** (*+2.0*)
Fatigue close-talk / reverberated	4-gram	65.5 (–2.7)	*76.6* (*+1.2*)	**77.2** (+0.4)
Fatigue close-talk / reverberated	0-gram	29.7 (–1.3)	*35.7* (*+1.6*)	**37.7** (*+0.9*)

Table 6.13: Average word accuracy for VERBMOBIL-based recognizers (μ-law features) across different acoustic situations; the values in parentheses are the difference to the corresponding result with MFCC (see Table 6.4). Results in italics are significantly better ($p \leq 0.01$) than on VM-base ($\mu = 10^5$) or on the corresponding recognizer with MFCC (in parentheses), respectively. The best results in each line are printed in boldface.

language model (49.1% with $\mu = 10^5$ vs. 46.7% on MFCC) show contrary behavior. Compared to MFCC, most of the results for the VM-base recognizer got worse with μ-law features.

The outcome of these experiments is that μ-law features in combination with artificially reverberated training data are beneficial for the recognition of reverberated speech while they also keep the recognition of clear speech at a high level.

6.2.5 Gaussianization of Feature Components

Gaussianization means the normalization of a set of values to match a Gaussian density function with a mean value of 0 and a standard deviation of 1. Applied to features, it follows the idea of cepstral mean subtraction [GM02] and was supposed to create more noise-robust features. For this thesis, the normalization was not applied to all of the 24 features that are computed per frame (cf. Chapter 5.1). The speech energy and its derivative were left untouched as they repre-

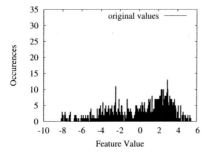 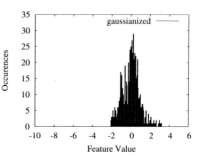

Figure 6.6: Gaussianization of the second MFCC of VERBMOBIL file 1G071A:HAH001A; the original file's mean value was 0.09 with a standard deviation of 3.17. The corresponding values of the gaussianized version were 0.05 and 0.88.

sent a completely different feature type and range. Only the 11 remaining components and their first derivatives were normalized with respect to the entire file. This was done for MFCC (Chapter 5.1.3), root cepstrum features (Chapter 5.2.2), and μ-law features (Chapter 5.2.3). Figure 6.6 illustrates the distribution of one feature component for one file before and after gaussianization. The normalization was combined with all the EMBASSI training scenarios *EMB-base* (Chapter 4.1.3), *EMB-12*, and *EMB-2* (Chapter 4.1.7). The three test sets from the close-talking microphone and the distant-talking microphone with 1 m or 2.5 m distance to the speaker, respectively, were the same as in the previously described experiments (see also Table 4.3).

There are not many experiments where the normalization was beneficial. Mostly the improvement was so small that it was not significant. Table 6.14 summarizes all these cases. Only an *EMB-12* recognizer with root cepstrum features ($n = 4$) received consistently and significantly better results than without gaussianization. Nevertheless, they are still far below the recognition rates that are reached with MFCC features.

Except for the mentioned exceptions, the feature normalization in general does not help to improve recognition. For this reason, it was no longer used in further experiments. The detailed results for all recognizers are subsumed in Appendix C.

The next section will describe a preprocessing operation that is commonly used to enhance the quality of noisy signals when more than one microphone is available. When they record synchronously, then their signals can be combined to a single one and attenuate noise in this way.

6.3   Results on Beamformed Test Data

In the previous sections, two different approaches for enhancing speech recognition in reverberated environment were introduced. The first one used artificially reverberated training data in order to integrate the acoustic environment into the phone models of the recognizer (Chapter 6.1). The second one was based on features that were supposed to be unaffected by reverberation. This means that they should allow to recognize distorted speech on a recognizer which was trained on undistorted signals (Chapter 6.2). In this section, a preprocessing operation will be applied in

recognizer	feature	mic. dist.	lang. model	WA_{gauss}	WA_{orig}
EMB-base	root, $n = 6$	1 m	4-gram	*89.6*	88.0
EMB-12	root, $n = 4$	close-talk	4-gram	*87.4*	81.6
EMB-12	root, $n = 4$	close-talk	0-gram	*42.9*	34.5
EMB-12	root, $n = 4$	1 m	0-gram	*36.9*	34.3
EMB-12	root, $n = 4$	2.5 m	4-gram	*73.8*	69.6
EMB-12	root, $n = 4$	2.5 m	0-gram	*28.6*	26.3
EMB-12	root, $n = 5$	close-talk	4-gram	90.8	89.9
EMB-12	root, $n = 5$	close-talk	0-gram	64.2	62.1
EMB-base	μ-law, $\mu = 10^4$	close-talk	0-gram	68.2	68.1
EMB-base	μ-law, $\mu = 10^4$	1 m	0-gram	51.8	51.7
EMB-base	μ-law, $\mu = 10^6$	2.5 m	4-gram	84.0	83.6
EMB-base	μ-law, $\mu = 10^8$	2.5 m	4-gram	85.7	84.5
EMB-base	μ-law, $\mu = 10^8$	2.5 m	0-gram	37.8	36.3
EMB-base	μ-law, $\mu = 10^9$	1 m	4-gram	90.9	90.2
EMB-base	μ-law, $\mu = 10^9$	2.5 m	4-gram	*86.3*	84.3

Table 6.14: Word accuracy for experiments where gaussianized features achieved better results than the non-converted features; numbers printed in italics denote improvements at least on a 0.01 significance level.

order to remove distortions from the test data and allow to process it with a recognizer for clean speech.

6.3.1 Removing Reverberation from Audio Signals

Dereverberation on a single microphone is very difficult [AH96, TLK93]. The use of several microphones is much more successful [OSM98, Jun00]. It offers for instance the method of Blind Deconvolution [MK88, Hay01, BAK04]. Convolutional noise can also be handled in the cepstral domain by Blind Equalization [Mau98, CLL03]. The quality of a speech signal is highly dependent on the type of the microphones. The use of a microphone array allows to separate signals from different spatial locations, even if their bandwidths overlap [OSM98]. When using more than one microphone, the microphones do not have to be expensive. Even with very cheap microphones, the error rate in far-field speech recognition can be substantially lowered [DGM03].

A completely different way to solve the problem is the application of an artificial neural network (ANN) which is trained with synchronously recorded close-talking speech and reverberated signals. The ANN learns to map a distorted signal to an undistorted one. This approach can be used on the time-domain signals [Sør91, Wei02] or in the feature domain [LCY+96]. For the EMBASSI corpus (see Chapter 4.1), this was examined in [Wei05].

6.3.2 Beamforming

If more than one microphone is available, then the quality of distorted recordings can be improved by combining several synchronously recorded audio files to a new one. The basic idea is that the desired signal, i.e. the speaker's voice, is amplified, and noise is canceled by appropriate addition of the single microphone outputs. A rather simple approach to achieve this is the delay-and-sum beamformer (DSB), sometimes also called delay-and-add beamformer. It introduces a time delay for each microphone in order to equalize the different runtimes from the sound source and adds up the signals using weighting factors (cf. e.g. [OSM98]). These conventional beam-formers do the runtime synchronization, the weighting and the summation one after the other. With noise reduction and adaptation of the acoustic models according to the preprocessing chan-nel, better improvement can be achieved [USB03]. However, this was not applied for this thesis. Examples for advanced beamformers are the General Sidelobe Canceller (GSC, [GJ82]) and the Frost beamformer [Fro72]. For an overview and further details, cf. [Her05].

6.3.3   Experiments with the EMBASSI Baseline System *EMB-base*

Beamforming was performed in order to combine one new signal out of several synchronously recorded signals of the EMBASSI microphone array (Figure 4.2). This was done at the Chair of Multimedia Communications and Signal Processing (LMS). The signals from session 10 of the EMBASSI corpus (see Chapter 4.1) served as the basis for the newly created data. In this session where the particular speaker was alone in a quiet room, the distance to the array microphones was 2.5 m, and the reverberation time T_{60} was 400 ms. Like for all other EMBASSI experiments, the test speaker group consisted of 3 male and 3 female speakers (see also Table 4.3).

The delay-and-sum approach was applied in combination with MFCC and μ-law features. The experiments were performed with training and test files containing one single sentence each. Note that the preprocessing was done on a recording of the entire session first (60 sentences), and the signal was cut into single sentences afterward. For the feature extraction, the mean feature files of the particular recognizers which had been computed on the respective training data were used for initialization.

The results for the *EMB-base* recognizer (Chapter 4.1.3) are shown in Table 6.15. There is only one case where beamforming could enhance the word accuracy on the test data ($\mu = 10^6$), and this improvement could only be achieved for the case where the 4-gram language model was applied. With a 0-gram model, the results on data from one single microphone without preprocessing were always better.

6.3.4   Beamforming and Artificially Reverberated EMBASSI Data

The recognizers *EMB-12* and *EMB-2* (Chapter 4.1.7) were also applied to the preprocessed data in order to find out whether the combination of artificial reverberation in the training data and beamforming of the natural reverberation in the test data has a positive effect on the recognition results. Table 6.16 shows that the beamforming is beneficial in the *EMB-12* scenario where only reverberated training data are used. For $\mu = 10^7$ and $\mu = 10^8$, the improvement almost reaches a 0.01 significance level when a 4-gram language model is used. The experiments were repeated with the *EMB-2* recognizer which is trained with close-talking and reverberated data (Table 6.17). Here the improvement was not as good and consistent among all tested values of μ. The advan-tage is clearly on the side of the *EMB-12* approach with the large training set. In order to exclude the effects of different amounts of training data, beamformed test data were also processed by the VERBMOBIL-based recognizers. The results will be presented in the next section.

EMB-base, μ-law features								
mic. dist.	lang. model	$\mu=10^4$	$\mu=10^5$	$\mu=10^6$	$\mu=10^7$	$\mu=10^8$	$\mu=10^9$	MFCC
2.5 m	4-gram	85.3	**87.0**	83.6	85.4	84.5	84.3	84.1
2.5 m	0-gram	35.9	**41.6**	41.0	40.6	36.3	38.6	37.5
2.5 m, DSB	4-gram	77.8	**86.0**	85.1	83.3	81.6	82.7	80.6
2.5 m, DSB	0-gram	27.9	**40.4**	33.9	36.1	34.2	36.1	32.8

Table 6.15: Word accuracy for *EMB-base* recognizers (μ-law features) with different values for μ on test data from one single distant-talking microphone and from 11 microphones after delay-and-sum beamforming (DSB); the best results in each line are printed in boldface.

EMB-12, μ-law features								
mic. dist.	lang. model	$\mu=10^4$	$\mu=10^5$	$\mu=10^6$	$\mu=10^7$	$\mu=10^8$	$\mu=10^9$	MFCC
2.5 m	4-gram	89.2	88.9	**90.0**	89.1	89.0	89.1	88.4
2.5 m	0-gram	54.6	**54.8**	54.6	54.3	53.5	53.9	52.4
2.5 m, DSB	4-gram	90.1	89.8	90.9	*91.6*	*91.4*	90.1	90.2
2.5 m, DSB	0-gram	52.1	52.2	**56.7**	55.2	56.1	54.1	53.9

Table 6.16: Word accuracy for *EMB-12* recognizers (μ-law features) with different values for μ on test data from one single distant-talking microphone and from 11 microphones after delay-and-sum beamforming (DSB); results in italics are significantly better ($p \le 0.01$) than on one single microphone. The best results in each line are printed in boldface.

EMB-2, μ-law features								
mic. dist.	lang. model	$\mu=10^4$	$\mu=10^5$	$\mu=10^6$	$\mu=10^7$	$\mu=10^8$	$\mu=10^9$	MFCC
2.5 m	4-gram	89.5	**90.7**	89.0	89.9	88.7	89.3	89.6
2.5 m	0-gram	53.9	52.1	**55.5**	54.7	54.2	54.9	55.3
2.5 m, DSB	4-gram	89.6	88.5	89.2	89.7	89.9	89.3	**90.8**
2.5 m, DSB	0-gram	50.6	49.7	51.7	52.3	**53.1**	51.0	**53.1**

Table 6.17: Word accuracy for *EMB-2* recognizers (μ-law features) with different values for μ on test data from one single distant-talking microphone and from 11 microphones after delay-and-sum beamforming (DSB); the best results in each line are printed in boldface.

6.3.5   Results on the VERBMOBIL-Based Recognizers

For the beamforming experiments with the VERBMOBIL-based recognizers, a simple delay-and-sum beamformer was implemented at the Chair of Pattern Recognition. To determine the time shift between two signals, this program randomly chooses 10 windows from the current speech signal with a length of 30 ms each. Since it could be assumed that the signals contain only the speaker's voice and no further noise source, it was sufficient to assume the presence of speech when a certain energy threshold is exceeded. In this case, the respective window is selected for further processing. Otherwise the window is removed from the selection list, and a new window is randomly chosen. Then each window of the current signal is compared to the corresponding window of a reference signal (here from array microphone #1; see Figure 4.5). The time shift between the signals is determined by the minimum difference between the energy integrals of both windows. The rounded shift average of all 10 windows is assumed to be the actual shift between current and reference signal. The current signal is then shifted by this value. In the end, all corresponding amplitude values of all synchronous signals are summed up and divided by the number of signals which is 13 here as the entire upper row of the Fatigue microphone array was involved.

Table 6.18 shows the results for the beamformed Fatigue test set (Chapter 4.2) on the recognizers trained with VERBMOBIL data and MFCC features. Table 6.19 shows the results when μ-law features were applied with $\mu = 10^5$ which has been the best value for μ on the former test sets (Chapter 6.2). Like for the signals from one single microphone, the *VM-base* recognizer cannot take advantage from the μ-law features. The word accuracy of 63.1% (with 4-gram language model) falls to 59.0% on the alternative features. For *VM-12* and *VM-2*, the μ-law features gain about one percent point which is significant on a 0.01 level. In comparison to the signals from a single, distant-talking microphone (Table 6.3 and 6.12), the beamforming yielded an unexpectedly large enhancement. For the best of the recognizers (*VM-12*, $\mu = 10^5$), the word accuracy rose from 71.7% and 31.7% (4-gram and 0-gram, respectively) for one array microphone to 77.4% and 37.0%, respectively, on the beamformed Fatigue test set. For the *VM-base* approaches, even a gain of 15% absolute for the 4-gram language model can be observed. Obviously the signal quality was substantially enhanced by adding up the 13 synchronous, reverberated distant-talking recordings. One of the reasons why the error reduction was so much less effective on the EM-BASSI data might be the larger microphone distance there (2.5 m).

An important note has to be made: The recordings in the Fatigue corpus are not equally modulated. Signals from microphone #1 to #9 reach only about 20% of the possible amplitude while microphones #10 to #13 reach 50–60%. The design of the array cannot be the reason. All of the microphones were in one line which excludes environmental influences during recording. Probably an error occurred during the composition of the 16 kHz version of the corpus. It had to be tested how strong the influence of this error was on the comparison between microphone #7 alone, i.e. the original distant-talking test set, and the beamformed data. For this purpose, all recordings were fully amplified by a sound processing program (*SoX* version 12.17.4). However, an experiment with the modified beamformed test set on the *VM-base* recognizer showed just an improvement of 0.1% word accuracy absolute. Nevertheless, it gave a helpful impression of the influence of different signal energies on beamforming and speech recognition: Recorded signals of different modulation are the usual case in a living-room scenario where the microphones are distributed within the room. Obviously weak signals do not need adjustment to be beneficial for speech recognition.

test set	lang. model	VM-base (MFCC)	VM-12 (MFCC)	VM-2 (MFCC)
Fatigue reverberated	4-gram	47.8	**69.8**	68.5
Fatigue reverberated	0-gram	12.4	**30.8**	28.1
Fatigue reverberated, DSB	4-gram	*63.1*	***76.5***	*76.3*
Fatigue reverberated, DSB	0-gram	*19.6*	***36.1***	*34.4*

Table 6.18: Word accuracy for VERBMOBIL-based recognizers (MFCC features) on test data from one single distant-talking microphone and from 11 microphones after delay-and-sum beam-forming (DSB); results in italics are significantly better ($p \leq 0.01$) than on one single microphone. The best results in each line are printed in boldface.

test set	lang. model	VM-base ($\mu = 10^5$)	VM-12 ($\mu = 10^5$)	VM-2 ($\mu = 10^5$)
Fatigue reverberated	4-gram	44.4 (–3.4)	***71.1*** *(+1.3)*	68.7 (+0.2)
Fatigue reverberated	0-gram	11.1 (–1.3)	***31.7*** *(+0.9)*	28.8 (+0.7)
Fatigue reverberated, DSB	4-gram	59.0 (–4.1)	***77.4*** *(+0.9)*	*77.0* (+0.7)
Fatigue reverberated, DSB	0-gram	17.6 (–2.0)	***37.0*** *(+0.9)*	*35.2* (+0.8)

Table 6.19: Word accuracy for VERBMOBIL-based recognizers (μ-law features) on test data from one single distant-talking microphone and from 11 microphones after delay-and-sum beamforming (DSB); the values in parentheses are the difference to the corresponding result with MFCC. Results in italics are significantly better ($p \leq 0.01$) than on VM-base ($\mu = 10^5$) or to the corresponding recognizer with MFCC (in parentheses), respectively. The best results in each line are printed in boldface.

6.3.6   Summary and Conclusion

In this chapter, different methods that are supposed to enhance the recognition results of reverberated test data have been introduced. The first one was the application of artificially reverberated training data. It was assumed that the test environment is not known at training time. For this reason, 12 different room impulse responses were measured at different positions in a room where the reverberation time could be changed by curtains at the walls. They were used to reverberate the close-talking training data of a speech recognizer. The results for the *EMB-2* and the *VM-2* recognizer showed that it is possible to process both close-talking and reverberated test data sufficiently when the training set is composed from close-talking recordings and artificially reverberated signals. On the Fatigue test set, the average word accuracy on clean and naturally reverberated signals rose from 68.2% on *VM-base* to 76.8% on *VM-2*.

The second kind of changes to the baseline system concerned the feature extraction. The root cepstrum did hardly perform as good as the standard MFCC features, but some improvements on μ-law features were significant on the EMBASSI data. On the Fatigue test set, the average word accuracy on clean and naturally reverberated signals reached 77.2% on the *VM-2* recognizer. Although this is just slightly better than with MFCC, the μ-law features can be recommended for the recognition of distant-talking speech.

Normalizing the features to a Gaussian distribution was beneficial for some of the root cepstrum features, but in general the gain in word accuracy occurred not consistently enough in order to regard the procedure as reliable for other data.

The third approach did not change the recognizer but the test data. Since several synchronous recordings of the EMBASSI and Fatigue set were available, these signals were combined by delay-and-sum beamforming in order to create a new signal with less noise. Indeed, for the *VM-base* recognizer (MFCC features), the word accuracy on the reverberated part of the Fatigue test set rose from 47.8% to 63.1%. Again, an artificially reverberated training set and μ-law features have a positive effect on the results. The best word accuracy achieved was 77.4% on the *VM-12* recognizer with $\mu = 10^5$.

Taking all results into account, the following conclusion is drawn: For a recording scenario in a room with distributed microphones where the test environment is not known at training time, a speech recognizer should be trained with a mixture of close-talking speech and artificially reverberated signals. It should apply beamforming as a preprocessing step and a μ-law companding function for the Mel spectrum during feature extraction.

The experiments in this chapter were performed in view of a speech therapy session where a patient should not be aware of the recording situation which might make him or her feel controlled. The experiments were not made with samples of pathologic speech because there were no speech corpora available that were large enough and recorded by distant-talking microphones. However, in Chapter 7.5 some of the results from this chapter will be verified on artificially reverberated recordings of tracheoesophageal substitute voices. The next chapter will present methods for the automatic evaluation of this kind of voice pathology, i.e. automatic measures that correlate with human evaluation criteria.

Chapter 7

Automatic Analysis of Tracheoesophageal Voices

This chapter will discuss the agreement between human and automatic rating. As a reference, 5 experts (denoted by K, L, R, S, and U) judged the 41 available recordings of the patients with tracheoesophageal (TE) substitute voice by 11 criteria (see Chapter 4.4). The recognizers which were used for the initial experiments were derived from the VERBMOBIL-based *VM-base* recognizer (Chapter 4.3). One of them is polyphone-based and is therefore called *NW-base-poly*; the other one is monophone-based (*NW-base-mono*). The recognition vocabulary for both of them was reduced to the words of the text "The North Wind and the Sun" (Chapter 4.4.1). For details see also Chapter 5.1.6.

7.1 Automatic Speech Recognition vs. Human Evaluation

7.1.1 Baseline Recognition Results on the *NW-base* Recognizers

The recognizers *NW-base-poly* and *NW-base-mono* were both trained on young normal speakers. One reason was that there were not enough data to train them with distorted speech from elderly people, and the other reason was that the recognizers were supposed to simulate a naïve listener who had never heard TE speech before. Hence, there is not only a mismatch between the degree of pathology in training and test speech but also in the age of the training speakers and the *laryng41* test speakers (Chapter 4.4.2). Already the age difference can cause a loss in recognition rate [WJ96]. For this reason, the recognizers were also tested with an older and a younger group of normal speakers (Chapter 4.5) in order to determine the degree of recognition error that is caused by age and by speech pathology. Because the word accuracy was assumed to express the speaker's pathology in some way, all recognizers used a unigram language model. In this way, the error correction by the language model was kept at a minimum The recognition results for all speaker groups are summarized in Table 7.1. All speakers read the text "The North Wind and the Sun". The lowest word accuracy for one TE speaker of the *laryng41* set on *NW-base-poly* was only –3.7% while the best one reached 71.6%; the average value was 36.9%. The control group of 16 young laryngeal speakers (*bas16*) showed an average of 83.3%. Since the *bas16* group is age-matched to the training speakers of the recognizers, this result is regarded as the maximum that can be reached by any of the considered test groups. Note that the two words that are different in the *bas16* variant of the text – "abzunehmen" instead of "auszuziehen" and "erwärmte" instead of

recognizer	speakers	μ(WA)	σ(WA)	min(WA)	max(WA)
NW-base-poly	bas16	83.3	5.7	69.4	92.6
NW-base-poly	kom18	67.3	9.1	49.1	81.7
NW-base-poly	laryng41	36.9	18.0	–3.7	71.6
NW-base-mono	bas16	69.1	9.6	52.8	88.0
NW-base-mono	kom18	58.0	7.2	40.7	72.2
NW-base-mono	laryng41	35.3	13.7	0.9	63.3

Table 7.1: Word accuracy for NW-base recognizers (normal and TE speakers)

recognizer	speakers	rater					all
		K	L	R	S	U	
NW-base-poly	laryng41	–0.74	–0.79	–0.82	–0.81	–0.75	–0.88
NW-base-mono	laryng41	–0.67	–0.71	–0.81	–0.75	–0.71	–0.82

Table 7.2: Correlation r between word accuracy of NW-base recognizers and human raters (intelligibility criterion, laryng41 data)

"wärmte" – were added to the recognition vocabulary of the recognizers (see also Appendix A.1). The influence of age in normal speakers can be seen in the recognition rates for the older kom18 group. Their mean word accuracy was 67.3%. The worst result was 49.1%, the best speaker reached only 81.7% WA. Neglecting minor influences by the microphone channel, the age of the elderly speakers causes a 15 percent points lower recognition rate than for the young speakers, and the speech pathology of the TE speakers is responsible for another 30 percent points.

The NW-base-mono recognizer was created because the more robust training of the monophones was supposed to have a positive effect on the recognition of substitute voices. For the laryng18 group, the mean word accuracy slightly rose (see Chapter 7.2), but on the laryng41 group this effect could not be observed. Figure 7.2 shows that the "low quality" voices were recognized better while the monophone models were disadvantageous for the clearer voices. One outlier appeared (file m000059s01; speaker 10 in the figure). The voice of this man had a gargling sound, and he breathed audibly very often. It is not clear whether this is the reason for his bad results.

7.1.2   Correlation between NW-base Recognizers and Human Rating

At the Department of Phoniatrics and Pedaudiology, 5 experienced phoniatricians and scientific engineers evaluated the voice and speech of the 41 test persons (see also Chapter 4.4.3). The scores given by the experts were represented by numbers between 1 ("very high") and 5 ("very low") for the respective criteria. The highest possible score for "quality" was 4, however. The "overall quality" had to be rated without regarding all the previous criteria on a continuous scale with values between 0.0 ("very good") and 10.0 ("very bad").

The possible maximum of the word accuracy is 100%, a lower bound does not exist. In order to compute the agreement between recognizers and human experts, for some agreement measures

WA interval	]−∞;0[	[0;15[	[15;25[	[25;40[	[40;100]
score	5	4	3	2	1

Table 7.3: Mapping for word accuracy (WA) conversion to the range of human rating criteria

introduced in Chapter 3 the word accuracy has to be mapped to the same number range as the raters' scores. Experiments on the first human evaluation of the *laryng18* group yielded the mapping of Table 7.3 (cf. [SHN$^+$06]) for the conversion of the recognition results. This scheme was afterward used for all further experiments with the *laryng41* data which also includes new human ratings for the *laryng18* subset (see Chapter 4.4.3). In Chapter 7.2.4, an optimization of the mapping with respect to the *laryng41* data will be addressed.

Table 7.4 and 7.5 contain the agreement between the word accuracy of *NW-base-poly* and *NW-base-mono*, respectively, and the criteria of the human raters. For the description and the abbreviations of the criteria, see Table 4.12. Note that κ and α were not computed for "overall quality" since this was marked on a continuous scale. Intelligibility, vocal tone, quality and use of prosody during speaking have the highest correlation to the word accuracy. This confirms also the findings summarized in Table 4.13 that these criteria correlate highly with each other. In the following, the intelligibility judgment will be focused on since it is an expression of the percentage of words the listener understood, just like the word accuracy.

The correlation between the average rater and the word accuracy for the intelligibility criterion was $r = -0.88$ for the *NW-base-poly* recognizer and $r = -0.82$ for *NW-base-mono*. The coefficient is negative because high recognition rates came from "good" voices with a low score number and vice versa. These values were compared to the inter-rater agreement among the expert group. For the files of the *laryng41* data set, the correlation of each single rater's intelligibility scores to the average scores across the other four persons was calculated (see Table 4.15). All correlation values were between 0.80 and 0.87, i.e. the word accuracy as an measure of intelligibility is as good as the average human rater. Table 4.14 shows the inter-rater correlation between single experts. It ranges from 0.69 to 0.82. Again, the agreement between the recognizers and single raters is almost the same, except for the negative sign due to the different domains (Table 7.2). The values for the weighted multi-rater $\kappa_{DF}(w)$ among the group of 5 raters and for the rater group vs. *NW-base-poly* are both 0.45, i.e. the agreement among the humans and the agreement between the human raters and the machine are identical. The $\kappa_{DF}(w)$ for the rater group vs. *NW-base-mono* is 0.41. Krippendorff's α, which was 0.66 for the rater group, shows the same tendency with $\alpha = 0.65$ for *NW-base-poly* and $\alpha = 0.61$ for *NW-base-mono*. The average score of the 5 raters and the word accuracy from the *NW-base-mono* recognizer are also depicted in Figure 7.1. The next section will describe how recognition and agreement change on recognizers that were adapted to TE speech.

7.2 Results of Recognizer Adaptation to TE Voices

The interpolation of the output weights of semi-continuous HMMs with a small data set was introduced in Chapter 5.3. The adaptation to the tracheoesophageal speakers was performed based upon the *NW-base-mono* recognizer. The vocabulary of the recognizers for the pilot experiments with the *laryng18* speakers group, however, consisted of the 71 words occurring in the

NW-base-poly, laryng41 data				
criterion	r	ρ	κ	$\kappa_{DF}(w)$	α
quality	−0.82	−0.81	+0.26	+0.45	+0.63
hoarse	+0.64	+0.66	+0.12	+0.17	+0.20
effort	+0.70	+0.69	+0.10	+0.16	+0.16
penetr	−0.71	−0.66	+0.15	+0.27	+0.39
proso	−0.80	−0.82	+0.15	+0.33	+0.49
brsense	−0.73	−0.76	+0.12	+0.31	+0.47
noise	+0.52	+0.43	+0.02	+0.08	+0.04
tone	−0.79	−0.80	+0.23	+0.44	+0.61
change	+0.39	+0.37	+0.01	+0.02	−0.08
intell	−0.88	−0.86	+0.20	+0.45	+0.65
overall	−0.85	−0.84	—	—	—

Table 7.4: Agreement between the word accuracy of the *NW-base-poly* recognizer and the human rating criteria (Table 4.12) averaged over 5 experts on the *laryng41* speaker group; given are Pearson's r, Spearman's ρ, Cohen's κ, the weighted multi-rater κ by Davies and Fleiss, and Krippendorff's α (see Chapter 3). For the "overall" criterion, no κ and α was computed due to its continuous range.

NW-base-mono, laryng41 data				
criterion	r	ρ	κ	$\kappa_{DF}(w)$	α
quality	−0.72	−0.75	+0.27	+0.44	+0.59
hoarse	+0.60	+0.64	+0.13	+0.20	+0.25
effort	+0.55	+0.54	+0.14	+0.22	+0.26
penetr	−0.62	−0.60	+0.14	+0.24	+0.34
proso	−0.68	−0.71	+0.15	+0.31	+0.45
brsense	−0.58	−0.64	+0.12	+0.28	+0.41
noise	+0.59	+0.51	+0.04	+0.11	+0.09
tone	−0.75	−0.77	+0.22	+0.42	+0.58
change	+0.33	+0.28	+0.01	+0.03	−0.07
intell	−0.82	−0.82	+0.19	+0.41	+0.61
overall	−0.76	−0.78	—	—	—

Table 7.5: Agreement between the word accuracy of the *NW-base-mono* recognizer and the human rating criteria (Table 4.12) averaged over 5 experts on the *laryng41* speaker group; given are Pearson's r, Spearman's ρ, Cohen's κ, the weighted multi-rater κ by Davies and Fleiss, and Krippendorff's α (see Chapter 3). For the "overall" criterion, no κ and α was computed due to its continuous range.

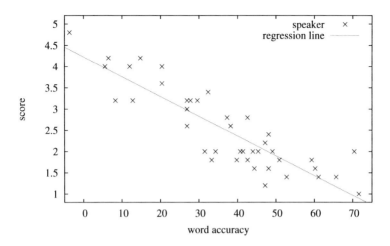

Figure 7.1: Word accuracy vs. intelligibility score for *NW-base-poly* recognizer (*laryng41* data, see also Table 7.1 and 7.4); the scores were averaged across 5 experienced raters. The patients are ordered with respect to their word accuracy.

text "The North Wind and the Sun" and the additional 32 words and word fragments uttered by these speakers (cf. [HSN$^+$04] and Chapter 4.4.2).

7.2.1 Adaptation to Single Speakers

The recordings of the *laryng18* test speakers showed a wide range in intelligibility and quality of the substitute voices. Therefore, the interpolation was first not done for the speaker group as a whole but to each single speaker separately. This lead to 18 different recognizers which will in the following be treated as if they were a single one. Each speaker was tested on "his own" recognizer only. The approaches where each HMM state was interpolated with one single interpolation partner for each HMM state will be together denoted as *NW-i1-mono*. The 18 recognizers interpolated with 40 interpolation partners will be called *NW-i40-mono* (see Chapter 5.3). The effects of the adaptation can be seen in Table 7.6 and Figure 7.2. Recognition rates were enhanced for almost all speakers where *NW-i40-mono* with its mean word accuracy of 36.4% outperformed *NW-i1-mono* by 3 percent points. The results cannot be compared directly to *NW-base-mono* because the new recognizers were adapted to single speakers, but they confirm the findings by Steidl et al. that a high number of HMM interpolation partners is better than a very small one [SSH$^+$03]. This is not the only conclusion that can be drawn. The main outcome of the experiments is that speech recognition on tracheoesophageal substitute voices can be improved already by a small amount of appropriate adaptation data.

Like in Chapter 7.1.2 for the baseline recognizers, the correlation between human and machine rating for the intelligibility rating was computed where the word accuracy of a particular speaker's entire utterance served as the automatically computed score. The results for the single

recognizer	speakers	μ(WA)	σ(WA)	min(WA)	max(WA)
NW-base-poly	laryng18	28.2	18.1	2.8	62.7
NW-base-mono	laryng18	28.7	12.1	10.0	50.0
NW-i1-mono	laryng18	33.5	13.2	10.0	54.1
NW-i40-mono	laryng18	36.4	14.7	9.2	55.6
NW-i1all-mono	laryng18	31.9	12.8	10.8	50.9
NW-i40all-mono	laryng18	33.8	13.4	8.3	52.7

Table 7.6: Word accuracy for NW-base recognizers and recognizers adapted to each single speaker or the entire group (laryng18 data), respectively

recognizer	speakers	rater					
		K	L	R	S	U	all
NW-base-poly	laryng18	–0.78	–0.61	–0.84	–0.81	–0.54	–0.83
NW-base-mono	laryng18	–0.81	–0.65	–0.81	–0.79	–0.55	–0.84
NW-i1-mono	laryng18	–0.82	–0.60	–0.78	–0.80	–0.49	–0.81
NW-i40-mono	laryng18	–0.81	–0.62	–0.73	–0.83	–0.56	–0.83
NW-i1all-mono	laryng18	–0.84	–0.60	–0.80	–0.80	–0.56	–0.84
NW-i40all-mono	laryng18	–0.81	–0.56	–0.73	–0.79	–0.52	–0.79

Table 7.7: Correlation r between word accuracy of NW recognizers and human raters (intelligibility criterion, laryng18 data)

raters and the overall correlation (average of the 5 experts) are shown in Table 7.7. Despite the adaptation of the derived recognizers with TE speech and the higher recognition rates (Table 7.6), the correlation between human and machine rating could not be enhanced.

7.2.2   Adaptation to the Entire laryng18 Speaker Group

The adaptation to single speakers will now be compared to one single recognizer which was adapted to the entire group of 18 speakers. The approach with one interpolation partner for each HMM state will be named NW-i1all-mono, and NW-i40all-mono is the recognizer adapted with 40 partners for each state. Both of them are monophone-based and use a unigram language model, like their competitors.

The results are worse than for the single speaker optimization but still better than for the baseline system (see Table 7.6 and Figure 7.3). Compared to both the polyphone- and the monophone-based baseline recognizer, an increase of 3 and 5 percent points of word accuracy was achieved, respectively. In order to confirm the positive effect of the adaptation with the laryng18 data, the NW-i40all-mono recognizer was also applied to the laryng41 group. The gain of word accuracy was the same. For the normal laryngeal speakers, the results are still in the same range as for NW-base-mono (Table 7.8 and 7.1).

For the laryng18 speakers, no significant improvement in the correlation of human and automatic evaluation of intelligibility was observed (Table 7.7). On the laryng41 data, the NW-

recognizer	speakers	μ(WA)	σ(WA)	min(WA)	max(WA)
NW-i40all-mono	bas16	67.7	10.0	50.0	87.0
NW-i40all-mono	kom18	59.3	6.2	48.1	74.1
NW-i40all-mono	laryng41	40.1	12.6	7.4	65.7

Table 7.8: Word accuracy for the NW-i40all-mono recognizer (normal and TE speakers); for the NW-base recognizers, see Table 7.1.

recognizer	speakers	rater					all
		K	L	R	S	U	
NW-i40all-mono	laryng41	–0.69	–0.72	–0.83	–0.76	–0.74	–0.84

Table 7.9: Correlation r between word accuracy of NW-i40all-mono recognizer and human raters (intelligibility criterion, laryng41 data); for the NW-base recognizers, see Table 7.2.

i40all-mono system was slightly better than the monophone-based baseline recognizer (Table 7.9 and 7.2). For criteria other than intelligibility, there was no improvement (see Table 7.10 and 7.5).

7.2.3 Correlation of the Word Accuracy Computed vs. the Reference Text

Usually the text reference for the calculation of the word accuracy was not the original written text that the test person had to read but a hand-labeled transliteration of the audio files in order to exclude an influence of reading errors on the intelligibility evaluation. This ensured that the word accuracy reflects merely the acoustic recognition errors which was important for these basic experiments. Nevertheless, reading errors by the patients have to be taken into account. The laryng41 speakers used 13 words that were not in the vocabulary of the text "The North Wind and the Sun" (see also Table 4.11). The transliteration of these data shows a word accuracy against the text reference of 98.7%, i.e. the rate of reading errors is very low. When the word accuracy between the recognized word sequence and the reference text is computed, then the values are hardly affected (Table 7.11; for the results using the transliteration, see Table 7.1 and 7.8). The correlation between the word accuracies computed on the text reference and the experts' average intelligibility scores (Table 7.12) was $r = -0.82$ for the baseline monophone-based recognizer NW-base-mono and $r = -0.84$ for the interpolated NW-i40all-mono, just like for the transliteration. The loss on the polyphone-based NW-base-poly from $r = -0.88$ to $r = -0.87$ is not significant (cf. Table 7.2 and 7.9). This means that the automatic evaluation of intelligibility works also for data with some reading errors. For a future clinical application where recordings with higher error rates might occur, however, the two types of error – by reading and by recognition – should be separated. Otherwise a patient with a high-quality voice might get bad evaluation results due to misread words.

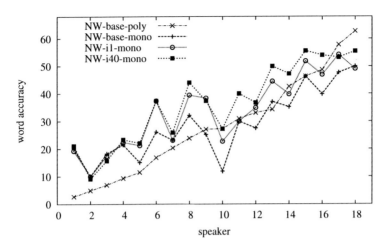

Figure 7.2: Word accuracy for *NW-base* and recognizers adapted to single speakers (*laryng18* data, see also Table 7.6); the speakers are ordered with respect to their result on *NW-base-poly*. Recordings processed by the same recognizer are connected by lines for the sake of clarity.

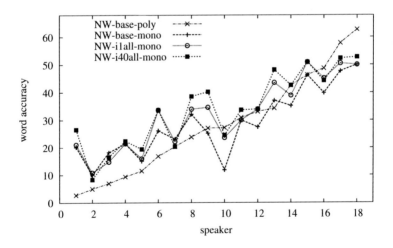

Figure 7.3: Word accuracy for *NW-base* and recognizers adapted to speaker group (*laryng18* data, see also Table 7.6); the speakers are ordered with respect to their result on *NW-base-poly*. Recordings processed by the same recognizer are connected by lines for the sake of clarity.

NW-i40all-mono, laryng41 data					
criterion	r	ρ	κ	$\kappa_{\mathrm{DF}}(w)$	α
quality	−0.71	−0.70	+0.24	+0.40	+0.55
hoarse	+0.58	+0.58	+0.11	+0.20	+0.27
effort	+0.54	+0.52	+0.13	+0.22	+0.25
penetr	−0.67	−0.62	+0.13	+0.22	+0.30
proso	−0.67	−0.67	+0.13	+0.28	+0.39
brsense	−0.57	−0.58	+0.09	+0.26	+0.38
noise	+0.59	+0.50	+0.04	+0.11	+0.07
tone	−0.73	−0.72	+0.21	+0.38	+0.52
change	+0.33	+0.30	+0.01	+0.03	−0.08
intell	−0.84	−0.80	+0.17	+0.39	+0.58
overall	−0.76	−0.73	—	—	—

Table 7.10: Agreement between the word accuracy of the *NW-i40all-mono* recognizer and the human rating criteria (Table 4.12) averaged over 5 experts on the *laryng41* speaker group; given are Pearson's r, Spearman's ρ, Cohen's κ, the weighted multi-rater κ by Davies and Fleiss, and Krippendorff's α (see Chapter 3). For the "overall" criterion, no κ and α was computed due to its continuous range. For the *NW-base* recognizers, see Table 7.4 and 7.5.

recognizer	speakers	μ(WA)	σ(WA)	min(WA)	max(WA)
NW-base-poly	*laryng41*	36.9	18.0	−3.7	71.3
NW-base-mono	*laryng41*	35.2	13.4	0.9	61.1
NW-i40all-mono	*laryng41*	40.0	12.4	7.4	66.7

Table 7.11: Word accuracy for *NW* recognizers (*laryng41* data); the word accuracy was computed against the reference text and **not** against the transliteration of the audio files (for those results, see Table 7.1 and 7.8).

recognizer	speakers	rater					
		K	L	R	S	U	all
NW-base-poly	*laryng41*	−0.73	−0.78	−0.81	−0.80	−0.73	−0.87
NW-base-mono	*laryng41*	−0.67	−0.71	−0.80	−0.76	−0.70	−0.82
NW-i40all-mono	*laryng41*	−0.68	−0.71	−0.82	−0.77	−0.72	−0.84

Table 7.12: Correlation r between word accuracy of *NW* recognizers and human raters (intelligibility criterion, *laryng41* data); the word accuracy was computed against the reference text and **not** against the transliteration of the audio files (for those results, see Table 7.2 and 7.9).

recognizer	score					$\kappa_{DF}(w)$
	5	4	3	2	1	
standard conversion						
NW-base-poly	]−∞;0[	[0;15[	[15;25[	[25;40[	[40;100]	0.47
NW-base-mono	]−∞;0[	[0;15[	[15;25[	[25;40[	[40;100]	0.36
NW-i40all-mono	]−∞;0[	[0;15[	[15;25[	[25;40[	[40;100]	0.24
optimal conversion						
NW-base-poly	]−∞;0[	[0;25[	[25;39[	[39;61[	[61;100]	0.79
NW-base-mono	]−∞;5[	[5;22[	[22;30[	[30;55[	[55;100]	0.78
NW-i40all-mono	]−∞;10[	[10;26[	[26;35[	[35;58[	[58;100]	0.78

Table 7.13: Standard and optimal mapping intervals for word accuracy conversion to human intelligibility scores on the *laryng41* data; the agreement (weighted multi-rater κ after Davies and Fleiss; see Chapter 3.2.4) was computed for the rounded average score of 5 experts and the respective recognizer.

7.2.4   Optimal Conversion of Word Accuracies to Integer Scores

The agreement of the automatic measures and the human scores was mainly described by means of Pearson's correlation coefficient r so far because of the following reasons: As described in Chapter 3, the agreement measures based upon Cohen's κ and Krippendorff's α weigh the difference between the automatic and human rating. This, however, requires a conversion of the continuous word accuracy or prosodic features (see Chapter 7.3) to the same integer range as the human rating criteria. Since different recognizers, e.g. polyphone- vs. monophone-based, yield different intervals of word accuracy on the same data, for each recognizer a particular conversion has to be determined. In the case of the prosodic features, each feature may have its own range, i.e. it needs its own specific mapping table. With the correlation coefficient, this is not necessary. It expresses how closely the human ratings can be approximated by the automatic measure except for a linear transformation. It was not the goal of this thesis to find this transformation for each used feature. For judging the ability of automatic measures to approximate human rating criteria, the correlation coefficient was sufficient.

In Table 7.3, a word accuracy mapping was introduced that was developed using the *laryng18* data. In Table 7.13, the conversion was optimized with respect to the multi-rater $\kappa_{DF}(w)$ for the special case of *laryng41* data and the intelligibility criterion. Note that $\kappa_{DF}(w)$ was computed for the rounded average score of the 5 experts and the respective recognizer. Therefore, its values deviate from those in the previous sections where the measure was computed for the entire group of 5 human raters and one recognizer. This example shows how the agreement can be tuned by optimization to certain data. This, however, strongly reduces the comparability to experiments with other data, recognizers, or other automatically computed evaluation measures. Hence, it is preferable to avoid the use of agreement measures that need this kind of range mapping.

7.2.5   Conclusion

There is a strong correlation between the results of the human and the automatic method of evaluating intelligibility. The word accuracy can obviously serve as a valid stand-alone measure for this criterion, even if the speech recognizer was trained with normal speakers only. In a communication situation between humans, the dialogue partners are able to adapt their hearing to the other person's voice. The same aspect was simulated by the HMM adaptation where the recognition system was adapted to the particular person. This improved recognition rates, but it corresponds to a human listener that knew the respective speaker before. Therefore, these approaches cannot be used in an objective evaluation method. A recognition system that was adapted to a group of pathologic speakers could be regarded as an expert who has listening experience with the respective type of speech pathology. However, the adaptation obviously just causes a shift of the word accuracy range towards higher values, so no positive effect on the correlation between word accuracy and human ratings could be observed. For this reason, the time-consuming adaptation is not necessary; later experiments were only performed with the baseline system. Furthermore, the adaptation incorporates knowledge that a naïve listener does not have, and it should be regarded how a person in everyday life can understand the patient.

The word accuracy is a very good measure for intelligibility. There are, however, evaluation criteria that cannot be expressed by the number of correctly understood or recognized words. In order to find appropriate automatic counterparts for them, prosodic features were computed. The results will be introduced in the next section.

7.3 Prosodic Analysis vs. Human Evaluation

Although there was a human rating criterion called "prosody" (Table 4.12), the prosodic features that were introduced in Chapter 5.5 were not expected to correlate highly with this particular criterion. One reason is that all patients read a standard text without questions or quotations, i.e. the occurrence of prosodic phenomena was not very likely. Second, the human auditory impression of prosodic phenomena is a complex combination of pause, signal energy and frequency features. Each of these feature groups contributes just a certain part to the overall impression. Single features were supposed to express other criteria, like e.g. F_0 values for the evaluation of "vocal tone". For the pause duration measures, it is important that silent pauses at the beginning or end of a file are not counted because they were often not caused by the patient's disability but by the therapist using the recording program.

7.3.1 Prosodic Features on TE Speakers and Laryngeal Speakers

In order to find out which prosodic features are particularly affected in tracheoesophageal speech, the prosodic feature values of TE speakers and laryngeal speakers were compared. Since only 18 elderly normal speakers were available, the *kom18* group (Chapter 4.5) and the *laryng18* group (Chapter 4.4.2) served as the databases for this experiment. The required word hypotheses graphs (WHGs, see Chapter 5.5.2) were provided by the *NW-base-mono* recognizer. In order to reduce the amount of word-based (local) and file-based (global) features, each feature was reduced to its mean value and standard deviation per speaker group. Table 7.14 contains the prosodic features whose average was at least 20% higher or lower for TE speakers. This threshold was chosen arbitrarily in order to find a reasonably small feature group to examine. If the threshold would have been at 10%, only 4 more features would have been selected. Note that the focus of this thesis is not to distinguish normal from substitute voices but to find the correlation to human rating criteria that were defined for pathologic voices only. For this reason, the comparison between the TE speakers and the control group will only be addressed shortly here. Large differences were expected in the duration of pauses and words and in the portions of voiced and unvoiced sections (cf. Chapter 2). Many word-based features yielded similar results in different word intervals, e.g. for the normalized energy EnNormWord-2,-1 and EnNormWord1,2 (cf. Chapter 5.5). Therefore, the table shows one word interval for each feature only.

Table 7.14 confirms that the articulation rate is lower with TE speakers (cf. Table 4.11) because pause and word durations are much longer than for the normal speakers. The higher absolute energy in an interval that contains words and the pause between them (EnAbsWord-2,-1; no. 4 in the table) might be caused by a higher perturbation level in speaking and breathing. The highest and lowest detected normalized F_0 values F0MaxWord0,0 and F0MinWord0,0 (no. 7 and 8) are the result of octave errors; for this aspect, see also Chapter 7.3.3. The voice onset position in the next word (F0OnPosWord1,1; no. 9) is so much higher for the pathologic speech ($\mu_{\text{laryng}18}/\mu_{\text{kom}18} = 1.80$) because it combines the longer pause between the reference point and the next word and the initial voiceless section of the following word (see Figure 5.8). For the current word, the ratio for F0OnPosWord0,0 is 0.93 ($\mu_{\text{laryng}18} = -26.6$, $\mu_{\text{kom}18} = -28.7$) which shows that the distance from the reference point back to the voice onset is smaller than in normal speech. This again reflects the long initial voiceless section. The global features show that the portion of unvoiced frames is much higher with the laryngectomees, and again that they speak slower. For jitter the difference between the speaker groups is not so clear. It might have been strongly affected by the unreliable F_0 detection.

The trajectory of the features gets lost when they are averaged over entire recordings. In order to obtain information whether a feature value shows a certain rise or decline over time, the covariance, correlation, regression coefficient, regression constant, and the mean square error, respectively, between the word numbers within the file and the feature values for the respective words were computed. However, these features did not show relevant differences between normal and pathologic speech.

The next section will compare prosodic features of pathologic speech to human rating scores.

7.3.2   Correlation between Prosodic Features and Human Rating

Finding the prosodic features that correlate with any of the rating criteria of the human raters introduced in Chapter 4.4.3 is difficult due to the high number of measures. All features have to be compared to one single score value given by the raters for a certain criterion. Since the local features are word-based, and the raters evaluated in a text-based manner, a similar method like in Chapter 7.3.1 was applied to quickly exclude the score-feature pairs probably least useful for automatic speech evaluation. First all values for each single feature in a file were reduced to their mean value and standard deviation as in the previous section. For each human rating criterion, they were then compared to the average score of all raters for each speaker of the *laryng41* group. Integrating information about the feature trajectory by measuring the interrelation between feature value and word number, like in Chapter 7.3.1, yielded substantially worse results and was therefore discarded after the first tests.

On the *laryng18* group, pilot experiments including also the statistical validity of this method were performed (see [HNT+07, HNS+06]). On the *laryng41* data set, several measures reached a correlation of $|r| \geq 0.7$. These results are summarized in Table 7.15 for the *NW-base-mono* and the *NW-base-poly* recognizer. The results of both recognizers are very similar; there are only few remarkable differences. While the standard deviation of the normalized word energy (EnNorm-

no.	feature name	μ_{kom18}	μ_{laryng18}	σ_{kom18}	σ_{laryng18}
1	Pause–beforeWord0,0	14.1	31.2	4.2	18.6
2	EnRegCoeffWord0,0	–5.6	–12.9	5.1	5.9
3	EnNormWord-2,-1	–0.55	–0.29	0.05	0.32
4	EnAbsWord-2,-1	95700	121940	23760	53370
5	DurNormWord-2,-1	0.23	0.92	0.15	0.70
6	F0MseRegWord-2,-1	64	210	17	87
7	F0MaxWord0,0	0.15	0.33	0.05	0.09
8	F0MinWord0,0	–0.14	–0.37	0.03	0.15
9	F0OnPosWord1,1	17.8	32.0	4.4	15.9
10	F0OffPosWord0,0	–3.6	–4.9	0.8	1.9
11	#+Voiced	1.74	2.53	0.20	0.67
12	#–Voiced	0.74	1.71	0.20	0.57
13	Dur+Voiced	21.6	15.2	3.1	6.5
14	Dur–Voiced	4.0	8.4	1.0	2.8
15	DurMax+Voiced	16.7	9.1	2.5	4.5
16	DurMax–Voiced	3.4	6.0	0.7	2.1
17	RelNum+/–Voiced	3.5	2.7	1.0	1.6
18	RelDur+Voiced/Sig	0.89	0.70	0.16	0.28
19	RelDur–Voiced/Sig	0.11	0.30	0.16	0.28
20	StandDevF0	0.15	0.40	0.03	0.13

Table 7.14: Prosodic features (Chapter 5.5) with mean values that differ at least by 20% between normal speakers (*kom18*) and TE speakers (*laryng18*); the upper part contains local, the lower part global features.

Word0,0; no. *10* in the table) reaches $r = 0.76$ for the intelligibility criterion on the monophone-based recognizer, the corresponding values on the polyphone-based approach drops to $r = 0.67$. No explanation for this phenomenon could be found. When the standard deviation of the maximum F_0 position in a word (F0MaxPosWord0,0; no. *15*) is compared to the human score describing the match of breath and sense units ("brsense"), then for *NW-base-mono* $r = 0.72$ and for *NW-base-poly* only $r = 0.61$ are reached. In general, the F_0 position features achieved worse results when then polyphone-based recognizer was used. The reason could be the less robust training of the polyphone models due to less amount of training data for each HMM. This might lead to less accurate detection of the phone positions when the word hypotheses graphs are created. For some of the rating criteria, some interesting findings should be noted:

- speech effort ("effort"): It is expressed by articulation rate, i.e. by the duration of words and pauses. Several features reach $|r| = 0.7$ and higher; among them is the standard deviation of DurAbsWord-2,-1 (no. *13* in Table 7.15), i.e. an interval containing two words and a pause. Obviously, it is hard for the affected persons to keep their articulation rate constant.

- prosody ("proso"): Several duration features reach $|r| = 0.6$ and higher, but the human "prosody" criterion describes complex phenomena and can actually not be expressed by single features.

- match of breath and sense units ("brsense"): The human ratings for this criterion can be mapped by the prosody module although it does not recognize the boundaries between sense units (see also Chapter 7.3.4). When a patient breathes within syntactic constituents and not only at phrase or sentence boundaries as a normal speaker would do it, the overall duration of pauses will get longer which influences many features. Word duration features get higher values as well when they are computed over more than one word because the pause between the words is also included.

- vocal tone ("tone"): It is expressed by energy features, mainly by the regression coefficient of the error between F_0 trajectory and its regression line (EnMseRegWord0,0; no. 2) and the absolute energy in two words and the pause between them (EnAbsWord-2,-1; no. 11).

- change of voice quality during reading ("change"): No reliable features were found which might be influenced by the fact that the information on the trajectory of the single features was lost by averaging over the entire files.

- overall intelligibility ("intell"): Duration features show the best correlations again, probably reflecting the fact that a slow speaker is understood better. However, intelligibility could be much easier and more reliably judged by the word accuracy (see Chapter 7.1).

- overall quality score ("overall"): The overall quality rating can be estimated from similar features like e.g. the intelligibility rating. It is not clear at first sight why the quality impression should be mostly dependent on some duration features, but the data from the rating session showed that the human ratings for intelligibility and overall quality are very similar (see Chapter 4.4.4). This explains the findings on the prosodic features.

Like for the comparison between the prosodic features of normal and pathologic speakers, the results concerning the voice onset position in the current word (F0OnPosWord0,0) are much worse than for the position in the following word (F0OnPosWord1,1; no. 5 and 14 in Table 7.15, cf. Chapter 7.3.1) and for the voice offset position in the previous word (F0OffPosWord-1,-1; no. 6). In both cases, the duration of the pause that is between the respective word and the reference point is essential for a good correlation to the rating criteria. Computed on the current word only, the best correlation is only about $|r| = 0.45$.

For the criteria of hoarseness ("hoarse") and distortions by insufficient occlusion of the tracheostoma ("noise"), no features were found that exceeded the given threshold of $|r| \geq 0.7$. For hoarseness the mean square error between F_0 trajectory and its regression curve yields values around $r = -0.6$. For the noise criterion, the normalized energy is the best feature with about $r = -0.56$, but the results are not reliable since the criterion was actually defined as "distortions by insufficient occlusion of tracheostoma", and there were not enough recordings that actually contained stoma noise. For the quality of the substitute voice ("quality"), the same features like for the overall quality show similar but still worse results. The agreement between those two criteria among the raters was $r = 0.97$ (see Table 4.13), so this result can easily be explained. For the voice penetration ("penetr") criterion, there was a correlation of $r = -0.71$ to the normalized energy EnNormWord1,2, but it was not clear how the raters defined "voice penetration" for themselves due to an unclear definition on the evaluation sheet (see also Chapter 4.4.3).

Nevertheless, the conclusion that can be drawn from these experiments is that some human rating criteria have reliable automatically computable correlates. These should be taken into account for a later refinement of the evaluation procedure.

no.	feature name		correl. r (*NW-base-mono*)	correl. r (*NW-base-poly*)
1	Pause–beforeWord0,0	(μ)	intell +0.70, overall +0.70, brsense +0.73, effort –0.75	intell +0.70, overall +0.70, brsense +0.72, effort –0.74
2	EnMseRegWord0,0	(μ)	tone +0.68	tone +0.71
3	DurNormWord-2,-1	(μ)	overall +0.70, intell +0.72	overall +0.69, intell +0.72
4	DurAbsWord-2,-1	(μ)	overall +0.70, brsense +0.75, effort –0.75	overall +0.70, brsense +0.75, effort –0.76
5	F0OnPosWord1,1	(μ)	quality +0.72, intell +0.73, overall +0.74, brsense +0.75	quality +0.66, intell +0.68, overall +0.69, brsense +0.69
6	F0OffPosWord-1,-1	(μ)	intell –0.70, proso –0.71, quality –0.71, overall –0.74, brsense –0.74	intell –0.67, proso –0.67, quality –0.69, overall –0.70, brsense –0.71
7	Pause–beforeWord0,0	(σ)	effort –0.72	effort –0.72
8	Pause–afterWord0,0	(σ)	overall +0.70, intell +0.70, effort –0.75	overall +0.70, intell +0.71, effort –0.75
9	EnMseRegWord0,0	(σ)	tone +0.71	tone +0.72
10	EnNormWord0,0	(σ)	intell +0.76	intell +0.67
11	EnAbsWord-2,-1	(σ)	tone +0.70	tone +0.69
12	DurNormWord0,0	(σ)	intell +0.74	intell +0.73
13	DurAbsWord-2,-1	(σ)	effort –0.72	effort –0.71
14	F0OnPosWord1,1	(σ)	overall +0.70	overall +0.69
15	F0MaxPosWord0,0	(σ)	brsense +0.72	brsense +0.62

Table 7.15: Correlation r between prosodic features (Chapter 5.5) and human ratings for TE speakers (*laryng41* group) on the *NW-base-mono* and *NW-base-poly* recognizer; the correlation was measured using the mean value (μ) or the standard deviation (σ) of all words per file. Given are criteria with a correlation of $|r| \geq 0.7$ for at least one of the recognizers. For the criteria names, see Table 4.12.

7.3.3   Analysis of the Fundamental Frequency

The final F_0 values from the Prosody module (Chapter 5.5) are only available in a normalized form and after application of a logarithmic function. For some experiments, however, the F_0 values from the basic feature computation of the prosody module were used. In the prosodic analysis described in the previous section, all features were computed for an interval containing at least one word, or for the entire file. The basic prosodic features, however, are computed per frame. The basic F_0 features are available as their original values computed in Hertz; if no F_0 could be detected, the value 0 is returned for the respective frame. The F_0 computation algorithm chosen for the task was a modification of the algorithm developed by Bagshaw and Medan [BHJ93, MYC91]; in the prosody module, it is denoted as Medan-Bagshaw-Nutt algorithm [Zei07]. Although it is very robust against distortions, the results on the TE speech recordings suffer from many octave errors, i.e. instead of the real fundamental frequency one of its harmonics one or more octaves higher is found. Figure 7.4 shows the distribution of the detected values for the *laryng18* speakers and their corresponding age-matched control group (*kom18*). The graphics shows only those frames where the F_0 could be computed, i.e. all voiced sections. In the case of the laryngectomees, these were 34809 of 127,546 frames (27.2%), and for the elderly laryngeal speakers 44010 of 93971 frames (46.8%). During reading the text "The North Wind and the Sun", no major F_0 changes were expected as the text doesn't contain questions or exclamations. Furthermore, both speaker groups consist of male persons only, and the voice of laryngectomees mostly have rather low F_0 (cf. Table 2.5). For these reasons, all detected values above 200 Hz for both groups were considered to be the result of octave errors and were excluded from further statistic analysis. This affected 1608 frames (3.7%) of the *kom18* recordings and 8988 frames (25.8%) of the *laryng18* signals. Interestingly, the maximum for both groups is in the interval between 110 and 120 Hz, although it should be higher for the laryngeal speakers. While, however, the *kom18* group shows an almost perfect Gaussian distribution, there is a significant peak for the laryngectomees between 60 and 70 Hz. The real portion of F_0 values is probably higher in the region below 100 Hz, but due to octave errors it might be distributed among higher frequencies. The minimum frequency to be detected was set to 50 Hz. Below 60 Hz, the detection algorithm has some problems discovered during earlier experiments in the working group which means that the results between 50 and 60 Hz should also not be considered for further analysis.

In order to achieve correlation measures between the detected F_0 values and the human ratings, the frame-based F_0 features had to be converted to word-based representation. This was done with the help of the word hypotheses graphs (WHGs, see Chapter 5.5.2) which contained the proposed start and end frame numbers for each word. For each word, the number of all frames with $60 < F_0 \leq 200$ Hz and their average F_0 were computed. The correlation between these numbers and the human ratings was computed for the TE speaker groups. Unfortunately, the best correlation values were substantially lower than for the prosodic features in the previous section for both the *laryng18* and the *laryng41* speakers, so no improvement over the "real" prosodic features was reached. These results allow the assumption that for highly pathological voices the automatic detection of exact F_0 values is less advantageous than the restriction to the binary voiced-unvoiced decision. This is supported by the findings in Table 7.15 where no F_0 feature could reach a high correlation to the rating criteria (note that the F0 position features represent durations, not F_0 values).

Figure 7.5 shows the detected F_0 values of the prosody module and the Hoarseness Dia-

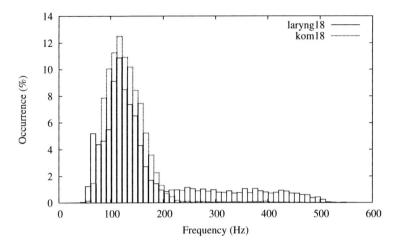

Figure 7.4: Distribution of automatically detected F_0 values for 18 laryngectomees (*laryng18*) and 18 laryngeal speakers (*kom18*); 14 erroneous values (0.04%) for *laryng18* between 600 and 863 Hz are not displayed.

gram (Chapter 2.5.4) in vowel recordings of a group of 24 TE speakers (cf. [TBS⁺06]). The number of octave errors by the Hoarseness Diagram is obviously much higher than for the prosody module because on highly pathologic voices the prosody module decides that the respective frame is unvoiced and returns 0. This again confirms that it is not always helpful to try to find an F_0 value under all circumstances and that the method of the prosody module is more suitable for this type of voices.

The next section will focus on the speech properties of the test persons. It will use not only quantitative information about pauses but also regard where in the text they were set.

7.3.4 Measuring the Match of Breath and Sense Units

For measuring the match of breath and sense units (abbreviated as "brsense", see Table 4.12) in the speech data of the *laryng41* group, segmental markers were added to the text "The North Wind and the Sun" (see Appendix A.1). These markers define the boundaries of text segments at which speaking pauses are usually tolerated by the listener. Table 7.16 shows the marker types used for the following experiments. For a detailed list and explanation, see [BKK⁺98].

For each test signal, a word hypotheses graph (WHG) was created using the *NW-base-mono* recognizer (Chapter 5.1.6). It was made by forced alignment based upon the text reference of the original text "The North Wind and the Sun". Afterwards, the WHG and the reference text with segmental markers were aligned, i.e. the differences between them were analyzed. The recognizer detects pauses with a minimum duration of 90 ms. However, such short pauses are not perceived by a human listener. The minimum time for a pause is often defined to 200 ms in order to avoid misinterpretation of the stopgap of voiceless plosives as pause, not only in the anal-

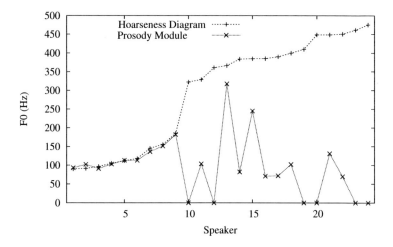

Figure 7.5: Automatically detected F_0 values by the prosody module and the Hoarseness Diagram (cf. [TBS$^+$06]); recordings of sustained vowels (/a/) were analyzed from a group of 24 TE speakers. The speakers are ordered with respect to their F_0 value obtained by the Hoarseness Diagram. They are connected by lines for the sake of clarity.

marker	at boundary between
SM3	main clause – main clause
SM2	main clause – subordinate clause
SC2	subordinate clause – subordinate clause
IC2	constituent – constituent

Table 7.16: Segmental markers denoting boundaries in the reference text

ysis of TE speakers [RFBS84a, PFKB89, BPH95, BLG01], but also for other speech patholo-
gies [NN06, NNH+00]. Examinations of stutterers' speech had revealed that delays shorter than
250 ms are only identifiable by a trained listener, and delays between 250 and 500 ms cannot
be identified uniquely as being pathologic or not [MOO79]. With respect to the fact that many
laryngectomees have similar problems speaking fluently, the minimum pause duration for the
automatic evaluation was set to 500 ms.

Three types of mismatches between the WHG and the text with segmental markers had to be
distinguished in the alignment:

- Segmental marker vs. detected pause: There is a pause at a segmental boundary; hence,
  it was placed correctly by the speaker.

- Segmental marker vs. "NIL" symbol in WHG: No pause was detected at a segmental
  boundary. This is not necessarily an error when the test person speaks fast, or the respective segments are on a lower hierarchical level, e.g. constituents (marker IC2).

- Pause in WHG but no segmental marker in the reference: This is an unwanted pause since
  no segmental boundary was defined.

These mismatch types can be evaluated for each of the defined markers. In order to find out
how the human "brsense" criterion is influenced by the occurrence of wanted ("w") and unwanted ("unw") pauses, the duration d, the number of pauses n, and the median duration m
for each of the test files and both pause classes were computed. The wanted pauses were also
separated into subtypes according to the segmental boundaries they represent. Several automatically computable measures were defined (see Table 7.17). The first one (φ_1) was the ratio of
the durations of unwanted pauses and all pauses in the audio files. Since the dialogue distortion
recognized by a listener is mostly dependent on the unwanted pauses, for φ_2 the duration of
unwanted pauses was weighted by their number n_{unw}. For φ_3 the weighting factor was n_{unw}^2 because the degree of perceived dialogue distortion might grow stronger than linearly with a higher
number of breaks. In order to control whether the median m or the mean value μ is more advantageous for the measures, the next experiment (φ_4) was performed with the median durations of
wanted and unwanted pauses instead of the average value as in φ_1. The median has the advantage that single, very long pauses do not affect it. Considering the different classes of syntactic
boundaries in Table 7.16, one might suggest that a longer break between constituents (IC2) is
likely to be "punished" harder by the raters than e.g. at boundaries between main or subordinate
clauses (SM3, SM2 or SC2). Therefore, the maximum $\max_{IC2}$, the median μ_{IC2}, and the mean μ_{IC2}
of the IC2 pauses were integrated into the definition of φ_5 and φ_6. For the final measure φ_7, the
idea was extended by regarding also the boundaries between subordinate clauses (SC2).

Table 7.17 shows the correlation of all measures to the average human rater's "brsense" score.
Different correlation coefficients for single raters might reflect the way how a listener judged for
the criterion. If a listener tolerates a few long pauses for deep breathing during the text, then
an automatic measure regarding the median pause length might be better than a measure based
upon the average pause durations. But obviously this was not true for the test data (φ_1 vs. φ_4).
The best correlation of $r = 0.62$ was reached for φ_2 that simply distinguishes between the two
classes of wanted and unwanted pauses; employing the IC2 and SC2 pauses is not necessary.
Further attempts using measures of SM3 and SM2 pauses were even less successful; the correlation dropped drastically.

measure	rater					all
	K	L	R	S	U	
$\varphi_1 = \frac{d_{unw}}{d_{unw}+d_w} = \frac{n_{unw}\cdot\mu_{unw}}{n_{unw}\cdot\mu_{unw}+n_w\cdot\mu_w}$	0.49	0.57	0.37	0.41	0.42	0.54
$\varphi_2 = \frac{d_{unw}\cdot n_{unw}}{d_{unw}+d_w}$	0.52	0.59	0.43	0.54	0.49	0.62
$\varphi_3 = \frac{d_{unw}\cdot n_{unw}^2}{d_{unw}+d_w}$	0.39	0.43	0.30	0.46	0.39	0.47
$\varphi_4 = \frac{n_{unw}\cdot m_{unw}}{n_{unw}\cdot m_{unw}+n_w\cdot m_w}$	0.46	0.55	0.37	0.42	0.40	0.53
$\varphi_5 = \frac{d_{unw}}{d_{unw}+d_w}\cdot\frac{max_{IC2}}{\mu_{IC2}}$	0.50	0.51	0.33	0.42	0.43	0.53
$\varphi_6 = \frac{d_{unw}}{d_{unw}+d_w}\cdot\frac{\mu_{IC2}}{m_{IC2}}$	0.50	0.52	0.32	0.39	0.42	0.51
$\varphi_7 = \frac{d_{unw}}{d_{unw}+d_w}\cdot\frac{\mu_{IC2}}{m_{IC2}}\cdot\frac{\mu_{SC2}}{m_{SC2}}$	0.51	0.54	0.35	0.40	0.43	0.54

Table 7.17: Correlation r between human raters and automatically computed measures for the criterion "match of breath and sense units" ("brsense") on the *laryng41* speaker group

A possible problem in the formulae is that the measures cannot be computed if the speaker speaks without any pause as several denominators in the equations would become zero. But in practical applications, this will not happen because a text for speech evaluation should have a certain length to produce reliable results. Reading the text "The North Wind and the Sun" without breathing is almost impossible for a laryngeal and even more for a TE speaker. However, the approach with the segmental markers was not further developed because the prosodic features described in Chapter 5.5 reached correlation coefficients beyond $|r|=0.7$ to the "brsense" criterion (see Table 7.15). They do not even need a text reference with syntactic annotations because they do not differentiate between different pause classes at all.

7.3.5 Summary

In this section, it was shown that the analysis of prosodic features reveals measures that show a high correlation to human rating criteria. TE speech is usually slower than normal speech, and the amount of voiced sections is strongly reduced. This affects many features measuring voice onset and offset, and also word and pause durations. These features show correlations of $|r| \geq 0.7$ to criteria like "intelligibility", "speech effort", "match of breath and sense units", or "overall quality". The criterion "vocal tone" is reflected by energy measures. Due to the high irregularity of substitute voices, it is not easy to detect correct values of F_0. This might be the reason why F_0 features do not match the rating criteria very well. For irregular voices, features based upon the decision whether a frame is voiced or unvoiced are the better choice. In order to measure whether a patient breathes only at syntactic boundaries where also a normal speaker would breathe, segmental markers were added to the text reference of the audio files. In this way, different pause types could be identified and measured. However, this approach was less successful than the prosodic features that simply contain the average pause durations in any place. Hence, the prosody module alone provides enough features to evaluate several of the human rating criteria. Only the word accuracy as a measure for intelligibility (Chapter 7.1.2) was better so far. The combination of prosody module and word accuracy will be addressed in Chapter 7.7.

The following section will introduce the automatic version of an intelligibility test for tracheoesophageal telephone speech.

7.4 The Post-Laryngectomy Telephone Test (PLTT)

7.4.1 Initial Experiments with Telephone Speech Data

For a human being, it is possible to recognize a person's voice over the telephone even when the fundamental frequency is cut off. The perceived pitch is reconstructed by the human brain from its harmonics ([Gol01] or [Gol02, pp. 407–408]). TE speakers are also able to do telephone communication although the percentage of voiced sections in their speech is very low. For initial experiments with "telephone" speech, the *laryng41* data were resampled with a sampling frequency of 8 kHz. The files of this new *laryng41_8kHz* set were then used to test speech recognizers for telephone data. In order to keep also the recognizers the same, the training data were downsampled to an 8 kHz version. The recognizers *NW-base-poly-8kHz* and *NW-base-mono-8kHz* correspond to *NW-base-poly* and *NW-base-mono*, respectively, which were trained with 16 kHz data (Chapter 5.1.5). Table 7.18 compares the recognition results of the 16 kHz and the 8 kHz recognizers and shows the influence of the sampling frequency. Not only the mean of the word accuracy is lower on the downsampled recordings, but also its standard deviation was reduced above average. This means that the range of the recognition rates was not just shifted to lower values; removing the frequencies above 4 kHz also removed a large portion of the noisy parts in the signals which caused e.g. the minimum word accuracy on *NW-base-mono-8kHz* to rise from 0.9% to 5.6%. The correlation between the single results of the 16 kHz and the 8 kHz version of the polyphone-based recognizer is higher ($r = 0.95$) than for both versions of the monophone-based recognizer ($r = 0.92$). The correlation of the word accuracy for the 8 kHz data to the human rating criterion "intelligibility" is shown in Table 7.19. It is only slightly lower than for the 16 kHz data (see also Table 7.4 and 7.5 or [RHS+06, RHN+06]).

7.4.2 Intelligibility Tests

In 1997, Lippmann stated that the recognition performance of human listeners on different tasks is by far better than that of machines [Lip97]. One decade later, there are still unsolved problems in this field especially when pathologic speech is examined. The recognition rate depends very much on the amount of training data [Moo03, LGA02]. A human listener of 50 years of age heard about 100,000 hours of speech in his or her life which can be seen as the "training data" for the human "recognizer". Moore [Moo03] states that it would require a "fantastic amount of speech" as training material for an automatic recognizer to achieve the same recognition rates as a human listener. Earlier studies revealed that in listening to laryngeal samples the dominant human recognition error is a misperception of manner of production while the dominant error for TE speech is the perception of voiceless instead of voiced phonemes [SCB01, SCO2].

A German sentence test for subjective and "objective" speech intelligibility assessment was developed by Kollmeier and Wesselkamp [KW97]. 20 test lists contain 10 sentences each whose phoneme frequency distribution approximates the distribution of the German language. This section will present a similar approach for automatic evaluation of the intelligibility of tracheoesophageal substitute voices on the telephone [Rie07, HRM+07]. It involved two factors that

recognizer	test set	μ(WA)	σ(WA)	min(WA)	max(WA)
NW-base-poly	laryng41	36.9	18.0	-3.7	71.6
NW-base-poly-8kHz	laryng41_8kHz	32.3	17.4	-7.4	69.4
NW-base-mono	laryng41	35.3	13.7	0.9	63.3
NW-base-mono-8kHz	laryng41_8kHz	33.4	12.1	5.6	62.0

Table 7.18: Recognition results on the *laryng41* speaker group for 16 kHz and 8 kHz recordings

recognizer	test set	r	ρ	κ	$\kappa_{DF}(w)$	α
NW-base-poly	laryng41	-0.88	-0.86	+0.20	+0.45	+0.65
NW-base-poly-8kHz	laryng41_8kHz	-0.85	-0.84	+0.23	+0.47	+0.68
NW-base-mono	laryng41	-0.82	-0.82	+0.19	+0.41	+0.61
NW-base-mono-8kHz	laryng41_8kHz	-0.81	-0.76	+0.19	+0.42	+0.63

Table 7.19: Agreement between word accuracy and intelligibility score of 5 experts on the *laryng41* speaker group for 16 kHz and 8 kHz recordings; given are Pearson's r, Spearman's ρ, Cohen's κ, the weighted multi-rater κ by Davies and Fleiss, and Krippendorff's α (see Chapter 3).

substantially influence the intelligibility: the telephone channel and the substitute voice.

7.4.3 PLTT Overview

The Post-Laryngectomy Telephone Test (PLTT, [Zen86, ZP86]; sometimes denoted as "Post-Laryngectomy Telephone Intelligibility Test") was developed in order to represent the communication situation outside the patient's usual environment, i.e. the family, by taking into account both voice and language. The patient calls a naïve rater over a standard landline telephone [Mad03]. The rater should not know about the text material of the test and may not have any hearing impairment.

The PLTT vocabulary consists of 400 monosyllabic words and 100 sentences, each of them written on an individual card. For one session, 22 words and 6 sentences are randomly chosen. The first two words and the first sentence are not taken into account for evaluation. Instead, they are supposed to allow the listener to adapt to the speaker. The speaker may only read what is written on the cards. Any further utterances, like articles (the German language has different ones for each grammatical gender), are not allowed. The test begins with reading the words. If the listener does not understand a word, he or she may say exactly once: "Please repeat the word." Further feedback about the intelligibility is not allowed. The sentences may not be repeated.

Three measures are computed from the experiment. The number of words w the listener understood correctly during the first attempt is multiplied by 5 and thus represents the word intelligibility i_{word} in percent. Words that were repeated do not get a point. Each sentence s gets a score c_s of 0 to 2 points. Two points are assigned when the sentence was understood completely correct. One point is given if one word is missing or not understood correctly. In all other cases, the reader gets no point. The sentence intelligibility i_{sent} in percent is the resulting sum of points multiplied with 10. The total intelligibility i_{total} in percent is then given by

$$i_{\text{total}} = \frac{i_{\text{word}} + i_{\text{sent}}}{2} = \frac{1}{2}\left(5w + 10\sum_{s=1}^{5} c_s\right) \quad . \tag{7.1}$$

The test was shown to be valid, reliable and objective [Zen86, ZP86], and it was also applied to patients with Provox® shunt valves before: Patients with voice prostheses reached an average PLTT result of about 70 while the results of esophageal speakers (Chapter 2.2.2) were just under 60 ([MZ96], see also Table 2.1). During the development of the test, words with two syllables were excluded from the test material as they could be guessed too easily by the listener even when the voice quality was very low [ZP86]. A reason why the test should be done via telephone was also given: A quiet room does not reflect a real-world communication situation as noise is present almost everywhere. In a noise-free environment, the voice rehabilitation progress would be overestimated. The telephone situation is easy to maintain and thus suitable for practical use. But like each evaluation that involves human raters, this test is subjective (see also Chapter 2.4). Therefore, an objective and automatic version of the PLTT was developed.

7.4.4 Words and Sentences in the PLTT

The PLTT vocabulary was originally defined for a test denoted as "Freiburger Sprachverständnistest" [Hah57, Bar01]. Six of the 400 words appeared twice ("Bart", "Feld", "Geld", "Schiff", "Schrift", "Tracht"). The electronic version of the 100 sentences ("Marburger Satzliste", [NB62]) was taken from the online resources of the Bavarian Archive for Speech Signals [BAS]. Words and sentences were available in the old German orthography that was valid until 2005. They were, however, not converted to the new orthography. On the one hand, the necessary changes were rather small. On the other hand, all the readers were elderly people mostly not familiar with the new way of writing (e.g. "Bass" instead of "Baß") which might have caused confusion and interruptions during reading.

For recording the PLTT, each patient got a unique sheet of paper with instructions and the texts to read on the telephone (see Appendix A.2). First of all, a sustained vowel (/a/) and the story of "The North Wind and the Sun" (see Appendix A.1) were recorded. The last part of the telephone session was the PLTT where each reader had 22 words and 6 sentences that were randomly extracted from the lists described above. The data were collected with a dialogue system provided by Sympalog Voice Solutions[1]. The speech therapist who was present when the patients called the system reported that some people had difficulties to listen to and follow the instructions and do the reading task alternately. For this reason, later recordings were not interrupted by the system any more (see Appendix A.2).

A speech recognition system can only recognize the words stored in its vocabulary list. This list had to be created from the words and sentences occurring in the PLTT. This, however, is not enough to simulate a human listener. A human being knows more words than those occurring in the test which might cause misperceptions. In order to simulate this in the automatic test, the vocabulary list of the recognizer had to be extended by words phonetically similar to those of the actual vocabulary. This was done in [Rie07] by the definition of a modified Levenshtein distance for phonetic transcriptions. It involved a weighting function which assigns

---

[1]http://www.sympalog.com

phoneme pairs that sound similar (e.g. /s/ and /z/) a low weight and thus finds the desired words. In this way, the basic PLTT vocabulary that consisted of 738 words (*PLTT-small*) was expanded to 1017 words (*PLTT-large*). The additional words and their transliterations were taken from the CELEX dictionary [BPG95]. The VERBMOBIL baseline training set *VM-base* (see Chapter 4.3) was downsampled at 8 kHz sampling frequency, a VERBMOBIL recognizer was trained and the vocabulary changed to the *PLTT-small* or *PLTT-large* word list, respectively. For both cases, a polyphone-based and a monophone-based version were created. A 0-gram language model was used so that the results are only dependent on the acoustic models.

7.4.5   Test Data and Automatic Evaluation Results

A test set of PLTT recordings (*pltt_8kHz*) from 31 TE speakers was available where each recording contained all words and sentences the respective speaker read out. The speakers were 25 men and 6 women (63.4 ± 8.7 years old); all of them were provided with a shunt valve of the Provox® type (Chapter 2.2.5). The files were also segmented so that each word and sentence was stored in a separate file. This was done in order to explore whether the automatic evaluation is influenced by noise or non-verbals between the words in the full recordings. This database is denoted as *pltt_mod_8kHz*. The human listeners were 8 male and 3 female students (average age: 22.5 ± 1.2 years). None of them had experience with voice and speech analysis. For recording the PLTT, each patient got a unique sheet of paper with instructions and 22 words and 6 sentences of the test that were randomly chosen. The first two words and the first sentence were neither used for human nor for automatic evaluation. The raters listened to the *pltt_seg_8kHz* data set. They could pause the play-back to write down the understood utterance.

Although the raters had never heard TE voices before, the inter-rater correlation between one rater and the remaining 10 for the total intelligibility i_{total} was greater than $r = 0.8$ for all persons. However, perceptive results varied strongly among the raters. The difference in the average of i_{total} for the "best" and the "worst" rater was more than 20 points which shows how strongly the test depends on the particular listener. The standard deviation was very similar for all raters, however (see [Rie07]).

The recognition results and the PLTT measures both for recognizers and human raters are displayed in Table 7.20. Since the first part of a PLTT session consists of single words, not only the word accuracy (WA) but also the word recognition rate (WR) was computed. It is based on the formula for the word accuracy (6.1), but the number of words n_{ins} that are wrongly inserted by the recognizer is not counted. In comparison to the human WA which reached 55%, the automatic recognition rates are much lower due to the following reasons: The speakers had read the text "The North Wind and the Sun" right before the PLTT and were therefore exhausted. The bad signal quality of the telephone transmission and the fact that the training data of the recognizers were just downsampled and not real telephone speech had also negative influence. No sentence was recognized completely correct according to the PLTT rules. For this reason, i_{sent} was 0 for all recognizers. Word accuracy and word recognition rate for the human raters were computed from their written transliteration of the audio files.

Although the automatic recognition yielded so bad results, the correlation to the human ratings was high (see Table 7.21). The best correlation between an automatic measure and the overall PLTT result i_{total} was reached for the word recognition rate on the polyphone-based recognizers. Both Pearson's and Spearman's correlation were about 0.9. Since a word that was not understood by the listener on first attempt does not get a point anyway, it is not necessary to

data set	pltt_8kHz				pltt_mod_8kHz				
vocabulary	PLTT-small		PLTT-large		PLTT-small		PLTT-large		raters
recog. units	mono	poly	mono	poly	mono	poly	mono	poly	
$\mu(\mathrm{WA})$	10.0	1.8	8.0	–0.1	9.2	0.3	7.4	–1.5	55.1
$\sigma(\mathrm{WA})$	14.8	20.4	13.5	19.9	14.7	21.4	12.9	20.2	21.4
$\mu(\mathrm{WR})$	17.3	16.6	14.4	13.7	16.4	15.6	14.2	13.2	55.3
$\sigma(\mathrm{WR})$	13.2	12.6	9.3	11.2	9.9	10.8	8.7	10.3	21.4
$\mu(i_{\mathrm{word}})$	17.8	13.1	14.5	10.9	14.1	11.1	12.0	9.4	41.4
$\sigma(i_{\mathrm{word}})$	15.1	13.0	12.8	10.9	13.8	11.6	12.7	11.1	21.3
$\mu(i_{\mathrm{sent}})$	0.0	0.0	0.0	0.0	0.0	0.0	0.0	0.0	52.8
$\sigma(i_{\mathrm{sent}})$	0.0	0.0	0.0	0.0	0.0	0.0	0.0	0.0	28.3
$\mu(i_{\mathrm{total}})$	8.9	6.6	7.3	5.5	7.0	5.5	6.0	4.7	47.1
$\sigma(i_{\mathrm{total}})$	7.5	6.5	6.4	5.8	6.9	5.8	6.4	5.6	22.0

Table 7.20: Average word accuracy (WA), word recognition rate (WR), and the PLTT measures i_{word}, i_{sent} and i_{total} for speech recognizers and human raters [Rie07]; pltt_8kHz denotes the recordings containing all words and sentences of one patient in one file; in the pltt_mod_8kHz data, the files were hand-segmented and contained one word or one sentence each.

data set	pltt_8kHz				pltt_mod_8kHz			
vocabulary	PLTT-small		PLTT-large		PLTT-small		PLTT-large	
recognition units	mono	poly	mono	poly	mono	poly	mono	poly
$r(\mathrm{WA}_{\mathrm{rec}}, i_{\mathrm{total, hum}})$	0.71	**0.72**	**0.72**	0.71	**0.72**	0.67	0.71	0.70
$\rho(\mathrm{WA}_{\mathrm{rec}}, i_{\mathrm{total, hum}})$	**0.84**	0.81	0.83	0.80	0.81	0.76	0.79	0.79
$r(\mathrm{WR}_{\mathrm{rec}}, i_{\mathrm{total, hum}})$	0.81	0.88	0.82	0.85	0.85	**0.89**	0.86	**0.89**
$\rho(\mathrm{WR}_{\mathrm{rec}}, i_{\mathrm{total, hum}})$	0.86	**0.93**	0.87	0.92	0.88	0.90	0.90	0.90

Table 7.21: Pearson's correlation r and Spearman's correlation ρ between the speech recognizers' results ("rec") and the human raters' average values ("hum"; [Rie07]); the best results in each line are printed in boldface.

consider word repetition in the automatic version at all. For more details, see [Rie07].

The outcome of these experiments is that the PLTT can be replaced by an objective, automatic approach. The question whether monophone-based or polyphone-based recognizers are better for the task could not be answered. When the word accuracy was compared to i_{total}, monophones were advantageous; when the word recognition rate was used instead, the polyphone-based recognizers were closer to the human rating. There were also some cases in which the correlation was slightly better when each word and sentence was processed separately, but in general the long pltt_8kHz recordings which contain the entire test can be used without prior segmentation.

The PLTT deals with speech that is – in addition to its pathology – also deteriorated by a telephone channel. The next section will address a similar problem, namely recordings within a room but with a certain distance between speaker and microphone.

7.5   Simulated Distant-Talking TE Recordings

In Chapter 5.2, the root cepstrum and the μ-law features were introduced in order to achieve better recognition results under reverberation. However, only the latter was successful. In this section, these features will be tested on substitute voices in (simulated) reverberant environment. The usual recording situation where a headset is used might have a negative influence on the patient. The patient might feel watched or controlled when he or she is aware that other people could get access to the recording. If the microphone is somewhere else in the room, this effect is attenuated. For patients after head or neck surgery, wearing a headset can also be painful. Furthermore, in everyday communication the listeners will also be at some distance to the speaker and thus get influenced by room reverberation. Therefore, the scenario with a distant microphone reflects the acquisition of more realistic data.

7.5.1   Test Data and Recognizers

As no real distant-talking data from laryngectomees were available, the experiments were made using artificially reverberated close-talking signals. Instead of the *laryng41* data sampled at 16 kHz, the *laryng41_8kHz* data set was examined because speech recognizers using different features were available for 8 kHz data already, and the correlation between the human intelligibility criterion and the word accuracy was almost the same on 16 kHz and 8 kHz data (Chapter 7.4). For testing, the *laryng41_8kHz* data were convolved with three room impulse responses (see Table 7.22) which were chosen from those which had been selected for the training data of some of the VERBMOBIL-based recognizers (see Table 4.4). The impulse responses were h411090 simulating a room with a reverberation time T_{60} of 250 ms, a microphone distance of 60 cm and a microphone in front of the speaker, i.e. at an angle of 90° to the microphone array, h413120 ($T_{60} - 250$ ms, distance 240 cm, angle 120°), and h422105 ($T_{60} - 400$ ms, distance 120 cm, angle 105°). They are depicted in Figure 7.6.

Three types of features were investigated following the experiments on normal voices in Chapter 6. The recognizer that used MFCC features was called *NW-base-mono-8kHz* as introduced in Chapter 7.4. Two further recognizers were available employing modified features and the respective parameter values that yielded the best results on the VERBMOBIL and Fatigue data. The root cepstrum recognizer which uses the 7th root in the feature companding function (see Chapter 5.2.2 and 6.2.1) will be denoted as *NW-root7-mono-8kHz*. For the μ-law features (Chapter 5.2.3), the factor $\mu = 10^5$ was chosen according to the findings in Chapter 6.2.2. The respective recognizer is called *NW-mule5-mono-8kHz*. All recognizers were trained with close-talking speech only. They were monophone-based and used a unigram language model.

7.5.2   Results

Table 7.23 shows the word accuracy computed using the transliteration of the respective data sets. When the word accuracy was computed against the text reference, the differences were marginal. Analogous to the findings in Chapter 6.2, the root cepstrum could not improve the results, the MFCC are always better. The μ-law features, however, are consistently better even on substitute voices and thus proof to be an alternative to the classic Mel-cepstrum approach also for pathologic speech. However, the improvement was not significant on the data used in this thesis. The degree of reverberation in the test signals does not only have an impact on the

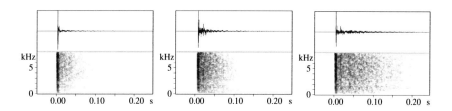

Figure 7.6: Waveform and spectrogram of the impulse responses h411090 (T_{60} = 250 ms, left), h413120 (T_{60} = 250 ms, middle), and h422105 (T_{60} = 400 ms, right)

word recognition but also on the correlation between word accuracy and human intelligibility score (Table 7.24). For close-talking speech, it was about $r = -0.8$ (Chapter 7.1.2). For the reverberated data, it is much worse. Note, however, that for this experiment the human ratings of the *laryng41* close-talking data had to be used since no human evaluation for the reverberated files was available. Nevertheless, the results show an interesting aspect: The same kind of reverberation must have different effects on different voices. Obviously the relation between the word accuracy on close-talking and deteriorated speech is not linear, otherwise they would yield the same correlation to the human ratings. This effect should be examined again on a database that contains real distant-talking data and human evaluation results for exactly these data.

7.6 Visualization of Results

The Sammon transform, introduced in Chapter 5.4, was applied to the speech data of the laryngectomees (Chapter 4.4) in order to achieve a graphical representation of the evaluation results. The "distance" between the speakers was determined by adapting the *NW-base-mono* recognizer (Chapter 5.1.6) to the single speakers and measuring how the Hidden Markov Models changed during this procedure. In the Sammon map (or "cosmos") of the *laryng18* speaker group and the normal-speaking elderly and younger control group (*kom18* and *bas16*; see Chapter 4.5), all speaker groups were separated from each other (Figure 7.7). It confirms the results of Zorn [Zor06] where in a similar setup also the groups with the highest and lowest speech pathology had the largest distance between them. The elderly normal speakers can be regarded as "slightly pathologic" due to natural changes in the voice at higher age. For this reason, they are located between the young, normal group and the TE group. Furthermore, the high-pitched voices among which are all women in the *bas16* set are located in the lower area of the cosmos while the low-pitched voices can be found in the upper region.

In order to find out whether the Sammon transform can also discriminate subgroups within one speaker group, the *laryng41* set was examined. Which voice or speech properties are expressed by the map can be visualized by assigning gray scale values to the markings representing the speakers ("stars"). In Figure 7.8, the word accuracy on the *NW-base-poly* and *NW-base-mono* is depicted. It shows that there is obviously a tendency that worse speakers – in terms of word accuracy – appear in the upper area of the map. This assumption is confirmed when the

test set	speakers	impulse response	T_{60} (ms)	dist. (cm)	angle ($^\circ$)
laryng41_8kHz_rev-a	*laryng41*	h411090	250	60	90
laryng41_8kHz_rev-b	*laryng41*	h413120	250	240	120
laryng41_8kHz_rev-c	*laryng41*	h422105	400	120	105

Table 7.22: Artificially reverberated TE speaker sets

recognizer	test set	μ(WA)	σ(WA)	min(WA)	max(WA)
NW-base-poly-8kHz	*laryng41_8kHz*	32.3	17.4	−7.4	69.4
NW-base-mono-8kHz	*laryng41_8kHz*	33.4	12.1	5.6	62.0
NW-base-mono-8kHz	*laryng41_8kHz_rev-a*	31.3	10.9	10.2	58.3
NW-root7-mono-8kHz	*laryng41_8kHz_rev-a*	28.3	10.6	5.6	51.4
NW-mu1e5-mono-8kHz	*laryng41_8kHz_rev-a*	31.8	11.0	11.1	57.4
NW-base-mono-8kHz	*laryng41_8kHz_rev-b*	24.8	8.6	9.3	46.3
NW-root7-mono-8kHz	*laryng41_8kHz_rev-b*	22.7	8.0	4.6	40.4
NW-mu1e5-mono-8kHz	*laryng41_8kHz_rev-b*	26.1	9.2	7.4	47.3
NW-base-mono-8kHz	*laryng41_8kHz_rev-c*	21.4	5.7	8.3	35.2
NW-root7-mono-8kHz	*laryng41_8kHz_rev-c*	20.1	6.2	6.5	35.2
NW-mu1e5-mono-8kHz	*laryng41_8kHz_rev-c*	22.0	6.0	12.0	36.1

Table 7.23: Word accuracy for different features on the original and artificially reverberated *laryng41_8kHz* data (computed against the transliteration of the test files)

recognizer	test set	r	ρ	κ	$\kappa_{\mathrm{DF}}(w)$	α
NW-base-poly-8kHz	*laryng41_8kHz*	−0.85	−0.84	+0.23	+0.47	+0.68
NW-base-mono-8kHz	*laryng41_8kHz*	−0.81	−0.76	+0.19	+0.42	+0.63
NW-base-mono-8kHz	*laryng41_8kHz_rev-a*	−0.73	−0.70	+0.20	+0.42	+0.62
NW-root7-mono-8kHz	*laryng41_8kHz_rev-a*	−0.75	−0.74	+0.23	+0.45	+0.64
NW-mu1e5-mono-8kHz	*laryng41_8kHz_rev-a*	−0.66	−0.64	+0.20	+0.42	+0.62
NW-base-mono-8kHz	*laryng41_8kHz_rev-b*	−0.58	−0.59	+0.18	+0.39	+0.59
NW-root7-mono-8kHz	*laryng41_8kHz_rev-b*	−0.55	−0.50	+0.19	+0.41	+0.61
NW-mu1e5-mono-8kHz	*laryng41_8kHz_rev-b*	−0.59	−0.62	+0.21	+0.42	+0.61
NW-base-mono-8kHz	*laryng41_8kHz_rev-c*	−0.56	−0.52	+0.14	+0.37	+0.57
NW-root7-mono-8kHz	*laryng41_8kHz_rev-c*	−0.61	−0.59	+0.18	+0.38	+0.57
NW-mu1e5-mono-8kHz	*laryng41_8kHz_rev-c*	−0.58	−0.58	+0.17	+0.39	+0.60

Table 7.24: Agreement between word accuracy and intelligibility score of 5 experts on the original and artificially reverberated *laryng41_8kHz* data; given are Pearson's r, Spearman's ρ, Cohen's κ, the weighted multi-rater κ by Davies and Fleiss, and Krippendorff's α (see Chapter 3). Note that the human ratings were actually made for the *laryng41* data set.

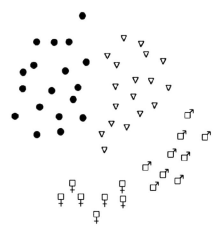

Figure 7.7: Sammon map of the *laryng18* data (•) and the normal-speaking control groups *kom18* (▽) and *bas16* (□ with gender symbol); basis of the map was the adaptation of the *NW-base-mono* recognizer to each speaker.

human evaluation results are coded by shades of grey. In the examples in Figure 7.9, a speaker was drawn the darker the better he or she was rated. In order to determine how good the Sammon transform mapped the respective rating criteria, the same procedure was applied as by Zorn in [Zor06, Chapter 3.5]: All speakers are orthogonally mapped to a line through the center of the graphics. The correlation of the positions of the projected stars on the axis and the respective human ratings is then used as a measure how good the rating criterion is represented in the map. Table 7.25 contains the best correlation for all criteria together with the angle of the axis in the cosmos where an angle of 0° means a horizontal line. For the word accuracy, the correlation values are in the same range as those that Zorn had achieved on the *laryng18* group. For *NW-base-poly*, it was $r = 0.74$ for an angle of $-60°$, for the *NW-base-mono* recognizer, $r = 0.63$ was reached at $-70°$. These results were also confirmed by multi-regression with the *Weka* package [WF05]. The absolute correlation values were exactly the same as with the line projection method.

Rating criteria like intelligibility and overall quality can be expressed better than the change of voice quality during reading, for instance (see Figure 7.9 and Table 7.25). This affects the same criteria as when the speaker is evaluated by means of the word accuracy (cf. Chapter 7.1). In this way, Sammon maps can provide a descriptive representation of speech data at least for several criteria which may be helpful for the medical personnel in clinical practice.

Up to now, the correlation of only one automatic measure to human evaluation results was examined at a time. A concluding experiment will reveal whether there is a group of features that can together represent human ratings better than single measures. This experiment will follow in the next section.

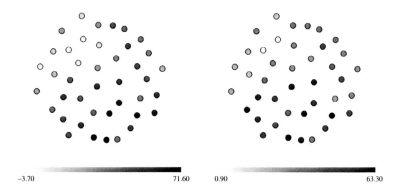

Figure 7.8: Sammon maps of the *laryng41* data; the shading denotes the word accuracy of the *NW-base-poly (left)* and the *NW-base-mono* recognizer *(right)*.

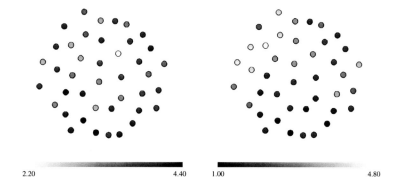

Figure 7.9: Sammon maps of the *laryng41* data; the shading denotes the experts' ratings on the change of voice quality during reading *(left)* and intelligibility *(right)*.

criterion	angle (°)	r
quality	–69	–0.60
hoarse	–80	+0.50
effort	–72	+0.70
penetr	–42	–0.52
proso	–63	–0.61
brsense	–69	–0.57
noise	–72	+0.51
tone	–75	–0.68
change	–90	+0.40
intell	–60	–0.66
overall	–68	–0.64

Table 7.25: Maximum correlation r between human rating criteria (see Table 4.12) and star positions in Sammon maps of *laryng41* data; lines are drawn through the center of the map at certain angles, and the position of the stars mapped on the lines is compared to the human rating.

7.7 Selection of a Set of Objective Measures

In Chapter 7.1, the word accuracy was introduced as a good automatic measure for the human rating criterion of intelligibility. On the *NW-base-poly* recognizer and the *laryng41* speech data, it reached a correlation of $r = -0.88$ to the averaged intelligibility score of 5 raters (Table 7.4). In Chapter 7.3, the correlation between human rating criteria and several prosodic features (Chapter 5.5) was presented. For the *laryng41* speakers, there were also correlations above $|r| = 0.7$ for the intelligibility criterion, mainly on features that represent word and pause durations but also – at least for the *NW-base-poly* recognizer – for the normalized word energy (EnNormWord0,0, see Table 7.15). In the frame of [Rie07], it was examined whether a combination of prosodic features and the word accuracy can improve the agreement between human and automatic evaluation.

The computation was done with PEAKS ("Program for Evaluation and Analysis of all Kinds of Speech disorders", [Mai06]) a client-server environment developed at the Chair of Pattern Recognition that allows to record and analyze speech recordings. Leave-one-speaker-out multi-correlation/regression analysis [CC83] was applied to the *laryng41* files in order to find the features with the best average rank among word accuracy and prosodic features. These features and the average expert rating were then the input data for Support Vector Regression (SVR; [Pla98, SS04]). The multi-correlation/regression analysis determined the following features as being most relevant for intelligibility analysis:

1. word accuracy; on average it had the best rank R for all configurations in the leave-one-out experiment ($R = 0$).

2. global F_0 mean (F0MeanG, $R = 1$)

3. position of the energy maximum in a word, averaged over all words (EnMaxPosWord0,0, $R = 3.2$)

4. mean square error computed between the F_0 curve and the regression line of the F_0 for word pairs (F0MseRegWord-1,0, $R = 3.6$)

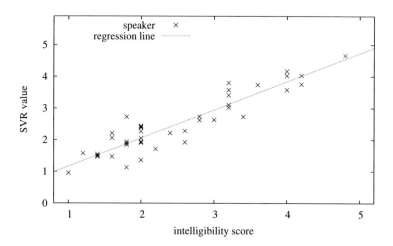

Figure 7.10: SVR value and human average intelligibility score from 5 human raters for the *laryng41* speakers

None of the three selected prosodic features had shown a high correlation to the human rating alone. For the position of the energy maximum, it was very low ($r = 0.15$); F0MseRegWord-1,0 reached $r = 0.34$, the global F_0 mean $r = 0.51$.

Given the average human intelligibility score as reference data, the SVR on the word accuracy and the three prosodic features for each speaker tried to predict the human score and produced the regression values shown in Figure 7.10 from the automatically computed measure. The correlation between these values and the human scores was $r = 0.92$. This is better than for the word accuracy alone with $|r| = 0.88$. However, the word accuracy was independent from the human evaluation while the SVR tried to match the human scores, i.e. the regression optimized the result with respect to the actual test data and only for the specific criterion. For this reason, it is not clear whether there was a real improvement by combining the prosodic features and the word accuracy.

No difference in the correlation between SVR and human rating was found when the word accuracy was not computed against the transliteration of the *laryng41* files but against the text reference. This supports the findings of Chapter 7.2.3, i.e. the rate of reading errors was so low that the time-consuming manual transliteration of the recording before the automatic analysis could be avoided by using the reference text instead. For more details, see [Rie07, NMH+07].

7.8   Conclusion

In this chapter, measures and features for the automatic evaluation of tracheoesophageal substitute voices were introduced. The examined methods and algorithms allow for the following conclusions: The speech data acquired from a patient should be a read out standard text in order to get comparable material for all readers. Usually in speech intelligibility tests, like the PLTT (Chapter 7.4), a naïve listener who does not know the words or texts in advance writes down the understood words. It was shown in this thesis, however, that the human-machine correlation for a known standard text evaluated by expert raters and a speech recognizer is in the same range (cf. Chapter 7.1 and 7.4). When the text is the same for all speakers, then the variance in the utterances among different speakers can be used to determine information about voice and speech pathology. Since intelligibility is the most important criterion in human evaluation, the word accuracy of a speech recognizer is an essential measure. For cooperative speakers, who keep to a given text, the word recognition rate yields almost identical results and can therefore be neglected. For non-cooperative speakers, like little children, it should be taken into account (see e.g. [MNNS06]).

The evaluation of other human rating criteria is not sufficiently possible without prosodic analysis based upon features computed from word and pause durations, speech energy, and fundamental frequency. Averaged across word or word-pause-word intervals, they serve as objective measures for criteria like the match of breath and sense units, vocal tone, or speech effort (Chapter 7.3). The speech recognizer for the analysis should contain the words from the standard text in its vocabulary list only. It was shown that the word accuracy can be computed with respect to the text reference, i.e. no transliteration of the speech data is necessary (see Chapter 7.2.3). Only a zerogram or unigram language model should be used. Otherwise the model eliminates too many recognition errors that might reflect a low degree of intelligibility for a particular voice.

The best results for human-machine correlation are achieved when the signal quality is high, i.e. when speech is recorded with 16 kHz sampling frequency and when a headset is used. Nevertheless, it was shown that for telephone-based evaluation as needed for the PLTT, for instance, the correlation is only slightly worse (Chapter 7.4). The setup of the speech recognizer does not have to be changed – except for the corresponding training data.

Instead of MFCC as features, μ-law features can be recommended for the recognition of all examined types of speech quality. For the telephone recordings of tracheoesophageal substitute speech, consistent improvement of word accuracy was achieved. However, the amount of available data was not large enough to determine whether the improvement was significant. Since it is desired to allow the patient to do a speech evaluation session from his or her home, future experiments on larger data sets will answer this question. In the experiments with the EMBASSI and VERBMOBIL corpus, significancy was confirmed (see Chapter 6.2). This means that μ-law features should be applied when the speech data are recorded by a distant-talking microphone which is a step towards therapy sessions that are more comfortable for the patients. Then the speech recognizer should also be trained with close-talking speech and artificially reverberated signals. When even a microphone array is available, beamforming as a preprocessing step will be beneficial (see Chapter 6.3 and 7.5).

For clinical practice, the developed methods have the advantage that they are objective and independent from single experts, and the measures can serve for the description of therapy progress because they are always based on the same algorithms and do not vary in their way of judging over time as a human being would do.

The next chapter will compare the findings of this thesis to those of other researchers.

Chapter 8

Discussion

The topic of this thesis is the automatic analysis of substitute voices where the focus is on speech-related criteria since current methods regard sustained vowels only.

Usually, automatic evaluation performs analysis of sustained vowels (see e.g. [GSO$^+$06, FMSK00] or Chapter 2.5). However, in everyday life it is important for the patient to speak fluently and intelligible. These properties cannot be evaluated on a single vowel recording. For this reason, speech recognition methods were applied in order to analyze a read-out standard text. The number of correctly recognized words alone, however, is not sufficient. It is also important to know how fast the patients speak, whether they have to breathe within a sentence, or if the speaking effort is high. In order to obtain information on these criteria, automatic prosodic analysis was performed on the same text recordings. Nishio and Niimi used the alternating motion rate (AMR) and the sequential motion rate (SMR) as measures for articulation abilities [NN06]. AMR involves the fast repetition of a single syllable, e.g. /pa/, while SMR is measured on repeated syllable sequences, e.g. /pataka/. For this thesis, these measures were not computed because the articulation rate is inherent in the word and pause duration features which are provided by the prosody module.

Still, a standard text does not represent a real communication situation. Read and spontaneous speech are significantly different. While the articulation rate of read speech is lower, it shows more pitch variation and less vowel reduction than spontaneous speech [BJKN92, Bla95, Laa97]. Nevertheless, a text is a much closer approximation of fluent, spontaneous speech than a single, sustained vowel. For the hoarseness criterion, Halberstam found that acoustic parameters from connected speech are more reliable than from sustained vowels [Hal04]. The study did not involve substitute voices, but it is likely that it also holds for them. A standard text is a necessary compromise because the evaluation of completely free speech would require much more effort in all components of the analysis framework. For instance, when different speakers use words of different length or with a different percentage of vowels, their results of the word duration analysis or voiced-voiceless decisions will become incomparable to other subjects. Furthermore, spoken words that are not in the vocabulary list of the speech recognizer will cause recognition errors. A bad intelligibility rating for the reader might be the result even when his or her voice sounds very natural. In order to avoid this, recordings of free speech would have to be transliterated by hand for each speaker.

Concerning the human evaluation reference of the recordings, the use of a standard text may mainly affect the intelligibility criterion. When the same text is used for every reader and it is too short, then the rater will know it by heart very quickly which might lead to better intelligibility scores than the speaker actually deserves. However, with free speech the raters' vocabulary must be a superset of the patients' vocabulary; otherwise it may happen that a speaker gets worse intelligibility scores when the listener does not know some of the words.

A study which was close to the approach used in this thesis was performed by the research group of Moerman et al. ([MPM$^+$04], see also Chapter 5.5). Among other pathologic speakers, 53 TE speakers were rated by semi-professional listeners. In agreement with the findings in Chapter 4.4.4, the criteria of "intelligibility" and the "general impression" correlated highly with each other ($r = 0.89$) when the files were evaluated by 10 speech pathology students. However, correlations to automatically computed measures were low. The best measure was the averaged voicing evidence (AVE) which denotes the degree of periodicity of the signal. For sustained vowels, it reached $r = 0.44$; for the syllables /apa/, /ipi/, and /upu/, it was slightly higher ($r = 0.49$). On the voiced frames of a Dutch 18-word phrase, it dropped to $r = 0.38$. The best measure on the short text was the percentage of voiced frames ($r = 0.46$). On the *laryng41* data (Chapter 4.4.2) where the text "The North Wind and the Sun" was read, the same feature reached a correlation of –0.24 on the *NW-base-mono* recognizer only. However, in Chapter 7.3 there are several prosodic features based upon pause durations and voice onset or offset positions that reach a correlation of about $|r| = 0.7$. Hence, the number of voiced sections alone is not sufficient for evaluation, and a more detailed prosodic analysis, like introduced in Chapter 5.5, should be a basic part of automatic evaluation for pathologic voices.

Moerman et al. also report difficulties in finding the fundamental frequency. Their pitch extractors often detected the first harmonic ($2F_0$) or subharmonic ($1/2F_0$) instead of the real F_0. They state that the classical acoustic methods of objective voice evaluation on the means of jitter, shimmer and harmonics-to-noise ratio are not suitable for substitute voices. These problems were confirmed in Chapter 7.3.3.

This thesis concentrated on the analysis of speech properties rather than on acoustic properties since the latter have been examined for several years by a large number of researchers. Although there are problems in finding periodic signals in TE speech, the frequency-based features should not be neglected completely in a future clinical evaluation method. They can, in case of less severe voices, give additional information and thus allow a more differentiated analysis. A speech recognizer and a prosody module are the other essential components of such a product.

In general, studies about voice quality can hardly be compared. Often, the number of patients is so small that the results are not reliable (see Table 2.5, 2.6 and 2.7). Further problems are caused by the different experience of the human raters. A large variability in intra- and inter-rater reliability in different studies was subsumed for instance in [KGK$^+$93].

When good results for automatic voice classification or evaluation methods are presented in the literature, then there are often strong restrictions concerning the data or the reference. Moran et al. examined 58 normal and 573 pathologic recordings of sustained /a/ that were transmitted by telephone. The automatic classification into the two classes "normal" or "pathologic" worked with an accuracy of 74.2% while it was 89.1% on clean speech that was not deteriorated by a telephone channel [MRCL06, RML04]. Different pitch and amplitude perturbation features were used for the classification. The results are interesting since they give an impression about the influence of the telephone line which is important for tests like the Post-Laryngectomy Telephone Test (PLTT, Chapter 7.4), but no substitute voices were examined, and the speech data consisted of a sustained vowel per speaker only. The most important aspect is, however, that the algorithm only distinguished between two classes. There is also no detailed human reference to which the automatic result could be compared.

In Chapter 5.3 and 7.2, the adaptation of speech recognizers to TE speakers was described. The achieved recognition rates were higher than for the baseline system that was trained with normal speech only, but the correlation to the human ratings were not improved. An assessment system for dysphonic voices based upon speaker recognition instead of speech recognition techniques was proposed by Fredouille et al. [FPB+05]. They used 2 minutes of speech per speaker to train a Gaussian mixture model from which pathologic class models were derived by maximum a posteriori (MAP) adaptation. With 32 MFCC and the respective derivatives, they achieved 85% of success rate on the two-class problem "normal" vs. "dysphonic". When the pathologic voices were classified into four categories according to the G parameter (grade of abnormality) of the GRBAS scale ([Hir81], see Chapter 2.4.2), the classification rate was 69%. In contrast to this thesis, 3 human raters did not evaluate the speech data separately, but they decided together for the human reference score. This eliminated the problem of inter-rater discrepancy already before the comparison of human and automatic results. Criteria like intelligibility, match of breath and sense units, etc., were not evaluated.

The analysis methods used in this thesis were also applied on telephone speech (Chapter 7.4). The evaluation of PLTT recordings was automated, the "objective" and time-consuming evaluation of intelligibility by a human listener was replaced by deterministic speech recognition methods. Morales et al. showed how it is possible to use a recognizer trained with data that was sampled with 16 kHz, i.e. which has a spectrum range from 0 to 8 kHz, and to apply it on band-limited data [MHT05]. They achieved this by introducing corrector terms in the Mel spectrum gained from the comparison of filtered and unfiltered speech material. Digit recognition for telephone band speech could be improved from 23.2% word accuracy to 73.0% which was very close to the result of the unfiltered speech data (75.3%). However, no pathologic voices were examined. In this thesis, the recognition rates and the correlation between automatic and human recognition do not substantially change when telephone speech is processed (Chapter 7.4). For this reason, this kind of preprocessing is not necessary. Unfortunately, many studies that examine new features for speech recognition or preprocessing steps perform digit recognition only, and it cannot be predicted how the algorithms behave on data with a much larger vocabulary.

Wilpon et al., who examined automatic recognition of elderly speakers via telephone, relied also on (Danish) digit recognition only [WJ96]. They found that the error rate rises for elderly speakers even if the recognizer is trained with speech from this group only, but they also state that for speakers up to 70 years there is no need for "special precautions". In Chapter 7.1, however, the word accuracy for the elderly *kom18* group was 67.3% while for the young *bas16* group it was 83.3% for the polyphone-based *NW-base-poly* recognizer. With a smaller vocabulary, this difference would have probably been less severe and regarded as non-significant.

One of the goals in speech therapy is to provide a situation for the affected persons where they can act and speak freely. Until now, the patients wear a headset during recording because otherwise the signal quality might not be sufficient. When the microphone is supposed to be further away from the speaker, many distortions deteriorate the audio file. The most important one is reverberation. For this reason, speech recognition in reverberated environment was examined in this thesis. It is very difficult to compare different studies in the literature on this topic. The audio data differ not only in the number of speakers but also in the acoustic conditions in which the data were collected. The room impulse response is dependent on the size and configuration of the room and also on the angle and position of the speaker relative to the microphone (Chapter 4.1 and 5.2). For instance, the reverberation time in the experiments of Stahl et al. (440 ms, [SFB01]) was comparable to the 400 ms in the virtual recording room defined for this thesis. Their "far" microphone (2.5 m distance) corresponds to the microphone array in the EMBASSI corpus and to the 2.4 m distance for measuring the room impulse responses in the virtual recording room (see Chapter 4.1). However, instead of a headset for synchronous recording they used a "near" microphone at a distance of 0.4 m and added also a stationary noise signal. The vocabulary was rather small since the speech data consisted of spoken numbers like "two thousand and three", so there were only 32 different words. Their second corpus consisted of short commands for consumer electronics, like in the EMBASSI corpus, but there were only 54 different words in contrast to 473 words in the EMBASSI sentences. The VERBMOBIL-based recognizers (Chapter 4.3) even had a vocabulary size of 6445 words, and the Fatigue data (Chapter 4.2) contain 865 different words. On the portion of the Fatigue corpus that was recorded with 1 m microphone distance, the word accuracy was about 70% (Chapter 6) when a 4-gram language model was used. With a 0-gram model, only approx. 30% word accuracy were achieved. Stahl et al. observed the highest recognition rates of approx. 86% when training was performed with recordings y_n obtained by

$$y_n = x_n * h_n^{-1} * h_f + n_c \qquad (8.1)$$

where x_n denotes the signal of the near microphone, h_n^{-1} is the inverse transfer function from the speaker to the near microphone, and h_f is the transfer function from the speaker to the far microphone. The added stationary noise signal n_c had the same power spectrum as the signal from the far microphone. In this thesis, the focus is on the robustness of speech features against reverberation, therefore the noise n_c was assumed to be non-existent in the available close-talking signals, and h_n was assumed to be the identity.

The simulated reverberation time of $T_{60} = 1.09$ s in the study of Couvreur et al. [CC00] was much higher than the 250 and 400 ms used in this thesis which makes the recognition task much more difficult in the first place. A word accuracy of approx. 93% word accuracy was reached when the training data were reverberated with many room impulse responses, like in the *VM-12* or *VM-2* recognizer (Chapter 4.3). However, the test data of Couvreur et al. were taken from the same corpus as the training data and artificially reverberated after selection. Furthermore, the vocabulary was very small since again only digit recognition was performed.

The conclusion from these experiments is that for the recognition of distant-talking speech from unknown environment at least a certain portion of the training data should be reverberated. It is not necessary to match the acoustic properties of the test data exactly when there are similar environments in the training data. The recognition error rate can be reduced slightly once more by using appropriate features, like the μ-law features based upon MFCC (Chapter 5.2), or beamforming as a preprocessing step (Chapter 6.3).

The overall outcome of this thesis is that the human speech evaluation which is affected by many possible sources of error or variation, like the raters' experience, can be supported by deterministic methods that enable to document a patient's progress during therapy and serve as objective means of description of pathologic voice. An automatic evaluation system should consist of a polyphone-based speech recognizer and a module for prosodic evaluation. For the determination of the agreement between the human rater and the machine, correlation coefficients are recommended when the numerical range of both evaluations is different. Otherwise, introduced chance-corrected measures for rater agreement, like Krippendorff's α, should be preferred.

The following chapter will give a short outlook on how these methods will be extended in future work.

Chapter 9

Outlook

Speech analysis, especially evaluation of pathologic speech for clinical purposes, is a very complex task. Despite the good results achieved in this thesis, there are some aspects that will have to be addressed in the future.

The problem of out-of-vocabulary (OOV) words was not examined yet because the number of reading errors was very small in the recordings of the laryngectomees (see Chapter 4.4.2). For a future clinical application, however, the two types of error – by reading and by recognition – must be separated. Otherwise a patient with a high-quality voice might get bad evaluation results due to misread words. By the application of confidence measures, the sections with reading errors could be detected in the recording [Ste01]. Then the remaining parts of the file are used for the computation of the voice quality only. Boros et al. suggested the distinction of OOV and *OOT (out-of-text)* words [BAG+97]. The latter are words that are likely to occur during reading errors when the patients read a text, for example in phrases like "Where did I stop?" In a category-based recognition system [GNN96], they could be included in the vocabulary list in advance and become a category of their own. In this way, they could be easily removed from the signal to be analyzed. In order to find words that are still not in the vocabulary list, it might also be helpful for distorted speech to introduce a language model which is not based upon words but upon smaller lexical units [Gal03].

A related problem are speech repairs, i.e. corrections after reading errors. The types of repairs that are relevant for a reading situation are *in-word repairs* where the reader corrects a part of a word, and *modification repairs* where a part of the whole sentence is repeated [SBN01]. The automatic evaluation of such events was examined with stutterers' speech [NNH+00]. However, the created repetition models are very complex and need conceptual revisions for the application with TE speech because the search trees become too large for low-quality voices during the decoding phase.

Although the correlation between human and automatic evaluation results is not enhanced when the speech recognizer is adapted to substitute voices (Chapter 7.2), there are some scenarios that make a better recognition of pathologic speech desirable. An example are patients where the quality of the substitute voice will permanently stay very bad due to anatomical or surgical reasons. These persons have severe problems in communication. Since TE speakers are elderly people in most of the cases, this will also have an impact on the listeners because they are usually elderly people, too, and their listening comprehension is often restricted [EB01]. For this reason, several research groups try to enhance the quality of pathologic voices not at its source but between speaker and listener. For instance, linear prediction analysis and a synthetic source for resynthesis were applied to enhance recorded samples of esophageal speech [MHKH02]. Reduction of breathiness in disordered speech is also an important topic. However, it cannot be reduced by usual noise reduction algorithms which assume that signal and noise are independent of each other because breathiness is highly correlated with the voice [HK04, MM02, MDB01].

This method cannot only help to improve the intelligibility in human-to-human conversation, but it may also enhance the automatic recognition of people with voice disorders, e.g. in dialogue systems. When these applications are supposed to be suited for the disabled, they will have to deal with many kinds of voice and speech disorders. The Sammon transform (Chapter 5.4 and 7.6) can support this. The idea is a pool of robust prototype recognizers trained on speech with different disorders. When confronted with a new speaker, the system would project the speaker into a cosmos of the prototype recognizers, determine the disorder and select the "closest" recognizer or combine a set of several close recognizers for further processing. Regarding the distribution of age in the population, a special focus on elderly speakers [BYY$^+$01] might also be advantageous.

For the application in dialogue systems and also for the communication among humans via telephone, the influence of different communication channels [Jun97] has to be further examined. Not only the speech effort but also the listening effort might be rated [HK04], and the evaluation attributes recommended for telephone transmission quality by the International Telecommunication Union [ITU96] should be taken into account.

Similarly, when distant-talking speech samples of TE speakers will be available, then the distortions by the acoustical environment will have to be regarded during the recognition phase. This does not only concern reverberation. There are multiple sources for sound that is not wanted in the recording, like noise from the street, a running computer, the present persons touching the text sheet or the furniture, etc. Short noise events might be eliminated by monitoring the spectrum of the signal and removing small sections with unusual phenomena. When longer parts of the therapy sessions are recorded, then also the patient's and the therapist's voice have to be separated by speaker recognition methods; only the laryngectomee should be analyzed. Nevertheless, reverberation will stay one of the main problems. A very successful solution might be the creation of an adaptive reverberation model at runtime. This model can be integrated into the decoding phase [SZK06, Zel06].

The evaluation experiments presented in this thesis are no long-term study. It is not easy to acquire speech data from one speaker group and the corresponding human evaluation data from one rater group over a longer time. However, this could confirm the assumption that the long-term evaluation of voice rehabilitation can be done more reliable by automatic methods than by humans. Additionally, a group of naïve raters should be involved because they represent the listeners the patients meet in everyday life (cf. [BSH$^+$06]). But not only listeners should judge a patient's voice, also the patients themselves should do this. There are self-evaluation scales (Chapter 2.4.3) that are used by the therapists to obtain how handicapped the patients feel by their impairment. This is an important aspect in modern therapy which should be regarded when the automatic evaluation methods are improved. However, it is not clear until now how these aspects can be modeled since the correlation between self-evaluation and evaluation by speech experts is low [SLH$^+$04].

The evaluation methods described in this thesis may not only be beneficial for patients after total laryngectomy. They will be revised and improved in a new research project about the evaluation of voice after partial laryngectomy which is funded by the German Cancer Aid from August 2007 on.

Chapter 10

Summary

In 20 to 40 percent of all cases of laryngeal cancer, total laryngectomy has to be performed, i.e. the removal of the entire larynx. After the procedure, the trachea and the esophagus stay separated. For the affected persons, this means the loss of the natural voice and thus the loss of the main means of communication. Modern surgery allows to establish a substitute voice which has to be evaluated from time to time by the therapist for the purpose of reporting therapy progress. This evaluation is subjective; it is therefore dependent on the particular expert's experience and other factors. In this thesis, it was examined how automatic methods can be used in order to provide an objective means of the evaluation of substitute voices.

There are many methods of voice restoration. In the esophageal substitute voice, a part of the esophagus serves as pseudoglottis, and the stomach can be used as an air reservoir. However, it takes several months or even years until laryngectomees can control this kind of voice. Several different surgical methods tried to allow the redirection of expiratory air from the trachea into the pharynx by means of fistulae or similar ways. However, the aspiration rate was very high, so most of these approaches are not used any more. The voicing function of the larynx can also be replaced by a sound generator. In most cases, it is electrically operated and is therefore called electrolarynx. The device is either held to the outside of the neck, to the floor of the mouth, or placed intraorally. The quality of these voices is often, however, not satisfactory as it sounds very "robot-like" and monotone.

A popular method of voice restoration involves a shunt valve ("voice prosthesis") between trachea and pharyngoesophageal (PE) segment which establishes the tracheoesophageal (TE) substitute voice. The valve allows redirection of expiratory air into the PE segment for voicing. The source of the voice is the same as in the esophageal voice, but the shunt valve allows the affected persons to use the entire lung volume for voicing again. Furthermore, the time for learning to speak with a TE voice is much shorter. For over 90% of laryngectomized persons, the shunt valve means an immediate restoration of their voicing function, and 65% of the patients keep on using the TE voice permanently. All patients examined for this thesis were provided with a Provox® shunt valve which was developed at the Netherlands Cancer Institute in 1988.

There are several established subjective analysis methods for the quality of pathologic voices. However, different therapists might evaluate a given voice differently according to their experience (inter-rater discrepancy), and also one single rater might have a different opinion if he or she listens to a voice recording some time later again (intra-rater discrepancy). This is avoided by automatic methods. They are deterministic and objective, their result will not change on the same data, and they can serve as a reference independent from a particular human expert's career.

Established methods for objective evaluation, however, analyze only recordings of sustained vowels in order to find irregularities in the voice. This does not reflect a real communication situation. The examination of speech is more important for the patient's daily life. Since the automatic processing of completely free speech is very difficult, for this thesis the test persons read out a standard text. This text was then analyzed by methods of automatic speech recognition.

When an automatic method and the human evaluation have to be compared, then the degree of agreement among the human raters and between human and automatically computed results has to be determined. Besides Pearson's correlation coefficient r, other measures used in medical and social sciences were applied. Two sources of agreement have to be differentiated. The first one is the agreement that occurs by competence, i.e. the agreement that arises from the experience of the raters with the patients and their (speech) data. The other portion is a certain amount of equal ratings possible already by chance which is called the expected agreement. Therefore, an agreement measure is needed which allows to see the proportion of agreement by competence alone, and a kind of "chance correction" has to be done. Extensions of Cohen's κ, like κ_{DF} by Davies and Fleiss, can do this for an arbitrary number of raters and rating categories. Krippendorff's α is even able to cope with the problem of missing ratings in the data. Both measures were used for the comparison of human and machine ratings.

The speech data for the experiments in this thesis were taken from several speech corpora. In a speech therapy session, a patient should not be aware of the recording situation which might make him or her feel controlled. For this reason, one of the goals was the improvement of speech recognition results in reverberated environment. The experiments were not made with samples of pathologic speech because there were no speech corpora available that were large enough and recorded by distant-talking microphones. The EMBASSI corpus was used for preliminary tests on this topic. If a recognizer is supposed to work sufficiently in many environments, the training data should provide recordings that were made in a lot of different places. By reverberating close-talking speech artificially with pre-defined room impulse responses, this problem can be avoided. Selected results were verified using the Fatigue corpus and the VERBMOBIL corpus. For the recognizer training, the original close-talking signals were partially or entirely replaced by their artificially reverberated versions. The VERBMOBIL recognizers were evaluated on the original and the artificially reverberated VERBMOBIL test set, the Fatigue close-talking set, and the Fatigue distant recordings.

The VERBMOBIL corpus was also the recognizer training base for the analysis of substitute voices. The test data for these experiments were recordings of 41 TE speakers and also 18 elderly and 16 younger normal speakers as control groups. Each test person read out the German version of "The North Wind and the Sun" which is a standard text that includes all phonemes of the German language. It consists of 108 words and is used in speech therapy. A human evaluation reference for the TE speech data was obtained from 5 speech pathology experts. 11 criteria, like e.g. "intelligibility", "hoarseness", and "speech effort" were rated on 5-point Likert scales, i.e. one out of 5 named alternatives had to be chosen. The overall quality was rated on a visual analog scale with values between 0.0 and 10.0. Between some of the criteria, high agreement was observed, e.g. for intelligibility and the overall quality ($r = +0.96$). This indicates the importance of intelligibility for the overall perceptive impression of TE speech. Vocal tone ($r = +0.96$) and ability for prosody ($r = +0.88$) seem to be further important aspects for human listeners.

Different methods were tested in order to enhance the recognition results of reverberated test data. The first one was the application of artificially reverberated training data. It was assumed that the test environment is not known at training time. For this reason, 12 different room impulse responses were used to reverberate the close-talking training data of the baseline speech recognizer. The results showed that it is possible to process both close-talking and reverberated test data sufficiently when the training set is composed from close-talking recordings and artificially reverberated signals. On the Fatigue test set, the average word accuracy on clean and naturally reverberated signals rose from 68.2% on the close-talking recognizer to 76.8% on a recognizer where one half of the training set consisted of artificially reverberated material. All recognizers were HMM-based.

The second kind of changes to the baseline system concerned the feature extraction. The basic features for speech recognition were Mel-Frequency Cepstrum Coefficients (MFCC). However, the logarithmic compression of the filterbank coefficients may be disadvantageous on noisy data. Therefore, alternative features were tested. The root cepstrum replaces the logarithm by a root function, and the "μ-law features" use a companding function instead which raises low values and compresses high values. The root cepstrum did hardly perform as good as the standard MFCC, but some improvements on μ-law features were significant on the EMBASSI data. On the Fatigue test set, the average word accuracy on clean and naturally reverberated signals reached 77.2%. Although this is just slightly better than with MFCC, the μ-law features can be recommended for the recognition of distant-talking speech.

Normalizing the features to a Gaussian distribution was beneficial for some of the root cepstrum features, but in general the gain in word accuracy occurred not consistently enough in order to regard the procedure as reliable for other data.

The third approach did not change the recognizer but the test data. Since several synchronous recordings of the EMBASSI and Fatigue data were available, these signals were combined by delay-and-sum beamforming in order to create a new signal with less noise. Indeed, for the VERBMOBIL baseline recognizer (MFCC features), the word accuracy on the reverberated part of the Fatigue test set rose from 47.8% to 63.1%. Again, an artificially reverberated training set and μ-law features had a positive effect on the results. The best word accuracy achieved was 77.4% when all the training data were reverberated.

Taking all results into account, the following conclusion is drawn: For a recording scenario in a room with distributed microphones where the test environment is not known at training time, a recognizer should be trained with close-talking speech and artificially reverberated signals. It should apply beamforming as a preprocessing step and μ-law features instead of MFCC.

The speech recognizers for the experiments with TE speakers were derived from the baseline VERBMOBIL recognizer. They were trained with young, normal-speaking persons because there were not enough training data from elderly or laryngectomized speakers. It was also important that the system simulates a naïve listener, i.e. a human being that never heard TE speech before because this is the situation that the patients face in their daily life. For the recordings of the TE speakers, the average word accuracy on a polyphone-based recognizer was 36.9%. The more robust training of monophone models was supposed to have a positive effect on the recognition of substitute voices. However, this could not be observed. Although the automatic recognition yielded so bad results, the correlation to the human ratings was high. The reason is that the crucial measure is not the average of the recognition rate but its range. Intelligibility, vocal tone, quality and use of prosody during speaking showed the highest correlation to the word accuracy ($|r| \geq 0.7$). This confirms also the findings that these criteria correlate highly with each other in the human evaluation results. The correlation between the average rater and the word accuracy of the polyphone-based recognizer for the intelligibility criterion was $|r| = 0.88$.

For the improvement of the recognition, the acoustic models of the VERBMOBIL-based recognizer were also interpolated with TE speech recordings. However, no positive impact on the correlation between word accuracy and human ratings could be observed. For this reason, the time-consuming adaptation can be omitted.

The word accuracy is a very good measure for intelligibility. There are, however, evaluation criteria that cannot be expressed by the number of correctly understood or recognized words. In order to find appropriate automatic counterparts for them, a prosody module was applied. Prosodic features are obtained by analyzing silent pauses, filled pauses, the signal energy, word and syllable durations, and the fundamental frequency F_0. The analysis of prosodic features revealed measures that showed a high correlation to human rating criteria. TE speech is usually slower than normal speech, and the amount of voiced sections is strongly reduced. This affects many features measuring voice onset and offset, and also word and pause durations. These features show correlations of up to $|r| = 0.76$ to criteria like intelligibility, overall quality, speech effort, or the match of breath and sense units. The criterion "vocal tone" is reflected by energy measures. Due to the high irregularity of substitute voices, it is not easy to detect correct values of F_0. This might be the reason why F_0 features do not match the rating criteria very well.

When the word accuracy of the speech recognizers and the prosodic features were processed together by leave-one-speaker-out multi-correlation/regression analysis, the word accuracy was again determined as the measure that represents intelligibility best. However, in the Post-Laryngectomy Telephone Test (PLTT) which was developed in order to represent the communication situation via telephone, the correlation to the human PLTT result was better for the word recognition rate ($r \approx 0.9$, polyphone-based recognizer).

Since no distant-talking data from laryngectomees were available, the root cepstrum and the μ-law features were tested on artificially reverberated TE speech signals in order to simulate a therapy session where no headset is used. The μ-law features achieved consistently better recognition results and thus proofed to be an alternative to the classic MFCC approach also for pathologic speech.

For speech therapists, it might be very helpful to get a graphical visualization of pathologic speech. The Sammon mapping performs a topology-preserving reduction of data dimension. It minimizes a "stress function" between the topology of the low-dimensional Sammon map and the high-dimensional original data. The latter topology is defined by a distance measure between utterances or speakers. In a Sammon map of TE speakers and the normal-speaking control groups, all speaker groups were separated from each other. In a Sammon map of the TE speakers alone, the positions of the single speakers reached correlations of up to $r = 0.74$ to the word accuracy and $|r| \approx 0.7$ for rating criteria like intelligibility and vocal tone.

Despite the good results achieved in this thesis, there are some aspects that will have to be addressed in the future. A standard text does not represent a real communication situation, but it is a much closer approximation of fluent, spontaneous speech than a single, sustained vowel. It is a necessary compromise because the evaluation of completely free speech would require substantial changes in all components of the analysis framework. The problem of out-of-vocabulary (OOV) words was not examined yet because the number of reading errors was very small in the available recordings. For a future clinical application, however, the two types of error – by reading and by recognition – must be separated. Additionally, the evaluation results should be confirmed by a long-term study. The methods described in this thesis may not only be beneficial for patients after total laryngectomy. They will be revised and improved in a new research project about the evaluation of voice after partial laryngectomy.

Bibliography

[AH91]   T.H. Applebaum and B.A. Hanson. Regression features for recognition of speech in
           quiet and in noise. In *Proc. Int. Conf. on Acoustics, Speech, and Signal Processing
           (ICASSP)*, volume 2, pages 985–988, Toronto (Canada), 1991.

[AH96]   C. Avendano and H. Hermansky. Study on the Dereverberation of Speech Based on
           Temporal Envelope Filtering. In *Proc. Int. Conf. on Spoken Language Processing
           (ICSLP)*, volume 2, pages 889–892, Philadelphia, PA (USA), 1996.

[AHA$^+$93] A.H. Ackerstaff, F.J.M. Hilgers, N.K. Aaronson, A.J.M. Balm, and N. van Zand-
           wijk. Improvements in respiratory and psychosocial functioning following total
           laryngectomy by the use of a heat and moisture exchanger (HME). *Ann Otol Rhi-
           nol Laryngol*, 102(11):878–883, 1993.

[AHAB94]   A.H. Ackerstaff, F.J.M. Hilgers, N.K. Aaronson, and A.J.M. Balm. Communi-
           cation, functional disorders and lifestyle changes after total laryngectomy. *Clin
           Otolaryngol Allied Sci*, 19(4):295–300, 1994.

[AHE04]   M. Athineos, H. Hermansky, and D.P.W. Ellis. LP-TRAP: Linear Predictive Tem-
           poral Patterns. In *Proc. Int. Conf. on Spoken Language Processing (ICSLP)*, vol-
           ume II, pages 949–953, Jeju Island (Rep. of Korea), 2004.

[AHG$^+$98] M. Aretoulaki, S. Harbeck, F. Gallwitz, E. Nöth, H. Niemann, J. Ivanecký, I. Ipšić,
           N. Pavešić, and V. Matoušek. SQEL: A Multilingual and Multifunctional Dialogue
           System. In *Proc. Int. Conf. on Spoken Language Processing (ICSLP)*, volume 1,
           pages 1119–1122, Sydney (Australia), 1998.

[AHKA98]   C.J. van As, F.J.M. Hilgers, F.J. Koopmans-van Beinum, and A.H. Ackerstaff.
           The Influence of Stoma Occlusion on Aspects of Tracheoesophageal Voice. *Acta
           Otolaryngol (Stockh)*, 118(5):732–738, 1998.

[AHM$^+$99] A.H. Ackerstaff, F.J.M. Hilgers, C.A. Meeuwis, L.A. van der Velden, F.J.A. van
           den Hoogen, H.A.M. Marres, G.C.M. Vreeburg, and J.J. Manni. Multi-institutional
           assessment of the Provox® 2 voice prosthesis. *Arch Otolaryngol Head Neck Surg*,
           125(2):167–173, 1999.

[AKPH03]   C.J. van As, F.J. Koopmans-van Beinum, L.C. Pols, and F.J.M. Hilgers. Perceptual
           evaluation of tracheoesophageal speech by naive and experienced judges through
           the use of semantic differential scales. *J Speech Lang Hear Res*, 46(4):947–959,
           2003.

[AL93]   P. Alexandre and P. Lockwood. Root cepstral analysis: A unified view. Appli-
            cation to speech processing in car noise environments. *Speech Communication*,
            12(3):277–288, 1993.

[ALB⁺99]   S.W. Anderson, N. Liberman, E. Bernstein, S. Foster, E. Cate, B. Levin, and
            R. Hudson. Recognition of elderly speech and voice-driven document retrieval. In
            Proc. Int. Conf. on Acoustics, Speech, and Signal Processing (ICASSP), volume 1,
            pages 145–148, Phoenix, AZ (USA), 1999.

[Alt91]   D.G. Altman. *Practical Statistics for Medical Research*. Chapman & Hall / CRC,
            London (England), 1991.

[Ars72]   M. Arslan. Reconstructive laryngectomy. Report on the first 35 cases. *Ann Otol*,
            81(4):479–487, 1972.

[AS67]   B.S. Atal and M.R. Schroeder. Predictive Coding of Speech Signals. In *Proc. IEEE
            Conf. on Communication and Processing*, pages 360–361, 1967.

[AS92]   W.A. Ainsworth and W. Singh. Perceptual Comparison of Neoglottal, Oesophageal
            and Normal Speech. *Folia Phoniatr (Basel)*, 44(6):297–307, 1992.

[Asa65]   R. Asai. Asai's new voice production method: substitution for human speech. In
            Proc. Int. Ear Nose Throat Conference, pages 730–735, Tokyo (Japan), 1965.

[ATH97]   C. Avendano, S. Tibrewala, and H. Hermansky. Multiresolution Channel Nor-
            malization for ASR in Reverberant Environments. In *Proc. European Conf. on
            Speech Communication and Technology (Eurospeech)*, volume 3, pages 1107–
            1110, Rhodes (Greece), 1997.

[BAG⁺97]   M. Boros, M. Aretoulaki, F. Gallwitz, H. Niemann, and E. Nöth. Semantic Process-
            ing of Out-of-Vocabulary Words in a Spoken Dialogue System. In *Proc. European
            Conf. on Speech Communication and Technology (Eurospeech)*, volume 4, pages
            1887–1890, Rhodes (Greece), 1997.

[Bak75]   J.K. Baker. The DRAGON System – an overview. *IEEE Trans. on Acoustics,
            Speech, and Signal Processing (ASSP)*, 23(1):24–29, 1975.

[BAK04]   H. Buchner, R. Aichner, and W. Kellermann. TRINICON: A Versatile Framework
            for Multichannel Blind Signal Processing. In *Proc. Int. Conf. on Acoustics, Speech,
            and Signal Processing (ICASSP)*, volume 3, pages 889–892, Montreal (Canada),
            2004.

[Bar01]   K. Barth. *Funktionelle postoperative Befunde bei Patienten mit oropharyn-
            gealen Tumoren*. PhD thesis, Medizinische Fakultät Charité der Humboldt-
            Universität zu Berlin, 2001. http://edoc.hu-berlin.de/dissertationen/barth-klaus-
            2001-01-26/HTML/barth.html, last visited May 30, 2007.

[BAS]   Bavarian Archive for Speech Signals (BAS).   http://www.phonetik.uni-
            muenchen.de/Bas/BasHomeeng.html; last visited May 30, 2007.

[Bau03]   S.R. Baum. Age differences in the influence of metrical structure on phonetic identification. *Speech Communication*, 39(3–4):231–242, 2003.

[BBH⁺99]   A. Batliner, J. Buckow, R. Huber, V. Warnke, E. Nöth, and H. Niemann. Prosodic Feature Evaluation: Brute Force or Well Designed? In *Proc. Int. Congress of Phonetic Sciences (ICPhS)*, volume 3, pages 2315–2318, San Francisco, CA (USA), 1999.

[BBH⁺01]   A. Batliner, J. Buckow, R. Huber, V. Warnke, E. Nöth, and H. Niemann. Boiling down Prosody for the Classification of Boundaries and Accents in German and English. In *Proc. European Conf. on Speech Communication and Technology (Eurospeech)*, volume 4, pages 2781–2784, Aalborg (Denmark), 2001.

[BBN⁺00]   A. Batliner, J. Buckow, H. Niemann, E. Nöth, and V. Warnke. The Prosody Module. In Wahlster [Wah00], pages 106–121.

[Ber58]   J. van den Berg. Myoelastic-Aerodynamic Theory of Voice Production. *J Speech Hear Res*, 1(3):227–244, 1958.

[BFH⁺00]   A. Batliner, K. Fischer, R. Huber, J. Spilker, and E. Nöth. Desperately Seeking Emotions: Actors, Wizards, and Human Beings. In R. Cowie, E. Douglas-Cowie, and M. Schröder, editors, *Proc. ISCA Workshop on Speech and Emotion: A Conceptual Framework for Research*, pages 195–200, Newcastle (Northern Ireland), 2000.

[BFH⁺03]   A. Batliner, K. Fischer, R. Huber, J. Spilker, and E. Nöth. How to Find Trouble in Communication. *Speech Communication*, 40(1–2):117–143, 2003.

[BHIB03]   D.H. Brown, F.J.M. Hilgers, J.C. Irish, and A.J.M. Balm. Postlaryngectomy Voice Rehabilitation: State of the Art at the Millennium. *World J Surg*, 27(7):824–831, 2003.

[BHJ93]   P.C. Bagshaw, S.M. Hiller, and M.A. Jack. Enhanced Pitch Tracking and the Processing of F0 Contours for Computer Aided Intonation Teaching. In *Proc. European Conf. on Speech Communication and Technology (Eurospeech)*, volume 2, pages 1003–1006, Berlin (Germany), 1993.

[BHM96]   H. Bourlard, H. Hermansky, and N. Morgan. Towards increasing speech recognition error rates. *Speech Communication*, 18(3):205–231, 1996.

[BHW⁺98]   M. Boros, J. Haas, V. Warnke, E. Nöth, and H. Niemann. How Statistics and Prosody can guide a Chunky Parser. In *Proc. of the AIII Workshop on Artificial Intelligence in Industry*, pages 388–398, Stará Lesná (Slovakia), 1998.

[BJKN92]   A. Batliner, B. Johne, A. Kießling, and E. Nöth. Zur prosodischen Kennzeichnung von spontaner und gelesener Sprache. In G. Görz, editor, *KONVENS 92*, Informatik aktuell, pages 29–38. Springer, New York, Berlin, 1992.

[BKG⁺96]   S. Bielamowicz, J. Kreiman, B.R. Gerratt, M.S. Dauer, and G.S. Berke. Comparison of voice analysis systems for perturbation measurement. *J Speech Hear Res*, 39(1):126–134, 1996.

[BKK+98] A. Batliner, R. Kompe, A. Kießling, M. Mast, H. Niemann, and E. Nöth. M = Syntax + Prosody: A syntactic-prosodic labelling scheme for large spontaneous speech databases. *Speech Communication*, 25(4):193–222, 1998.

[Bla95]   E. Blaauw. *On the Perceptual Classification of Spontaneous and Read Speech*. PhD thesis, Research Institute for Language and Speech, Faculty of Humanities, Utrecht University, Utrecht (The Netherlands), 1995.

[BLG01]   M.H. Bellandese, J.W. Lerman, and H.R. Gilbert. An Acoustic Analysis of Excellent Female Esophageal, Tracheoesophageal, and Laryngeal Speakers. *J Speech Lang Hear Res*, 44(6):1315–1320, 2001.

[Blo84]   G.W. Blood. Fundamental Frequency and Intensity Measurements in Laryngeal and Alaryngeal Speakers. *J Commun Disord*, 17(5):319–324, 1984.

[Blo95]   E.D. Blom. Tracheoesophageal speech. *Semin Speech Lang*, 16(3):191–204, 1995.

[Blo00]   E.D. Blom. Tracheoesophageal voice restoration: origin – evolution – state-of-the-art. *Folia Phoniatr Logop*, 52(1–3):14–23, 2000.

[BMD58]   J. van den Berg, A.J. Moolenaar-Bijl, and P.H. Damsté. Oesophageal Speech. *Folia Phoniatr (Basel)*, 10(2):65–84, 1958.

[Bor01]   M. Boros. *Partielles robustes Parsing spontansprachlicher Dialoge am Beispiel von Zugauskunftdialogen*, volume 2 of *Studien zur Mustererkennung*. Logos Verlag, Berlin (Germany), 2001.

[BP83]   T.W. Baggs and S.J. Pine. Acoustic Characteristics: Tracheoesophageal Speech. *J Commun Disord*, 16(4):299–307, 1983.

[BPC91]   N.R. Bleach, A.R. Perry, and A.D. Cheesman. Surgical voice restoration with the Blom-Singer prosthesis following laryngopharyngoesophagectomy and pharyngogastric anastomosis. *Ann Otol Rhinol Laryngol*, 100(2):142–147, 1991.

[BPG95]   R.H. Baayen, R. Piepenbrock, and L. Gulikers. The CELEX Lexical Database (Release 2). Linguistic Data Consortium, Philadelphia, PA (USA), 1995.

[BPH95]   E.D. Blom, B.R. Pauloski, and R.C. Hamaker. Functional Outcome after Surgery for Prevention of Pharyngospasms in Tracheoesophageal Speakers. Part I: Speech Characteristics. *Laryngoscope*, 105(10):1093–1103, 1995.

[BPSW70] L.E. Baum, T. Petrie, G. Soules, and N. Weiss. A maximization technique occurring in the statistical analysis of probabilistic functions of Markov chains. *Ann Math Statist*, 41(1):164–171, 1970.

[Bra84]   R.N. Bracewell. The fast Hartley transform. *Proc. IEEE*, 72(8):1010–1018, 1984.

[BSC92]   H.G. Beniers and H.J. Schultz-Coulon. Langzeitergebnisse der stimmlichen Sofortrehabilitation nach Laryngektomie. *Eur Arch Otorhinolaryngol Suppl II*, pages 183–184, 1992.

[BSH82]   E.D. Blom, M.I. Singer, and R.C. Hamaker. Tracheostoma valve for postlaryngec-
            tomy voice rehabilitation. *Ann Otol Rhinol Laryngol*, 91(6 Pt 1):576–578, 1982.

[BSH86]   E.D. Blom, M.I. Singer, and R.C. Hamaker. A prospective study of Tracheoeso-
            phageal Speech. *Arch Otolaryngol Head Neck Surg*, 112(4):440–447, 1986.

[BSH+06]   M. Bellanova, M. Schuster, T. Haderlein, E. Nöth, U. Eysholdt, and F. Rosanowski.
            Die tracheoösophageale Ersatzstimme: Evaluation durch Experten, naive Hörer
            und automatische Spracherkennung. In M. Gross and E. Kruse, editors, *Ak-
            tuelle phoniatrisch-pädaudiologische Aspekte 2006*, pages 48–50, Norderstedt
            (Germany), 2006. Book on Demand GmbH.

[Bud00]   E.H. Buder. Acoustic Analysis of Voice Quality: A Tabulation of Algorithms
            1902–1990. In R.D. Kent and M.J. Ball, editors, *Voice Quality Measurement*, chap-
            ter 9, pages 119–244. Singular Publishing Group, San Diego, CA (USA), 2000.

[Bul95]   M. Bullinger. German translation and psychometric testing of the SF-36® Health
            Survey: Preliminary results from the IQOLA project. *Soc Sci Med*, 41(10):1359–
            1366, 1995.

[BYY+01]   A. Baba, S. Yoshizawa, M. Yamada, A. Lee, and K. Shikano. Elderly Acous-
            tic Model for Large Vocabulary Speech Recognition. In *Proc. European Conf.
            on Speech Communication and Technology (Eurospeech)*, volume 3, pages 1657–
            1660, Aalborg (Denmark), 2001.

[CAP58]   J.J. Conley, F. de Amesti, and M.K. Pierce. A new surgical technique for the
            vocal rehabilitation of the laryngectomized patient. *Ann Otol Rhinol Laryngol*,
            67(3):655–664, 1958.

[CC83]   J. Cohen and P. Cohen. *Applied Multiple Regression/Correlation Analysis for the
            Behavioral Sciences*. Lawrence Erlbaum Associates, Hillsdale, NJ (USA), 2nd edi-
            tion, 1983.

[CC00]   L. Couvreur and C. Couvreur. On the Use of Artificial Reverberation for ASR in
            Highly Reverberant Environments. In *Proc. of 2nd IEEE Benelux Signal Process-
            ing Symposium (SPS-2000)*, Hilvarenbeek (The Netherlands), 2000.

[CCR00]   L. Couvreur, C. Couvreur, and C. Ris. A Corpus-Based Approach for Robust ASR
            in Reverberant Environments. In *Proc. Int. Conf. on Spoken Language Processing
            (ICSLP)*, volume 1, pages 397–400, Beijing (China), 2000.

[CDJ+98]   K. Claßen, G. Dogil, M. Jessen, K. Marasek, and W. Wokurek. Stimmqualität und
            Wortbetonung im Deutschen. *Linguistische Berichte*, 174:202–245, 1998.

[CF90]   D.V. Cicchetti and A.R. Feinstein. High agreement but low kappa: II. Resolving
            the paradoxes. *J Clin Epidemiol*, 43(6):551–558, 1990.

[CFM92]   J.M. Christensen, S.G. Fletcher, and M.J. McCutcheon. Esophageal speaker articu-
            lation of /s,z/: a dynamic palatometric assessment. *J Commun Disord*, 25(1):65–76,
            1992.

[CG00]   R.A. Cummins and E. Gullone. Why we should not use 5-point Likert scales: The case for subjective quality of life measurement. In *Proc. Second International Conference on Quality of Life in Cities*, volume 1, pages 74–93, Singapore, 2000. National University of Singapore.

[Cic76]   D.V. Cicchetti. Assessing inter-rater reliability for rating scales: Resolving some basic issues. *British Journal of Psychiatry*, 129(5):452–456, 1976.

[Cla85]   J.G. Clark. Alaryngeal speech intelligibility and the older listener. *J Speech Hear Disord*, 50(1):60–65, 1985.

[CLL03]   K.F. Chow, S.C. Liew, and K.T. Lua. Thin client front-end processor for distributed speech recognition. In *Proc. Int. Conf. on Acoustics, Speech, and Signal Processing (ICASSP)*, volume II, pages 29–32, Hong Kong, 2003.

[CMG01]   T. Cervera, J.L. Miralles, and J. González-Àlvarez. Acoustical Analysis of Spanish Vowels Produced by Laryngectomized Subjects. *J Speech Lang Hear Res*, 44(5):988–996, 2001.

[Coh60]   J. Cohen. A Coefficient of Agreement for Nominal Scales. *Educational and Psychological Measurement*, XX(1):37–46, 1960.

[Coh88]   J. Cohen. *Statistical Power Analysis for the Behavioral Sciences*. Lawrence Erlbaum Associates, Hillsdale, NJ (USA), 2nd edition, 1988.

[Cre01]   P.E. Crewson. A Correction for Unbalanced Kappa Tables. In *Proc. Twenty-Sixth Annual SAS® Users Group International Conference*, Cary, NC (USA), 2001. SAS Institute Inc. Paper 194-26, http://www2.sas.com/proceedings/sugi26/p194-26.pdf, last visited May 30, 2007.

[Cro51]   L.J. Cronbach. Coefficient alpha and the internal structure of tests. *Psychometrika*, 16(3):297–334, 1951.

[CW76]   J.M. Christensen and B. Weinberg. Vowel duration characteristics of esophageal speech. *J Speech Hear Res*, 19(4):678–689, 1976.

[CZM04]   B. Chen, Q. Zhu, and N. Morgan. Learning Long-Term Temporal Features in LVCSR Using Neural Networks. In *Proc. Int. Conf. on Spoken Language Processing (ICSLP)*, volume II, pages 925–928, Jeju Island (Rep. of Korea), 2004.

[DBC+01]   P.H. Dejonckere, P. Bradley, P. Clemente, G. Cornut, L. Crevier-Buchman, G. Friedrich, P. van de Heyning, M. Remacle, V. Woisard, and The Committee on Phoniatrics of the European Laryngological Society (ELS). A basic protocol for functional assessment of voice pathology, especially for investigating the efficacy of (phonosurgical) treatments and evaluating new assessment techniques. Guideline elaborated by the Committee on Phoniatrics of the European Laryngological Society (ELS). *Eur Arch Otorhinolaryngol*, 258(2):77–82, 2001.

[DDRS98]   D.G. Deschler, E.T. Doherty, C.G. Reed, and M.I. Singer. Quantitative and qualitative analysis of tracheoesophageal voice after pectoralis major flap reconstruction of the neopharynx. *Otolaryngol Head Neck Surg*, 118(6):771–776, 1998.

[DDWU94] F. Debruyne, P. Delaere, J. Wouters, and P. Uwents. Acoustic analysis of tracheo-esophageal speech. *J Laryngol Otol*, 108(4):325–328, 1994.

[DF82] M. Davies and J.L. Fleiss. Measuring agreement for multinomial data. *Biometrics*, 38(4):1047–1051, 1982.

[DGM03] L. Docio-Fernandez, D. Gelbart, and N. Morgan. Far-Field ASR on Inexpensive Microphones. In *Proc. European Conf. on Speech Communication and Technology (Eurospeech)*, volume 3, pages 2141–2144, Geneva (Switzerland), 2003.

[DHH+02] M. Döllinger, U. Hoppe, F. Hettlich, J. Lohscheller, S. Schuberth, and U. Eysholdt. Vibration parameter extraction from endoscopic image series of the vocal folds. *IEEE Trans. on Biomedical Engineering*, 49(8):773–781, 2002.

[Die68] W.M. Diedrich. The mechanism of esophageal speech. *Annals of the New York Academy of Science*, 155:303–317, 1968.

[Dim89] S. Dimolitsas. Objective speech distortion measures and their relevance to speech quality assessments. *Communications, Speech and Vision; IEE Proceedings I*, 136, Pt. I(5):317–324, 1989.

[DIN00] *DIN EN ISO 3382: Messung der Nachhallzeit von Räumen mit Hinweisen auf andere raumakustische Parameter*. Beuth Verlag, Berlin (Germany), 2000.

[DM80] S.B. Davis and P. Mermelstein. Comparison of Parametric Representation for Monosyllabic Word Recognition in Continuously Spoken Sentences. *IEEE Trans. on Acoustics, Speech, and Signal Processing (ASSP)*, 28(4):357–366, 1980.

[Döl02] M. Döllinger. *Parameter Estimation of Vocal Fold Dynamics by Inversion of a Biomechanical Model*, volume 10 of *Berichte aus Phoniatrie und Pädaudiologie*. Shaker Verlag, Aachen (Germany), 2002.

[DRF+96] P.H. Dejonckere, M. Remacle, E. Fresnel-Elbaz, V. Woisard, L. Crevier-Buchman, and B. Millet. Differentiated perceptual evaluation of pathological voice quality: reliability and correlations with acoustic measurement. *Revue de Laryngologie - Otologie - Rhinologie*, 117(3):219–224, 1996.

[DSK94] G.M. Devins, H.J. Stam, and J.P. Koopmans. Psychosocial impact of laryngectomy mediated by perceived stigma and illness intrusiveness. *Canadian Journal of Psychiatry*, 39(10):608–616, 1994.

[Dun92] G. Dunn. *Design and Analysis of Reliability Studies: Statistical Evaluation of Measurement Errors*. Edward Arnold, London (England), 1992.

[DY66] W.M. Diedrich and K.A. Youngstorm. *Alaryngeal speech*. Charles C. Thomas, Springfield, IL (USA), 1966.

[EB01] M. Eskenazi and A.W. Black. A Study on Speech Over Telephone and Aging. In *Proc. European Conf. on Speech Communication and Technology (Eurospeech)*, volume 1, pages 171–174, Aalborg (Denmark), 2001.

[Eck96]   W. Eckert. *Gesprochener Mensch-Maschine-Dialog*. Berichte aus der Informatik. Shaker Verlag, Aachen (Germany), 1996.

[ESVB01]   S.E. Eerenstein, P.F. Schouwenburg, L.A. van der Velden, and M.F. de Boer. First results of the VoiceMaster prosthesis in three centres in the Netherlands. *Clin Otolaryngol Allied Sci*, 26(2):99–103, 2001.

[EWP⁺85]   K. Ehrenberger, W. Wicke, H. Piza, R. Roka, M. Grasl, and H. Swoboda. Jejunal grafts for reconstructing a phonatory neoglottis in laryngectomized patients. *Arch Otorhinolaryngol*, 242(2):217–223, 1985.

[Fai44]   G. Fairbanks. *Practical voice practice*. Harper & Brothers, New York, NY (USA), 1944.

[Fai60]   G. Fairbanks. *Voice and articulation drillbook*. Harper, New York, NY (USA), 2nd edition, 1960.

[FBMP96]   J.M. Festen, J.H.M. van Beek, H.F. Mahieu, and A.J. Parker. Acoustic analysis of tracheoesophageal voice. In J. Algaba, editor, *Surgery and Prosthetic Voice Restoration after Total and Subtotal Laryngectomy*, pages 171–175. Elsevier Science, Amsterdam (The Netherlands), 1996.

[FC90]   A.R. Feinstein and D.V. Cicchetti. High agreement but low kappa: I. The problems of two paradoxes. *J Clin Epidemiol*, 43(6):543–549, 1990.

[FCE69]   J.L. Fleiss, J. Cohen, and B.S. Everitt. Large sample standard errors of kappa and weighted kappa. *Psychological Bulletin*, 72(5):323–327, 1969.

[Fei85]   A.R. Feinstein. A bibliography of publications on observer variability. *J Chronic Dis*, 38(8):619–632, 1985.

[Fer02]   C.T. Ferrand. Harmonics-to-noise ratio: An index of vocal aging. *J Voice*, 16(4):480–487, 2002.

[Fle71]   J.L. Fleiss. Measuring Nominal Scale Agreement Among Many Raters. *Psychological Bulletin*, 76(5):378–382, 1971.

[Fle81]   J.L. Fleiss. *Statistical Methods for Rates and Proportions*. John Wiley & Sons, New York, NY (USA), 2nd edition, 1981.

[FLL85]   G. Fant, J. Liljencrants, and Q. Lin. A four-parameter model of glottal flow. *STL-QPSR (KTH, Stockholm)*, 26(4):1–13, 1985.

[FMSK00]   M. Fröhlich, D. Michaelis, H.-W. Strube, and E. Kruse. Acoustic voice analysis by means of the hoarseness diagram. *J Speech Lang Hear Res*, 43(3):706–720, 2000.

[For73]   G.D. Forney. The Viterbi Algorithm. *Proc. IEEE*, 61(3):268–278, 1973.

[FPB⁺05]   C. Fredouille, G. Pouchoulin, J.-F. Bonastre, M. Azzarello, A. Giovanni, and A. Ghio. Application of Automatic Speaker Recognition techniques to pathological voice assessment (dysphonia). In *Proc. Interspeech*, pages 149–153, Lisbon (Portugal), 2005.

[Fre23]   M. Freyd. The graphic rating scale. *Journal of Educational Psychology*, 14:83–102, 1923.

[Fro72]   O.L. Frost III. An algorithm for linearly constrained adaptive array processing. *Proc. IEEE*, 60(8):926–935, 1972.

[Fur81]   S. Furui. Cepstral Analysis Technique for Automatic Speaker Verification. *IEEE Trans. on Acoustics, Speech, and Signal Processing (ASSP)*, 29(2):254–272, 1981.

[Fur86]   S. Furui. Speaker-Independent Isolated Word Recognition Using Dynamic Features of Speech Spectrum. *IEEE Trans. on Acoustics, Speech, and Signal Processing (ASSP)*, ASSP-34(1):52–59, 1986.

[GAB+98] F. Gallwitz, M. Aretoulaki, M. Boros, J. Haas, S. Harbeck, R. Huber, H. Niemann, and E. Nöth. The Erlangen Spoken Dialogue System EVAR: A State-of-the-Art Information Retrieval System. In *Proceedings of 1998 International Symposium on Spoken Dialogue (ISSD-98)*, pages 19–26, Sydney (Australia), 1998.

[Gal02]   F. Gallwitz. *Integrated Stochastic Models for Spontaneous Speech Recognition*, volume 6 of *Studien zur Mustererkennung*. Logos Verlag, Berlin (Germany), 2002.

[Gal03]   L. Galescu. Recognition of Out-of-Vocabulary Words with Sub-Lexical Language Models. In *Proc. European Conf. on Speech Communication and Technology (Eurospeech)*, volume 1, pages 249–252, Geneva (Switzerland), 2003.

[GBB+97] W. Grolman, E.D. Blom, R. Branson, P.F. Schouwenburg, and R.C. Hamaker. An Efficiency Comparison of Four Heat and Moisture Exchangers Used in the Laryngectomized Patient. *Laryngoscope*, 107(6):814–820, 1997.

[GFV+05] C.D.L. van Gogh, J.M. Festen, I.M. Verdonck-de Leeuw, A.J. Parker, L. Traissac, A.D. Cheesman, and H.F. Mahieu. Acoustical analysis of tracheoesophageal voice. *Speech Communication*, 47(1–2):160–168, 2005.

[GHSS05] L. Gu, J. Harris, R. Shrivastav, and C. Sapienza. Disordered Speech Evaluation Using Objective Quality Measures. In *Proc. Int. Conf. on Acoustics, Speech, and Signal Processing (ICASSP)*, volume I, pages 321–324, Philadelphia, PA (USA), 2005.

[GJ82]   L.J. Griffiths and C.W. Jim. An Alternative Approach to Linearly Constrained Adaptive Beamforming. *IEEE Trans. on Antennas and Propagation*, AP-30(1):27–34, 1982.

[GK97]   S. Greenberg and B.E.D. Kingsbury. The Modulation Spectrogram: In Pursuit of an Invariant Representation of Speech. In *Proc. Int. Conf. on Acoustics, Speech, and Signal Processing (ICASSP)*, volume 2, pages 1647–1650, Munich (Germany), 1997.

[GK03]   H. Gölzer and M. Kleinschmidt. Importance of early and late reflections for automatic speech recognition in reverberant environments. In *Proc. Elektronische Sprachsignalverarbeitung (ESSV)*, pages 98–105, Karlsruhe (Germany), 2003.

[GL94]   J.-L. Gauvain and C.-H. Lee. Maximum a-posteriori estimation for multivariate
            Gaussian mixture observations of Markov chains. *IEEE Trans. on Speech and
            Audio Processing*, 2(2):291–298, 1994.

[GM98]   D. Giuliani and R. de Mori. Speaker adaptation. In R. de Mori, editor, *Spoken
            Dialogues with Computers*, pages 363–404. Academic Press, London (England),
            1998.

[GM02]   D. Gelbart and N. Morgan. Double the Trouble: Handling Noise and Reverber-
            ation in Far-Field Automatic Speech Recognition. In *Proc. Int. Conf. on Spoken
            Language Processing (ICSLP)*, volume 3, pages 2185–2188, Denver, CO (USA),
            2002.

[GNN96]   F. Gallwitz, E. Nöth, and H. Niemann. A Category Based Approach for Recog-
            nition of Out-of-Vocabulary Words. In *Proc. Int. Conf. on Spoken Language Pro-
            cessing (ICSLP)*, volume 1, pages 228–231, Philadelphia, PA (USA), 1996.

[GNNW02]   F. Gallwitz, H. Niemann, E. Nöth, and V. Warnke. Integrated Recognition of Words
            and Prosodic Phrase Boundaries. *Speech Communication*, 36(1–2):81–95, 2002.

[Gol01]   E.B. Goldstein. *Sensation and Perception*. Wadsworth Publishing Company, Bel-
            mont, CA (USA), 6th edition, 2001.

[Gol02]   E.B. Goldstein. *Wahrnehmungspsychologie: Eine Einführung*. Spektrum Aka-
            demischer Verlag, Heidelberg (Germany), 2nd edition, 2002. German edition of
            Sensation and Perception.

[Gon95]   Y. Gong. Speech recognition in noisy environments: A survey. *Speech Communi-
            cation*, 16(3):261–291, 1995.

[GRS+05]   J. Guinness, B. Raj, B. Schmidt-Nielsen, L. Turicchia, and R. Sarpeshkar. A Com-
            panding Front End for Noise-Robust Automatic Speech Recognition. In *Proc. Int.
            Conf. on Acoustics, Speech, and Signal Processing (ICASSP)*, volume 1, pages
            249–253, Philadelphia, PA (USA), 2005.

[GS79]   S.A. Gelfand and S. Silman. Effects of small room reverberation upon the recog-
            nition of some consonant features. *J Acoust Soc Am*, 66(1):22–29, 1979.

[GSN96]   F. Gallwitz, E.G. Schukat-Talamazzini, and H. Niemann. Integrating Large Context
            Language Models into a Real Time Word Recognizer. In N. Pavešić and H. Nie-
            mann, editors, *3rd Slovenian-German and 2nd SDRV Workshop*, pages 105–114.
            Faculty of Electrical and Computer Engineering, University of Ljubljana (Slove-
            nia), 1996.

[GSO+06]   J.I. Godino-Llorente, N. Sáenz-Lechón, V. Osma-Ruiz, S. Aguilera-Navarro, and
            P. Gómez-Vilda. An integrated tool for the diagnosis of voice disorders. *Med Eng
            Phys*, 28(3):276–289, 2006.

[Gus74]   C. Gussenbauer. Ueber die erste durch Th. Billroth am Menschen ausgeführte
            Kehlkopf-Exstirpation und die Anwendung eines künstlichen Kehlkopfes. *Archiv
            für klinische Chirurgie*, 17:343–356, 1874.

[Gut09]   H. Gutzmann. Stimme und Sprache ohne Kehlkopf. *Zeitschrift für Laryngologie, Rhinologie und ihre Grenzgebiete*, 1:221–242, 1909.

[Gut32]   M.R. Guttman. Rehabilitation of the voice in laryngectomized patients. *Arch Otolaryngol*, 15(3):478–479, 1932.

[Gut35]   M.R. Guttman. Tracheopharyngeal fistulization: a new procedure in the laryngectomized patient. *Trans Am Laryngol Rhinol Otol Soc*, 41:219–226, 1935.

[GW83]   J. Gandour and B. Weinberg. Perception of Intonational Contrasts in Alaryngeal Speech. *J Speech Hear Res*, 26(1):142–148, 1983.

[Gwe02]   K. Gwet. Kappa Statistic is not Satisfactory for Assessing the Extent of Agreement Between Raters. *Statistical Methods For Inter-Rater Reliability Assessment*, No. 1:1–6, 2002. STATAXIS Consulting, Gaithersburg, MD (USA).

[HA90]   B.A. Hanson and T.H. Applebaum. Robust speaker-independent word recognition using static, dynamic and acceleration features. In *Proc. Int. Conf. on Acoustics, Speech, and Signal Processing (ICASSP)*, volume 2, pages 857–860, Albuquerque, NM (USA), 1990.

[HAA+90]   F.J.M. Hilgers, A.H. Ackerstaff, N.K. Aaronson, P.F. Schouwenburg, and N. van Zandwijk. Physical and psychosocial consequences of total laryngectomy. *Clin Otolaryngol*, 15(5):421–425, 1990.

[Haa01]   J. Haas. *Probabilistic Methods in Linguistic Analysis*, volume 1 of *Studien zur Mustererkennung*. Logos Verlag, Berlin (Germany), 2001.

[HAA+03]   F.J.M. Hilgers, A.H. Ackerstaff, C.J. van As, A.J.M. Balm, M.W. van den Brekel, and I.B. Tan. Development and clinical assessment of a heat and moisture exchanger with a multi-magnet automatic tracheostoma valve (Provox® FreeHands HME) for vocal and pulmonary rehabilitation after total laryngectomy. *Acta Otolaryngol*, 123(1):91–99, 2003.

[HAB+97]   F.J.M. Hilgers, A.H. Ackerstaff, A.J.M. Balm, I.B. Tan, N.K. Aaronson, and J.O. Persson. Development and clinical evaluation of a second generation voice prosthesis (Provox® 2) designed for anterograde and retrograde insertion. *Acta Otolaryngol*, 117(6):889–896, 1997.

[HABG96]   F.J.M. Hilgers, A.H. Ackerstaff, A.J.M. Balm, and R.T. Gregor. A new heat and moisture exchanger with speech valve (Provox® stomafilter). *Clin Otolaryngol*, 21(5):414–418, 1996.

[Hac01]   C. Hacker. Optimierung der Merkmalberechnung für die automatische Spracherkennung. Student's thesis, Lehrstuhl für Mustererkennung (Chair for Pattern Recognition), Universität Erlangen–Nürnberg, Erlangen (Germany), 2001.

[Had02]   T. Haderlein. Using the ISADORA System for Analyzing Fatigue Symptoms and Robustness of Features against Reverberation. Technical report, Chair of Multimedia Communications and Signal Processing, Universität Erlangen–Nürnberg, Erlangen (Germany), 2002.

[Hag90a]   R. Hagen. Stimmrehabilitation nach totaler Laryngektomie in der Bundesrepublik
            Deutschland. *HNO*, 38(11):417–420, 1990.

[Hag90b]   R. Hagen. Stimmrehabilitation nach totaler Laryngektomie: Mikrovaskuläre La-
            rynxersatzplastik (Laryngoplastik) statt Stimmprothese. *Laryngo-Rhino-Otologie*,
            69(4):213–216, 1990.

[Hag97]   R. Hagen. Operative Verfahren zur Wiederherstellung des Sprechvermögens nach
            totaler Laryngektomie. *Sprache - Stimme - Gehör*, 21(1):7–12, 1997.

[Hah57]   K.H. Hahlbrock. *Sprachaudiometrie*. Georg Thieme Verlag, Stuttgart (Germany),
            1957.

[Hal04]   B. Halberstam. Acoustic and Perceptual Parameters Relating to Connected Speech
            Are More Reliable Measures of Hoarseness than Parameters Relating to Sustained
            Vowels. *ORL - Journal for Oto-Rhino-Laryngology and Its Related Specialties*,
            66(2):70–73, 2004.

[Hay01]   S. Haykin. *Adaptive Filter Theory*. Prentice-Hall, Englewood Cliffs, NJ (USA),
            4th edition, 2001.

[HB93]   F.J.M. Hilgers and A.J.M. Balm. Long-term results of vocal rehabilitation after
            total laryngectomy with the low-resistance, indwelling Provox™ voice prosthesis
            system. *Clin Otolaryngol*, 18(6):517–523, 1993.

[HC99]   H.M. Hanson and E.S. Chuang. Glottal characteristics of male speakers: acoustic
            correlates and comparison with female data. *J Acoust Soc Am*, 106(2):1064–1077,
            1999.

[HCB93]   F.J.M. Hilgers, M.W. Cornelissen, and A.J.M. Balm. Aerodynamic characteristics
            of the Provox® low-resistance indwelling voice prosthesis. *Eur Arch Otorhino-
            laryngol*, 250(7):375–378, 1993.

[HCK01]   F.S. Hodge, R.H. Colton, and R.T. Kelley. Vocal intensity characteristics in normal
            and elderly speakers. *J Voice*, 15(4):503–511, 2001.

[Her86]   I.F. Herrmann. *Speech restoration via voice prosthesis*. Springer, Berlin, Heidel-
            berg, New York, 1986.

[Her90]   H. Hermansky. Perceptual Linear Predictive (PLP) Analysis of Speech. *J Acoust
            Soc Am*, 87(4):1738–1752, 1990.

[Her97]   J. Hernando. Maximum likelihood weighting of dynamic speech features for
            CDHMM speech recognition. In *Proc. Int. Conf. on Acoustics, Speech, and Signal
            Processing (ICASSP)*, volume 2, pages 1267–1270, Munich (Germany), 1997.

[Her05]   W. Herbordt. *Sound Capture for Human/Machine Interfaces. Practical Aspects of
            Microphone Array Signal Processing*. Springer, Berlin (Germany), 2005.

[HG90]   M.A. Hughes and D.E. Garrett. Intercoder Reliability Estimation – Approaches in
           Marketing: A Generalizability Theory Framework for Quantitative Data. *Journal
           of Marketing Research*, 27(2):185–195, 1990.

[Hir74]   M. Hirano. Morphological structure of the vocal cord as a vibrator and its varia-
           tions. *Folia Phoniatr (Basel)*, 26(2):89–94, 1974.

[Hir81]   M. Hirano. *Clinical Examination of Voice*. Springer, New York, NY (USA), 1981.

[HK04]   M. Hagmüller and G. Kubin. Voice enhancement of male speakers with laryngeal
           neoplasm. In *Proc. Int. Conf. on Spoken Language Processing (ICSLP)*, volume I,
           pages 541–544, Jeju Island (Rep. of Korea), 2004.

[HM94]   H. Hermansky and N. Morgan. RASTA Processing of Speech. *IEEE Trans. on
           Speech and Audio Processing*, 2(4):578–589, 1994.

[HN03]   T. Haderlein and E. Nöth. The EMBASSI Speech Corpus. Technical report,
           Lehrstuhl für Mustererkennung (Chair for Pattern Recognition), Universität Erlan-
           gen–Nürnberg, Erlangen (Germany), 2003.

[HNH⁺05]   T. Haderlein, E. Nöth, W. Herbordt, W. Kellermann, and H. Niemann. Using Ar-
           tificially Reverberated Training Data in Distant-Talking ASR. In V. Matoušek,
           P. Mautner, and T. Pavelka, editors, *Proc. Text, Speech and Dialogue; 8th Int. Conf.,
           TSD 2005; Karlovy Vary (Czech Republic)*, volume 3658 of *Lecture Notes in Arti-
           ficial Intelligence*, pages 226–233, Berlin, Heidelberg, 2005. Springer.

[HNS⁺05]   T. Haderlein, E. Nöth, M. Schuster, U. Eysholdt, and F. Rosanowski. Objek-
           tive Bewertung der tracheo-ösophagealen Ersatzstimme. In *22. Wissenschaftliche
           Jahrestagung der Deutschen Gesellschaft für Phoniatrie und Pädaudiologie*,
           Berlin (Germany), 2005.

[HNS⁺06]   T. Haderlein, E. Nöth, M. Schuster, U. Eysholdt, and F. Rosanowski. Evaluation of
           Tracheoesophageal Substitute Voices Using Prosodic Features. In R. Hoffmann and
           H. Mixdorff, editors, *Proc. Speech Prosody, 3rd International Conference*, pages
           701–704, Dresden (Germany), 2006. TUDpress.

[HNT⁺07]   T. Haderlein, E. Nöth, H. Toy, A. Batliner, M. Schuster, U. Eysholdt, J. Hornegger,
           and F. Rosanowski. Automatic Evaluation of Prosodic Features of Tracheoesopha-
           geal Substitute Voice. *Eur Arch Otorhinolaryngol*, 2007. To appear.

[Hor79]   Y. Horii. Fundamental frequency perturbation observed in sustained phonation.
           J Speech Hear Res, 22(1):5–19, 1979.

[Hor80]   Y. Horii. Vocal shimmer in sustained phonation. *J Speech Hear Res*, 23(1):202–
           209, 1980.

[HP98]   J.H.L. Hansen and B.L. Pellom. An Effective Quality Evaluation Protocol for
           Speech Enhancement Algorithms. In *Proc. Int. Conf. on Spoken Language Pro-
           cessing (ICSLP)*, volume 7, pages 2819–2822, Sydney (Australia), 1998.

160

BIBLIOGRAPHY

ed at the top right: BIBLIOGRAPHY

[HRM+07] T. Haderlein, K. Riedhammer, A. Maier, E. Nöth, H. Toy, and F. Rosanowski. An Automatic Version of the Post-Laryngectomy Telephone Test. In *Proc. Text, Speech and Dialogue; 10th Int. Conf., TSD 2007; Pilsen (Czech Republic)*, Lecture Notes in Artificial Intelligence, Berlin, Heidelberg, 2007. Springer. To appear.

[HS90] F.J.M. Hilgers and P.F. Schouwenburg. A new low-resistance, self-retaining prosthesis (Provox™) for voice rehabilitation after total laryngectomy. *Laryngoscope*, 100(11):1202–1207, 1990.

[HS98] H. Hermansky and S. Sharma. TRAPS – classifiers of temporal patterns. In *Proc. Int. Conf. on Spoken Language Processing (ICSLP)*, volume 3, pages 1003–1006, Sydney (Australia), 1998.

[HS99] N.D. Hogikyan and G. Sethuraman. Validation of an instrument to measure voice-related quality of life (V-RQOL). *J Voice*, 13(4):557–569, 1999.

[HSN03] T. Haderlein, G. Stemmer, and E. Nöth. Speech Recognition with μ-Law Companded Features on Reverberated Signals. In V. Matoušek and P. Mautner, editors, *Proc. Text, Speech and Dialogue; 6th Int. Conf., TSD 2003; České Budějovice (Czech Republic)*, volume 2807 of *Lecture Notes in Artificial Intelligence*, pages 173–180, Berlin (Germany), 2003. Springer.

[HSN+04] T. Haderlein, S. Steidl, E. Nöth, F. Rosanowski, and M. Schuster. Automatic Recognition and Evaluation of Tracheoesophageal Speech. In P. Sojka, I. Kopeček, and K. Pala, editors, *Proc. Text, Speech and Dialogue; 7th Int. Conf., TSD 2004; Brno (Czech Republic)*, volume 3206 of *Lecture Notes in Artificial Intelligence*, pages 331–338, Berlin, Heidelberg, 2004. Springer.

[HSNS05] T. Haderlein, S. Steidl, E. Nöth, and M. Schuster. Menschliche und automatische Verständlichkeitsbewertung bei tracheoösophagealen Ersatzstimmen. In *Fortschritte der Akustik – DAGA 2005*, pages 243–244, Munich (Germany), 2005.

[HTW+97] H. Höge, H.S. Tropf, R. Winski, H. van den Heuvel, R. Haeb-Umbach, and K. Choukri. European Speech Databases for Telephone Applications. In *Proc. Int. Conf. on Acoustics, Speech, and Signal Processing (ICASSP)*, volume 3, pages 1771–1774, Munich (Germany), 1997.

[Hub02] R. Huber. *Prosodisch-linguistische Klassifikation von Emotion*, volume 8 of *Studien zur Mustererkennung*. Logos Verlag, Berlin (Germany), 2002.

[Hum99] J. Hummel. *Stimmprothesen in der sprachlichen und sozialen Rehabilitation nach Laryngektomie*. PhD thesis, Universität Hamburg, Hamburg (Germany), 1999.

[Hun99] M.J. Hunt. Spectral Signal Processing for ASR. In *Proc. IEEE Workshop on Automatic Speech Recognition and Understanding (ASRU)*, volume 1, pages 17–25, Keystone, CO (USA), 1999.

[HZN+06] T. Haderlein, D. Zorn, E. Nöth, H. Toy, U. Eysholdt, and F. Rosanowski. Die tracheoösophageale Ersatzstimme: Grafische Darstellung von Sprechstörungen mithilfe der Sammon-Transformation. In M. Gross and E. Kruse, editors, *Aktuelle phoniatrisch-pädaudiologische Aspekte 2006*, pages 56–58, Norderstedt (Germany), 2006. Book on Demand GmbH.

[HZS⁺06] T. Haderlein, D. Zorn, S. Steidl, E. Nöth, M. Shozakai, and M. Schuster. Visualization of Voice Disorders Using the Sammon Transform. In P. Sojka, I. Kopeček, and K. Pala, editors, *Proc. Text, Speech and Dialogue; 9th Int. Conf., TSD 2006; Brno (Czech Republic)*, volume 4188 of *Lecture Notes in Artificial Intelligence*, pages 589–596, Berlin, Heidelberg, 2006. Springer.

[IF72] K. Ishizaka and J.L. Flanagan. Synthesis of Voiced Sounds from a Two-Mass Model of the Vocal Cords. *Bell Systems Technical Journal*, 51(6):1233–1268, 1972.

[InH00] InHealth company website, 2000. http://www.inhealth.com, last visited May 30, 2007; InHealth Technologies, Carpinteria, CA (USA).

[IPA99] Handbook of the International Phonetic Association. Cambridge University Press, Cambridge (England), 1999.

[ITU96] Methods for Subjective Determination of Transmission Quality; ITU-T Recommendation P.800. International Telecommunication Union (ITU), 1996. Series P: Telephone Transmission Quality.

[Jan03] M. Janke. *Erste klinische Erfahrungen mit dem neuen Tracheostomaventil Window® (Adeva)*. PhD thesis, Julius-Maximilians-Universität, Würzburg (Germany), 2003.

[JBM75] F. Jelinek, L.R. Bahl, and R.L. Mercer. Design of a Linguistic Statistical Decoder for the Recognition of Continuous Speech. *IEEE Trans. on Information Theory*, IT-21(3):250–256, 1975.

[JJG⁺97] B.H. Jacobson, A. Johnson, C. Grywalski, A. Silbergleit, G. Jacobson, M.S. Benninger, and C.W. Newman. The Voice Handicap Index (VHI): Development and Validation. *Am J Speech-Language Path*, 6(3):66–70, 1997.

[JM80] F. Jelinek and R.L. Mercer. Interpolated estimation of markov source parameters from sparse data. In E.S. Gelesma and L.N. Kanal, editors, *Proc. Workshop on Pattern Recognition in Practice*, pages 381–397, Amsterdam (The Netherlands), 1980. North-Holland.

[Jon01] R.B. Jones. Impairment, disability and handicap – old fashioned concepts? *J Med Ethics*, 27(6):377–379, 2001.

[Jun97] J.-C. Junqua. Impact of the Unknown Communication Channel on Automatic Speech Recognition: A Review. In *Proc. European Conf. on Speech Communication and Technology (Eurospeech)*, volume 1, pages KN29–KN32, Rhodes (Greece), 1997.

[Jun00] J.-C. Junqua. *Robust Speech Recognition in Embedded Systems and PC Applications*. Kluwer Academic Publishers, Boston, MA (USA), 2000.

[KA86]   M. Kinishi and M. Amatsu.   Aerodynamic Studies of Laryngectomees after
            the Amatsu Tracheoesophageal Shunt Operation. *Ann Otol Rhinol Laryngol*,
            95(2 Pt 1):181–184, 1986.

[KD99]   C. Kapusta-Shemie and C. Dromey. Acoustic and Perceptual Improvements in Tra-
            cheoesophageal Voice Using a Neck Strap. *J Otolaryngol*, 28(2):102–104, 1999.

[KF93]   T. Klauer and S.-H. Filipp.   Trierer Skalen zur Krankheitsbewältigung (TSK).
            Hogrefe Verlag, Göttingen (Germany), 1993. Manual.

[KGK+93]   J. Kreiman, B.R. Gerratt, G.B. Kempster, A. Erman, and G.S. Berke. Perceptual
            evaluation of voice quality: review, tutorial, and a framework for future research.
            J Speech Hear Res, 36(1):21–40, 1993.

[Kir98]   K. Kirchhoff.   Combining Articulatory and Acoustic Information for Speech
            Recognition in Noisy and Reverberant Environments. In *Proc. Int. Conf. on Spo-
            ken Language Processing (ICSLP)*, volume 3, pages 891–894, Sydney (Australia),
            1998.

[Kli91]   F. Klingholz. Jitter. *Sprache - Stimme - Gehör*, 15(3):79–85, 1991.

[KLP+94]   K. Kohler, G. Lex, M. Pätzold, M. Scheffers, A. Simpson, and W. Thon. Handbuch
            zur Datenaufnahme und Transliteration in TP14 von Verbmobil, V3.0. Verbmobil
            Technisches–Dokument 11, Institut für Phonetik und digitale Sprachverarbeitung,
            Universität Kiel, Kiel (Germany), 1994.

[KM97]   B.E.D. Kingsbury and N. Morgan. Recognizing Reverberant Speech with RASTA-
            PLP. In *Proc. Int. Conf. on Acoustics, Speech, and Signal Processing (ICASSP)*,
            volume 2, pages 1259–1262, Munich (Germany), 1997.

[KMH+94]   J. Köhler, N. Morgan, H. Hermansky, H.G. Hirsch, and G. Tong. Integrating
            RASTA-PLP into Speech Recognition. In *Proc. Int. Conf. on Acoustics, Speech,
            and Signal Processing (ICASSP)*, volume 1, pages 421–424, Adelaide (Australia),
            1994.

[KMZB97]   E. Kruse, D. Michaelis, P. Zwirner, and E. Bender.   Stimmfunktionelle Quali-
            tätssicherung in der kurativen Mikrochirurgie der Larynxmalignome. *HNO*,
            45(9):712–718, 1997.

[Kom97]   R. Kompe. *Prosody in Speech Understanding Systems*, volume 1307 of *Lecture
            Notes in Artificial Intelligence*. Springer, Berlin (Germany), 1997.

[Kri02]   K. Krippendorff.   Computing   Krippendorff's Alpha-Reliability,   2002.
            http://www.asc.upenn.edu/usr/krippendorff/webreliability2.pdf;   last   visited
            May 30, 2007.

[Kri03]   K. Krippendorff. *Content Analysis, an Introduction to Its Methodology*. Sage
            Publications, Thousand Oaks, CA (USA), 2nd edition, 2003.

[Kro93]   G. de Krom. A cepstrum-based technique for determining a harmonics-to-noise
            ratio in speech signals. *J Speech Hear Res*, 36(2):254–266, 1993.

[Kro95]   G. de Krom. Some spectral correlates of pathological breathy and rough voice quality for different types of vowel fragments. *J Speech Hear Res*, 38(4):794–811, 1995.

[Kru99]   F. Krummenauer. Erweiterungen von Cohen's kappa-Maß für Multi-Rater-Studien: Eine Übersicht. *Informatik, Biometrie und Epidemiologie in Medizin und Biologie*, 30(1):3–20, 1999.

[KSE77]   D.N. Kalikow, K.N. Stevens, and L.L. Elliot. Development of a test of speech intelligibility in noise using sentence materials with controlled word predictability. *J Acoust Soc Am*, 61(5):1337–1351, 1977.

[Kuh95]   T. Kuhn. *Die Erkennungsphase in einem Dialogsystem*, volume 80 of *Dissertationen zur Künstlichen Intelligenz*. Infix, St. Augustin (Germany), 1995.

[KW97]   B. Kollmeier and M. Wesselkamp. Development and evaluation of a German sentence test for objective and subjective speech intelligibility assessment. *J Acoust Soc Am*, 102(4):2412–2421, 1997.

[Kyt64]   J. Kyttä. Finnish oesophageal speech after laryngectomy: Sound spectrographic and cineradiographic studies. *Acta Otolaryngol (Stockh)*, Suppl. 195, 1964.

[LA94]   P. Lockwood and P. Alexandre. Root Adaptive Homomorphic Deconvolution Schemes for Speech Recognition in Noise. In *Proc. Int. Conf. on Acoustics, Speech, and Signal Processing (ICASSP)*, volume 1, pages 441–444, Adelaide (Australia), 1994.

[Laa97]   G.P.M. Laan. The Contribution of Intonation, Segmental Durations, and Spectral Features to the Perception of a Spontaneous and a Read Speaking Style. *Speech Communication*, 22(1):43–65, 1997.

[LCY+96]   Q. Lin, C.W. Che, D.-S. Yuk, L. Yin, B. de Vries, J. Pearson, and J.L. Flanagan. Robust Distant-Talking Speech Recognition. In *Proc. Int. Conf. on Acoustics, Speech, and Signal Processing (ICASSP)*, volume 1, pages 21–24, Atlanta, GA (USA), 1996.

[LDR+02]   J. Lohscheller, M. Döllinger, F. Rosanowski, U. Eysholdt, and U. Hoppe. Image Processing and Modeling of the Laryngectomee Substitute Voice. In *7th International Workshop Vision, Modeling, and Visualization (VMV)*, pages 447–454, Erlangen (Germany), 2002.

[LDS+03]   J. Lohscheller, M. Döllinger, M. Schuster, U. Eysholdt, and U. Hoppe. The laryngectomee substitute voice: image processing of endoscopic recordings by fusion with acoustic signals. *Methods Inf Med*, 42(3):277–281, 2003.

[LE97]   S.B. Leder and M.C. Erskine. Voice restoration after laryngectomy: Experience with the Blom-Singer extended-wear indwelling tracheoesophageal voice prosthesis. *Head & Neck*, 19(6):487–493, 1997.

[Lev66]   V.I. Levenshtein. Binary Codes Capable of Correcting Deletions, Insertions and Reversals. *Soviet Physics Doklady*, 10(8):707–710, 1966.

[LGA02]   L. Lamel, J.-L. Gauvain, and G. Adda. Unsupervised Acoustic Model Training. In *Proc. Int. Conf. on Acoustics, Speech, and Signal Processing (ICASSP)*, volume I, pages 877–880, Orlando, FL (USA), 2002.

[LGM+96]   P. Lavertu, M.E. Guay, S.S. Meeker, J.R. Kmiecik, M. Secic, J.R. Wanamaker, I. Eliachar, and B.G. Wood. Secondary tracheoesophageal puncture: factors predictive of voice quality and prosthesis use. *Head & Neck*, 18(5):393–398, 1996.

[Lik32]   R. Likert. A technique for the measurement of attitudes. *Archives of Psychology*, No. 140, 1932. Columbia University, New York, NY (USA).

[Lim79]   J.S. Lim. Spectral Root Homomorphic Deconvolution System. *IEEE Trans. on Acoustics, Speech, and Signal Processing (ASSP)*, 27(3):223–233, 1979.

[Lip97]   R.P. Lippmann. Speech recognition by machines and humans. *Speech Communication*, 22(1):1–15, 1997.

[LJR01]   G. Lawson, J. Jamart, and M. Remacle. Improving the functional outcome of Tucker's reconstructive laryngectomy. *Head & Neck*, 23(10):871–878, 2001.

[LJW+04]   T. Li, C. Jo, S.-G. Wang, B.-G. Yang, and H.-S. Kim. Classification of Pathological Voice including Severely Noisy Cases. In *Proc. Int. Conf. on Spoken Language Processing (ICSLP)*, volume I, pages 77–80, Jeju Island (Rep. of Korea), 2004.

[LK75]   J.R. Landis and G.G. Koch. A review of statistical methods in the analysis of data arising from observer reliability studies (parts I and II). *Statistica Neerlandica*, 29:101–123 and 151–161, 1975.

[Loh03]   J. Lohscheller. *Dynamics of the Laryngectomee Substitute Voice Production*, volume 14 of *Berichte aus Phoniatrie und Pädaudiologie*. Shaker Verlag, Aachen (Germany), 2003.

[LSS03]   Y. Liu, E. Shriberg, and A. Stolcke. Automatic Disfluency Identification in Conversational Speech Using Multiple Knowledge Sources. In *Proc. European Conf. on Speech Communication and Technology (Eurospeech)*, volume 2, pages 957–960, Geneva (Switzerland), 2003.

[LW94]   C.J. Leggetter and P.C. Woodland. Speaker adaptation of continuous density HMMs using multivariate linear regression. In *Proc. Int. Conf. on Spoken Language Processing (ICSLP)*, volume 1, pages 451–454, Yokohama (Japan), 1994.

[Mac67]   J.B. MacQueen. Some Methods for Classification and Analysis of Multivariate Observations. In L.M. Le Cam and J. Neyman, editors, *Proc. Fifth Berkeley Symposium on Mathematical Statistics and Probability*, volume I, pages 281–297, Berkeley, CA (USA), 1967. University of California Press.

[Mad03]   H. de Maddalena. Vorbereitung des PLTT – Durchführung des PLTT. Unpublished instruction sheet for preparing and performing the Postlaryngectomy Telephone Test; Universität Tübingen, Tübingen (Germany), 2003.

[Mah36]   P.C. Mahalanobis. On the generalised distance in statistics. *Proceedings of the National Institute of Science of India*, 2:49–55, 1936.

[Mai06]   A. Maier. PEAKS – Programm zur Evaluation und Analyse Kindlicher Sprachstörungen. Technical report, Lehrstuhl für Mustererkennung (Chair for Pattern Recognition), Universität Erlangen–Nürnberg, Erlangen (Germany), 2006.

[Mau98]   L. Mauuray. Blind Equalization in the Cepstral Domain for Robust Telephone Based Speech Recognition. In *Proc. European Signal Processing Conference (EU-SIPCO)*, volume 1, pages 359–363, Rhodes (Greece), 1998.

[MDB01]   C. Manfredi, M. D'Aniello, and P. Bruscaglioni. A simple subspace approach for speech denoising. *Logoped Phoniatr Vocol*, 26(4):179–192, 2001.

[MFP+98]   D. McColl, D. Fucci, L. Petrosino, D.E. Martin, and P. McCaffrey. Listener Ratings of the Intelligibility of Tracheoesophageal Speech in Noise. *J Commun Disord*, 31(4):279–288, quiz 288–289, 1998.

[MFS98]   D. Michaelis, M. Fröhlich, and H.-W. Strube. Selection and combination of acoustic features for the description of pathologic voices. *J Acoust Soc Am*, 103(3):1628–1639, 1998.

[MGS97]   D. Michaelis, T. Gramß, and H.-W. Strube. Glottal to noise excitation ratio – a new measure for describing pathological voices. *Acustica/acta acustica*, 83(4):700–706, 1997.

[MH92]   N. Morgan and H. Hermansky. RASTA Extensions: Robustness to Additive and Convolutional Noise. In *Proc. ESCA Workshop on Speech Processing in Adverse Conditions*, pages 115–118, Cannes (France), 1992.

[MHKH02]   K. Matsui, N. Hara, N. Kobayashi, and H. Hirose. Enhancement of esophageal speech using formant synthesis. *Acoustical Science and Technology*, 23(2):69–76, 2002.

[MHT05]   N. Morales, J.H.L. Hansen, and D.T. Toledano. MFCC Compensation for Improved Recognition of Filtered and Band-Limited Speech. In *Proc. Int. Conf. on Acoustics, Speech, and Signal Processing (ICASSP)*, volume I, pages 521–524, Philadelphia, PA (USA), 2005.

[Mic00]   D. Michaelis. *Das Göttinger Heiserkeitsdiagramm – Entwicklung und Prüfung eines akustischen Verfahrens zur objektiven Stimmgütebeurteilung pathologischer Stimmen*. PhD thesis, Universität Göttingen, Göttingen (Germany), 2000. Published online: http://webdoc.sub.gwdg.de/diss/2000/michaelis/index.html.

[MK88]   M. Miyoshi and Y. Kaneda. Inverse Filtering of Room Acoustics. *IEEE Trans. on Acoustics, Speech, and Signal Processing (ASSP)*, 36(2):145–152, 1988.

[MM02]   L. Matassini and C. Manfredi. Software Corrections of Vocal Disorders. *Computer Methods and Programs in Biomedicine*, 68(2):135–145, 2002.

[MMB⁺06]   M.B.J. Moerman, J.P. Martens, M.J. van der Borgt, M. Peleman, and M. Gillis and P.H. Dejonckere. Perceptual evaluation of substitution voices: development and evaluation of the (I)INFVo rating scale. *Eur Arch Otorhinolaryngol*, 263(2):183–187, 2006.

[MMG93]   M. Mendelsohn, M. Morris, and R. Gallagher. Speaking proficiency after primary tracheoesophageal puncture. *J Otolaryngol*, 22(6):435–437, 1993.

[MMW⁺03]   K. Manickam, C.J. Moore, T. Willard, S. Jones, and N. Slevin. A Comparison of Voice Quality Classification in Male Larnyx Cancer Radiotherapy by Speech Therapists & Complexity Analysis. In A. Wendemuth, editor, *Proc. Speech Processing Workshop*, pages 41–48, Magdeburg (Germany), 2003.

[MNNS06]   A. Maier, E. Nöth, E. Nkenke, and M. Schuster. Automatic Assessment of Children's Speech with Cleft Lip and Palate. In T. Erjavec and J. Žganec Gros, editors, *Proc. 5th Slovenian and 1st International Conference Language Technologies (IS-LTC 2006)*, pages 31–35, Ljubljana (Slovenia), 2006.

[MOO79]   D.E. Metz, J. Onufrak, and R.S. Ogburn. An Acoustical Analysis of Stutterers' Speech Prior to and at the Termination of Therapy. *J Fluency Disord*, 4(4):249–254, 1979.

[Moo03]   R.K. Moore. A Comparison of the Data Requirements of Automatic Speech Recognition Systems and Human Listeners. In *Proc. European Conf. on Speech Communication and Technology (Eurospeech)*, volume 4, pages 2581–2584, Geneva (Switzerland), 2003.

[MPM⁺04]   M.B.J. Moerman, G. Pieters, J.P. Martens, M.J. van der Borgt, and P.H. Dejonckere. Objective evaluation of the quality of substitution voices. *Eur Arch Otorhinolaryngol*, 261(10):541–547, 2004.

[MRCL06]   R.J. Moran, R.B. Reilly, P. de Chazal, and P.D. Lacy. Telephony-based voice pathology assessment using automated speech analysis. *IEEE Trans. on Biomedical Engineering*, 53(3):468–477, 2006.

[MSK97]   D. Michaelis, H.-W. Strube, and E. Kruse. Reliabilität und Validität des Heiserkeits-Diagramms. In *Aktuelle phoniatrisch-pädaudiologische Aspekte 1996 (4)*, pages 25–26. Verlag Abteilung Phoniatrie Universitäts-HNO-Klinik Göttingen, Göttingen (Germany), 1997.

[MTM00]   T. Most, Y. Tobin, and R.C. Mimran. Acoustic and perceptual characteristics of esophageal and tracheoesophageal speech production. *J Commun Disord*, 33(2):165–180; quiz 180–181, 2000.

[MW87]   J.B. Moon and B. Weinberg. Aerodynamic and Myoelastic Contributions to Tracheoesophageal Voice Production. *J Speech Hear Res*, 30(3):387–395, 1987.

[MW94] H. Maier and H. Weidauer. Chirurgische Stimmrehabilitation nach Laryngektomie durch eine Modifikation des Verfahrens nach Asai. *HNO*, 42(2):99–103, 1994.

[MYC91] Y. Medan, E. Yair, and D. Chazan. Super Resolution Pitch Determination of Speech Signals. *IEEE Trans. on Acoustics, Speech, and Signal Processing (ASSP)*, 39(1):40–48, 1991.

[MZ96] H. de Maddalena and H.-P. Zenner. Evaluation of speech intelligibility after prosthetic voice restoration by a standardized telephone test. In J. Algaba, editor, *Proc. 6th International Congress on Surgical and Prosthetic Voice Restoration After Total Laryngectomy*, pages 183–187, San Sebastian (Spain), 1996. Elsevier Science.

[NASL82] H.F. Nijdam, A.A. Annyas, H.K. Schutte, and H.F. Leever. A new prosthesis for voice rehabilitation after laryngectomy. *Arch Otolaryngol*, 237(1):27–33, 1982.

[NAW94] T. Nawka, L.-C. Anders, and J. Wendler. Die auditive Beurteilung heiserer Stimmen nach dem RBH-System. *Sprache - Stimme - Gehör*, 18(3):130–133, 1994.

[NB62] W. Niemeyer and G. Beckmann. Ein sprachaudiometrischer Satztest. *Archiv für Ohren-, Nasen- und Kehlkopfheilkunde*, 180:742–749, 1962.

[NBK⁺00] E. Nöth, A. Batliner, A. Kießling, R. Kompe, and H. Niemann. VERBMOBIL: The Use of Prosody in the Linguistic Components of a Speech Understanding System. *IEEE Trans. on Speech and Audio Processing*, 8(5):519–532, 2000.

[NHW⁺99] E. Nöth, J. Haas, V. Warnke, F. Gallwitz, and M. Boros. A Hybrid Approach to Spoken Dialogue Understanding: Prosody, Statistics and Partial Parsing. In *Proc. European Conf. on Speech Communication and Technology (Eurospeech)*, volume 5, pages 2019–2022, Budapest (Hungary), 1999.

[Nie90] H. Niemann. *Pattern Analysis and Understanding*, volume 4 of *Springer Series in Information Sciences*. Springer, Heidelberg (Germany), 1990.

[Nie03] H. Niemann. *Klassifikation von Mustern.* available online, 2nd edition, 2003. http://www5.informatik.uni-erlangen.de/Personen/niemann/klassifikation-von-mustern/m00links.html; last visited May 30, 2007.

[NK88] E. Nöth and R. Kompe. Der Einsatz prosodischer Information im Spracherkennungssystem EVAR. In H. Bunke, O. Kübler, and P. Stucki, editors, *Mustererkennung 1988 (10. DAGM-Symposium)*, volume 180 of *Informatik-Fachberichte*, pages 2–9, Berlin (Germany), 1988. Springer.

[NMH⁺07] E. Nöth, A. Maier, T. Haderlein, K. Riedhammer, F. Rosanowski, and M. Schuster. Automatic Evaluation of Pathologic Speech – from Research to Routine Clinical Use. In *Proc. Text, Speech and Dialogue; 10th Int. Conf., TSD 2007; Pilsen (Czech Republic)*, Lecture Notes in Artificial Intelligence, Berlin, Heidelberg, 2007. Springer. To appear.

[NN06] M. Nishio and S. Niimi. Comparison of Speaking Rate, Articulation Rate and Alternating Motion Rate in Dysarthric Speakers. *Folia Phoniatr Logop*, 58(2):114–131, 2006.

[NNH+00] E. Nöth, H. Niemann, T. Haderlein, M. Decher, U. Eysholdt, F. Rosanowski, and T. Wittenberg. Automatic Stuttering Recognition using Hidden Markov Models. In *Proc. Int. Conf. on Spoken Language Processing (ICSLP)*, volume 4, pages 65–68, Beijing (China), 2000.

[Nöt91] E. Nöth. *Prosodische Information in der automatischen Spracherkennung – Berechnung und Anwendung*. Niemeyer, Tübingen (Germany), 1991.

[NR78] A.K. Nabelek and L.N. Robinette. Reverberation as a parameter in clinical testing. *Audiology*, 17(3):239–259, 1978.

[NS87] G.L.J. Nieboer and H.K. Schutte. The Groningen button: results of in vivo measurements. *Revue de Laryngologie - Otologie - Rhinologie*, 108(2):121–122, 1987.

[NW79] H. Niemann and J. Weiß. A Fast-Converging Algorithm for Nonlinear Mapping of High-Dimensional Data to a Plane. *IEEE Trans. on Computers*, C-28(2):142–147, 1979.

[OKNF94] K. Omori, H. Kojima, M. Nonomura, and H. Fukushima. Mechanism of tracheoesophageal shunt phonation. *Arch Otolaryngol Head Neck Surg*, 120(6):648–652, 1994.

[ON93] M. Oerder and H. Ney. Word graphs: An efficient interface between continuous speech recognition and language understanding. In *Proc. Int. Conf. on Acoustics, Speech, and Signal Processing (ICASSP)*, volume II, pages 119–122, Minneapolis, MN (USA), 1993.

[OS68] A.V. Oppenheim and R.W. Schafer. Homomorphic Analysis of Speech. *IEEE Trans. on Audio and Electroacoustics*, AU-16(2):221–226, 1968.

[OS75] A.V. Oppenheim and R.W. Schafer. *Digital Signal Processing*. Prentice-Hall, Englewood Cliffs, NJ (USA), 1975.

[OSM98] M. Omologo, P. Svaizer, and M. Matassoni. Environmental conditions and acoustic transduction in hands-free speech recognition. *Speech Communication*, 25(1–3):75–95, 1998.

[PC89] R.H. Pindzola and B.H. Cain. Duration and frequency characteristics of tracheoesophageal speech. *Ann Otol Rhinol Laryngol*, 98(12 Pt 1):960–964, 1989.

[PDP01] J. Pahn, R. Dahl, and E. Pahn. Beziehung zwischen Messung der stimmlichen Durchdringungsfähigkeit, Stimmstatus nach Pahn und ausgewählten Parametern des Stimmanalyseprogramms MDVP (Kay). *Folia Phoniatr Logop*, 53(6):308–316, 2001.

[Pea01] K. Pearson. On Lines and Planes of Closest Fit to Systems of Points in Space. *Philosophical Magazine*, 2(6th series):559–572, 1901.

[Pet27] E. Petzold. *Elementare Raumakustik*. Bauwelt-Verlag, Berlin (Germany), 1927.

[PFKB89]   B.R. Pauloski, H.B. Fisher, G.B. Kempster, and E.D. Blom. Statistical Differentiation of Tracheoesophageal Speech Produced under Four Prosthetic/Occlusion Speaking Conditions. *J Speech Hear Res*, 32(3):591–599, 1989.

[Pin91]   S.M. Pincus. Approximate entropy as a measure of system complexity. *Proc. National Academy of Sciences of the United States of America (PNAS)*, 88(6):2297–2301, 1991.

[PJ01]   V. Parsa and D.G. Jamieson. Acoustic discrimination of pathological voice: sustained vowels versus continuous speech. *J Speech Lang Hear Res*, 44(2):327–339, 2001.

[Pla98]   J.C. Platt. Fast Training of Support Vector Machines using Sequential Minimal Optimization. In B. Schölkopf, C.J.C. Burges, and A.J. Smola, editors, *Advances in Kernel Methods – Support Vector Learning*, pages 41–65. MIT Press, Cambridge, MA (USA), 1998.

[QBC88]   S.R. Quackenbush, T.P. Barnwell III, and M.A. Clements. *Objective Measures of Speech Quality*. Prentice-Hall, New York, NY (USA), 1988.

[QW95]   Y. Qi and B. Weinberg. Characteristics of Voicing Source Waveforms Produced by Esophageal and Tracheoesophageal Speakers. *J Speech Hear Res*, 38(3):536–548, 1995.

[RCK86]   J. Robbins, J.M. Christensen, and G.B. Kempster. Characteristics of speech production after tracheoesophageal puncture: voice onset time and vowel duration. *J Speech Hear Res*, 29(4):499–504, 1986.

[RFBS84a] J. Robbins, H.B. Fisher, E.D. Blom, and M.I. Singer. A Comparative Acoustic Study of Normal, Esophageal, and Tracheoesophageal Speech Production. *J Speech Hear Disord*, 49(2):202–210, 1984.

[RFBS84b] J. Robbins, H.B. Fisher, E.D. Blom, and M.I. Singer. Selected Acoustic Features of Tracheoesophageal, Esophageal, and Laryngeal Speech. *Arch Otolaryngol*, 110(10):670–672, 1984.

[RHN+06]   K. Riedhammer, T. Haderlein, E. Nöth, H. Toy, U. Eysholdt, and F. Rosanowski. Die tracheoösophageale Ersatzstimme: Automatische Verständlichkeitsbewertung über das Telefon. In M. Gross and E. Kruse, editors, *Aktuelle phoniatrisch-pädaudiologische Aspekte 2006*, pages 51–53, Norderstedt (Germany), 2006. Book on Demand GmbH.

[RHS+06]   K. Riedhammer, T. Haderlein, M. Schuster, F. Rosanowski, and E. Nöth. Automatic Evaluation of Tracheoesophageal Telephone Speech. In T. Erjavec and J. Žganec Gros, editors, *Proc. 5th Slovenian and 1st International Conference Language Technologies (IS-LTC 2006)*, pages 17–22, Ljubljana (Slovenia), 2006.

[Rie95]   S. Rieck. *Parametrisierung und Klassifikation gesprochener Sprache*, volume 353 of *VDI Fortschrittberichte Reihe 10: Informatik/Kommunikationstechnik*. VDI Verlag, Düsseldorf (Germany), 1995.

[Rie07]   K. Riedhammer. An Automatic Intelligibility Test Based on the Post-Laryngec-
            tomy Telephone Test. Student's thesis, Lehrstuhl für Mustererkennung (Chair for
            Pattern Recognition), Universität Erlangen–Nürnberg, Erlangen (Germany), 2007.

[RKNQ02]   M.A. van Rossum, G. de Krom, S.G. Nooteboom, and H. Quené. "Pitch" accent in
            alaryngeal speech. *J Speech Lang Hear Res*, 45(6):1106–1118, 2002.

[RLKB03]   V. Roth, J. Laub, M. Kawanabe, and J.M. Buhmann. Optimal Cluster Preserving
            Embedding of Nonmetric Proximity Data. *IEEE Trans. on Pattern Analysis and
            Machine Intelligence (PAMI)*, 25(12):1540–1551, 2003.

[RML04]   R.B. Reilly, R.J. Moran, and P.D. Lacy. Voice Pathology Assessment Based on a
            Dialogue System and Speech Analysis. In T. Bickmore, editor, *Proc. AAAI Fall
            Symposium on Dialogue Systems for Health Communication October 2004*, pages
            104–109, Washington, DC (USA), 2004.

[Rob84]   J. Robbins. Acoustic Differentiation of Laryngeal, Esophageal, and Tracheoeso-
            phageal Speech. *J Speech Hear Res*, 27(4):577–585, 1984.

[Sab64]   W.C. Sabine. Reverberation. In *Collected Papers on Acoustics*. Dover Publications,
            New York, NY (USA), 1964. Originally published in The American Architect,
            1900.

[Sam69]   J.W. Sammon Jr. A Nonlinear Mapping for Data Structure Analysis. *IEEE Trans.
            on Computers*, C-18(5):401–409, 1969.

[Sat05]   R.T. Sataloff, editor. *Professional Voice – The Science and Art of Clinical Care*.
            Plural Publishing Inc., San Diego, CA (USA), 3rd edition, 2005.

[SB80]   M.I. Singer and E.D. Blom. An Endoscopic Technique for Restoration of the Voice
            after Laryngectomy. *Ann Otol Rhinol Laryngol*, 89(6 Pt 1):529–533, 1980.

[SBN01]   J. Spilker, A. Batliner, and E. Nöth. How to Repair Speech Repairs in an End-
            to-End System. In R. Lickley and L. Shriberg, editors, *Proc. ISCA Workshop on
            Disfluency in Spontaneous Speech*, pages 73–76, Edinburgh (Scotland), 2001.

[SC02]   J.P. Searl and M.A. Carpenter. Acoustic Cues to the Voicing Feature in Tracheo-
            esophageal Speech. *J Speech Lang Hear Res*, 45(2):282–294, 2002.

[SCB01]   J.P. Searl, M.A. Carpenter, and C.L. Banta. Intelligibility of stops and fricatives in
            tracheoesophageal speech. *J Commun Disord*, 34(4):305–321, 2001.

[Sch95]   E.G. Schukat-Talamazzini. *Automatische Spracherkennung – Grundlagen, statis-
            tische Modelle und effiziente Algorithmen*. Vieweg, Braunschweig (Germany),
            1995.

[Sch97a]   R. Schönweiler. Hilfsmittel für laryngektomierte Patienten. *Sprache - Stimme -
            Gehör*, 21(1):30–34, 1997.

[Sch97b]   H.-J. Schultz-Coulon. Die Stimmprothese. *Sprache - Stimme - Gehör*, 21(1):13–
            19, 1997.

[Sco55]   W. Scott. Reliability of Content Analysis: The Case of Nominal Scale Coding.
            Public Opinion Quarterly, 19(3):321–325, 1955.

[SD01]   M.I. Singer and C. DeLassus Gress. Voice Rehabilitation after Laryngectomy. In
            B.J. Bailey and G.B. Healy et al., editors, *Head and Neck Surgery – Otolaryngol-
            ogy*, pages 1505–1523. Lippincott Williams & Wilkins, Philadelphia, PA (USA),
            3rd edition, 2001.

[See22]   M. Seeman. Speech and voice without larynx. *Časopis lékařů českých*, 61:369–
            372, 1922.

[SFB01]   V. Stahl, A. Fischer, and R. Bippus. Acoustic Synthesis Of Training Data For
            Speech Recognition In Living Room Environments. In *Proc. Int. Conf. on Acous-
            tics, Speech, and Signal Processing (ICASSP)*, volume 1, pages 21–24, Salt Lake
            City, UT (USA), 2001.

[SG97]   E. Schmitz and M. Glunz. Shuntventil – Ein Weg zur Stimme. *Sprache - Stimme -
            Gehör*, 21(1):23–25, 1997.

[SGO91]   P.M. Sloane, J.F. Griffin, and T.P. O'Dwyer. Esophageal insufflation and videoflu-
            oroscopy for evaluation of esophageal speech in laryngectomy patients: clinical
            implications. *Radiology*, 181(2):433–437, 1991.

[SH81]   J.R. Smitheran and T.J. Hixon. A clinical method for estimating laryngeal airway
            resistance during vowel production. *J Speech Hear Disord*, 46(2):138–146, 1981.

[SH87]   F. Schön and I.F. Herrmann. Ein neuer Qualitätstest der Sprache nach funktioneller
            Kehlkopfchirurgie. *Arch Otorhinolaryngol Suppl II*, pages 96–97, 1987.

[SH95a]   I. Steinecke and H. Herzel. Bifurcations in an asymmetric vocal fold model.
            J Acoust Soc Am, 97(3):1874–1884, 1995.

[SH95b]   K.N. Stevens and H.M. Hanson. Classification of glottal vibration from acoustic
            measurements. In O. Fujimura and M. Hirano, editors, *Vocal Fold Physiology:
            Voice Quality Control*, pages 147–170. Singular Publishing Group, San Diego, CA
            (USA), 1995.

[SHC89]   S.E. Sedory, S.L. Hamlet, and N.P. Connor. Comparisons of Perceptual and
            Acoustic Characteristics of Tracheoesophageal and Excellent Esophageal Speech.
            J Speech Hear Disord, 54(2):209–214, 1989.

[SHN⁺06]   M. Schuster, T. Haderlein, E. Nöth, J. Lohscheller, U. Eysholdt, and F. Rosanowski.
            Intelligibility of laryngectomees' substitute speech: automatic speech recognition
            and subjective rating. *Eur Arch Otorhinolaryngol*, 263(2):188–193, 2006.

[SHSN03]   G. Stemmer, C. Hacker, S. Steidl, and E. Nöth. Acoustic Normalization of Chil-
            dren's Speech. In *Proc. European Conf. on Speech Communication and Technology
            (Eurospeech)*, volume 2, pages 1313–1316, Geneva (Switzerland), 2003.

[SKA00]   M. Saito, M. Kinishi, and M. Amatsu. Acoustic Analyses Clarify Voiced–Voiceless
            Distinction in Tracheoesophageal Speech. *Acta Otolaryngol*, 120(6):771–777,
            2000.

[SKER03]   M. Schuster, P. Kummer, U. Eysholdt, and F. Rosanowski. Quality of life in laryn-
            gectomees after prosthetic voice restoration. *Folia Phoniatr Logop*, 55(5):211–219,
            2003.

[SLH+04]   M. Schuster, J. Lohscheller, U. Hoppe, P. Kummer, U. Eysholdt, and F. Rosa-
            nowski. Voice handicap of laryngectomees with tracheoesophageal speech. *Folia
            Phoniatr Logop*, 56(1):62–67, 2004.

[Slu95]   A.M.C. Sluijter. *Phonetic Correlates of Stress and Accent*. Holland Academic
            Graphics, The Hague (The Netherlands), 1995.

[SN93]   E.G. Schukat-Talamazzini and H. Niemann. ISADORA – A Speech Modelling
            Network Based on Hidden Markov Models. Technical report, Universität
            Erlangen–Nürnberg, Erlangen (Germany), 1993. http://www.minet.uni-
            jena.de/fakultaet/schukat/MYPUB/SchukatTalamazzini93:IAS.ps; last visited
            May 30, 2007.

[SN02]   H.K. Schutte and G.L.J. Nieboer. Aerodynamics of esophageal voice production
            with and without a Groningen voice prosthesis. *Folia Phoniatr Logop*, 54(1):8–18,
            2002.

[SN04]   M. Shozakai and G. Nagino. Analysis of Speaking Styles by Two-Dimensional
            Visualization of Aggregate of Acoustic Models. In *Proc. Int. Conf. on Spoken Lan-
            guage Processing (ICSLP)*, volume I, pages 717–720, Jeju Island (Rep. of Korea),
            2004.

[SNE+92]   E.G. Schukat-Talamazzini, H. Niemann, W. Eckert, T. Kuhn, and S. Rieck. Acous-
            tic Modelling of Subword Units in the ISADORA Speech Recognizer. In *Proc.
            Int. Conf. on Acoustics, Speech, and Signal Processing (ICASSP)*, volume 1, pages
            577–580, San Francisco, CA (USA), 1992.

[SNE+93]   E.G. Schukat-Talamazzini, H. Niemann, W. Eckert, T. Kuhn, and S. Rieck. Auto-
            matic Speech Recognition without Phonemes. In *Proc. European Conf. on Speech
            Communication and Technology (Eurospeech)*, volume 1, pages 129–132, Berlin
            (Germany), 1993.

[SNH+05]   M. Schuster, E. Nöth, T. Haderlein, S. Steidl, A. Batliner, and F. Rosanowski. Can
            You Understand Him? Let's Look at His Word Accuracy – Automatic Evaluation
            of Tracheoesophageal Speech. In *Proc. Int. Conf. on Acoustics, Speech, and Signal
            Processing (ICASSP)*, volume I, pages 61–64, Philadelphia, PA (USA), 2005.

[Sør91]   H.B.D. Sørensen. A Cepstral Noise Reduction Multi-Layer Neural-Network. In
            Proc. Int. Conf. on Acoustics, Speech, and Signal Processing (ICASSP), volume 2,
            pages 933–936, Toronto (Canada), 1991.

[Spe04]   C. Spearman. The Proof and Measurement of Association between Two Things. *Am J Psychol*, 15(1):72–101, 1904.

[SRS+05]   M. Schuster, F. Rosanowski, R. Schwarz, U. Eysholdt, and J. Lohscheller. Quantitative Detection of the Substitute Voice Generator During Phonation in Patients Undergoing Laryngectomy. *Arch Otolaryngol Head Neck Surg*, 131(11):945–952, 2005.

[SS04]   A.J. Smola and B. Schölkopf. A Tutorial on Support Vector Regression. *Statistics and Computing*, 14(3):199–222, 2004.

[SSE+01]   M. Strome, J. Stein, R. Esclamado, D. Hicks, R.R. Lorenz, W. Braun, R. Yetman, I. Eliachar, and J. Mayes. Laryngeal Transplantation and 40-Month Follow-up. *N Engl J Med*, 344(22):1676–1679, comment 1712–1714, 2001.

[SSH+03]   S. Steidl, G. Stemmer, C. Hacker, E. Nöth, and H. Niemann. Improving Children's Speech Recognition by HMM Interpolation with an Adults' Speech Recognizer. In B. Michaelis and G. Krell, editors, *Pattern Recognition, 25th DAGM Symposium*, volume 2781 of *Lecture Notes in Computer Science*, pages 600–607, Berlin, Heidelberg, 2003. Springer.

[SSHN04]   S. Steidl, G. Stemmer, C. Hacker, and E. Nöth. Adaption in the Pronunciation Space for Non-Native Speech Recognition. In *Proc. Int. Conf. on Spoken Language Processing (ICSLP)*, volume IV, pages 2901–2904, Jeju Island (Rep. of Korea), 2004.

[SSN+02]   G. Stemmer, S. Steidl, E. Nöth, H. Niemann, and A. Batliner. Comparison and Combination of Confidence Measures. In P. Sojka, I. Kopeček, and K. Pala, editors, *Proc. Text, Speech and Dialogue; 5th Int. Conf., TSD 2002; Brno (Czech Republic)*, volume 2448 of *Lecture Notes in Artificial Intelligence LNCS/LNAI*, pages 181–188, Berlin (Germany), 2002. Springer.

[Sta81]   M. Staffieri. Phonatory neoglottis surgery. *Ear Nose Throat J*, 60(6):254–258, 1981.

[Ste01]   S. Steidl. Konfidenzbewertung von Worthypothesen. Student's thesis, Lehrstuhl für Mustererkennung (Chair for Pattern Recognition), Universität Erlangen–Nürnberg, Erlangen (Germany), 2001.

[Ste05]   G. Stemmer. *Modeling Variability in Speech Recognition*, volume 19 of *Studien zur Mustererkennung*. Logos Verlag, Berlin (Germany), 2005.

[Stu83]   A. Stuart. Kendall's tau. In S. Kotz and N.L. Johnson, editors, *Encyclopedia of Statistical Sciences*, volume 4, pages 367–369. John Wiley & Sons, New York, NY (USA), 1st edition, 1983.

[STW+06]   L.Q. Schwandt, H.-J. Tjong-Ayong, R. van Weissenbruch, H.C. van der Mei, and F.W.J. Albers. Differences in aerodynamic characteristics of new and dysfunctional Provox® 2 voice prostheses in vivo. *Eur Arch Otorhinolaryngol*, 263(6):518–523, 2006.

[SW72]   N.L. Sisty and B. Weinberg. Formant frequency characteristics of esophageal speech. *J Speech Hear Res*, 15(2):439–448, 1972.

[SZK06]   A. Sehr, M. Zeller, and W. Kellermann. Distant-talking Continuous Speech Recognition based on a novel Reverberation Model in the Feature Domain. In *Proc. Interspeech*, pages 769–772, Pittsburgh, PA (USA), 2006.

[SZNN01]   G. Stemmer, V. Zeißler, E. Nöth, and H. Niemann. Towards a Dynamic Adjustment of the Language Weight. In *Proc. Text, Speech and Dialogue; 4th Int. Conf., TSD 2001; Železná Ruda (Czech Republic)*, volume 2166 of *Lecture Notes in Artificial Intelligence*, pages 323–328, Berlin (Germany), 2001. Springer.

[Tau75]   S. Taub. Air bypass voice prosthesis for vocal rehabilitation of laryngectomees. *Ann Otol Rhinol Laryngol*, 84(1 Pt 1):45–48, 1975.

[TBS⁺06]   H. Toy, T. Bocklet, M. Schuster, U. Eysholdt, E. Nöth, and F. Rosanowski. Die tracheoösophageale Ersatzstimme: objektive Messung mit dem Göttinger Heiserkeitsdiagramm. In M. Gross and E. Kruse, editors, *Aktuelle phoniatrisch-pädaudiologische Aspekte 2006*, pages 54–55, Norderstedt (Germany), 2006. Book on Demand GmbH.

[Tit76]   I.R. Titze. On the mechanics of vocal-fold vibration. *J Acoust Soc Am*, 60(6):1366–1380, 1976.

[TKMA95]   M. Teraoka, M. Kinishi, M. Mohri, and M. Amatsu. Neoglottic articulatory adjustment in tracheoesophageal speech. *Larynx Japan*, 7:35–42, 1995.

[TLK93]   M. Tohyama, R.H. Lyon, and T. Koike. Source Waveform Recovery in a Reverberant Space by Cepstrum Dereverberation. In *Proc. Int. Conf. on Acoustics, Speech, and Signal Processing (ICASSP)*, volume I, pages 157–160, Minneapolis, MN (USA), 1993.

[TMF01]   M. van der Torn, H.F. Mahieu, and J.M. Festen. Aero-acoustics of silicone rubber lip reeds for alternative voice production in laryngectomees. *J Acoust Soc Am*, 110(5 Pt 1):2548–2559, 2001.

[TMP⁺84]   T. Todisco, M. Maurizi, G. Paludetti, M. Dottorini, and F. Merante. Laryngeal cancer: long-term follow-up of respiratory functions after laryngectomy. *Respiration*, 45(3):303–315, 1984.

[TQ90]   M.D. Trudeau and Y. Qi. Acoustic Characteristics of Female Tracheoesophageal Speech. *J Speech Hear Disord*, 55(2):244–250, 1990.

[TS72]   S. Taub and R.H. Spiro. Vocal rehabilitation of laryngectomees: Preliminary report of a new technique. *American Journal of Surgery*, 124(1):87–90, 1972.

[TS97]   I.R. Titze and B.H. Story. Acoustic interactions of the voice source with the lower vocal tract. *J Acoust Soc Am*, 101(4):2234–2243, 1997.

[TY99]   L. Thorpe and W. Yang. Performance of Current Perceptual Objective Speech
             Quality Measures. In *Proc. IEEE Workshop on Speech Coding*, pages 144–146,
             Porvoo (Finland), 1999.

[Ueb87]   J.S. Uebersax. Diversity of decision-making models and the measurement of inter-
             rater agreement. *Psychological Bulletin*, 101(1):140–146, 1987.

[USB03]   G. Uhlrich, D. Schuchardt, and H. Baesekow. Untersuchungen zum Einsatz von
             Mikrofonarrays in Verbindung mit Spracherkennungssystemen. In *Proc. Elektro-
             nische Sprachsignalverarbeitung (ESSV)*, pages 146–153, Karlsruhe (Germany),
             2003.

[VGS01]   G.J. Verkerke, A.A. Geertsema, and H.K. Schutte. Airflow resistance of airflow-
             regulating devices described by independent coefficients. *Ann Otol Rhinol Laryn-
             gol*, 110(7 Pt 1):639–645, 2001.

[Vit67]   A.J. Viterbi. Error Bounds for Convolutional Codes and an Asymptotically Opti-
             mum Decoding Algorithm. *IEEE Trans. on Information Theory*, IT-13(2):260–269,
             1967.

[Wah00]   W. Wahlster, editor. *Verbmobil: Foundations of Speech-to-Speech Translation*.
             Springer, Berlin (Germany), 2000.

[Wah06]   W. Wahlster, editor. *SmartKom: Foundations of Multimodal Dialogue Systems*.
             Springer, Berlin (Germany), 2006.

[War03]   V. Warnke. *Integrierte Segmentierung und Klassifikation von Äußerungen und Dia-
             logakten mit heterogenen Wissensquellen*, volume 9 of *Studien zur Mustererken-
             nung*. Logos Verlag, Berlin (Germany), 2003.

[WBJR94]   P.S. Wilson, F.J. Bruce-Lockhart, A.P. Johnson, and P.H. Rhys Evans. Speech
             restoration following total laryngo-pharyngectomy with free jejunal repair. *Clin
             Otolaryngol Allied Sci*, 19(2):145–148, 1994.

[WdM+00]   F.L. Wuyts, M.S. de Bodt, G. Molenberghs, M. Remacle, L. Heylen, B. Millet,
             K. van Lierde, J. Raes, and P.H. van de Heyning. The Dysphonia Severity In-
             dex: An Objective Measure of Vocal Quality Based on a Multiparameter Approach.
             J Speech Lang Hear Res, 43(3):796–809, 2000.

[Wei02]   R. Weiß. Anwendung von KNN zur Beseitigung der raumbedingten Störungen in
             einem Sprachsignal. Student's thesis, Lehrstuhl für Mustererkennung (Chair for
             Pattern Recognition), Universität Erlangen–Nürnberg, Erlangen (Germany), 2002.

[Wei05]   R. Weiß. Untersuchung zur Beseitigung von hallbedingten Störungen in der
             Spracherkennung. Technical report, Lehrstuhl für Mustererkennung (Chair for Pat-
             tern Recognition), Universität Erlangen–Nürnberg, Erlangen (Germany), 2005.

[WF05]   I.H. Witten and E. Frank. *Data Mining: Practical Machine Learning Tools and
             Techniques*. Morgan Kaufmann Series in Data Management Systems. Morgan
             Kaufmann Publishers, San Francisco, CA (USA), 2nd edition, 2005.

[WH96]   E.J. Wallen and J.H.L. Hansen. A Screening Test for Speech Pathology Assessment Using Objective Quality Measures. In *Proc. Int. Conf. on Spoken Language Processing (ICSLP)*, volume 2, pages 776–779, Philadelphia, PA (USA), 1996.

[WHBS82]   B. Weinberg, Y. Horii, E.D. Blom, and M.I. Singer. Airway resistance during esophageal phonation. *J Speech Hear Disord*, 47(2):194–199, 1982.

[WHO80]   International Classification of Impairments, Disabilities and Handicaps: A Manual of Classification Relating to the Consequences of Disease. World Health Organization, Geneva (Switzerland), 1980.

[WHO01]   International Classification of Functioning, Disability and Health. World Health Organization, Geneva (Switzerland), 2001.

[WJ96]   J.G. Wilpon and C.N. Jacobsen. A Study of Speech Recognition for Children and the Elderly. In *Proc. Int. Conf. on Acoustics, Speech, and Signal Processing (ICASSP)*, volume 1, pages 349–352, Atlanta, GA (USA), 1996.

[WKMG98]   S.-L. Wu, B.E.D. Kingsbury, N. Morgan, and S. Greenberg. Incorporating information from syllable-length time scales into automatic speech recognition. In *Proc. Int. Conf. on Acoustics, Speech, and Signal Processing (ICASSP)*, volume 2, pages 721–724, Seattle, WA (USA), 1998.

[WM95]   T.L. Watterson and S.C. McFarlane. The artificial larynx. *Semin Speech Lang*, 16(3):205–214, 1995.

[WP03]   W. Wokurek and M. Pützer. Automated Corpus Based Spectral Measurements of Voice Quality Parameters. In *Proc. Int. Congress of Phonetic Sciences (ICPhS)*, pages 2173–2176, Barcelona (Spain), 2003.

[WRM+85]   S.J. Wetmore, S.P. Ryan, J.C. Montague, K. Krueger, K. Wesson, R. Tirman, and W. Diner. Location of the vibratory segment in tracheoesophageal speakers. *Otolaryngol Head Neck Surg*, 93(3):355–361, 1985.

[WS92]   J.E. Ware and C.D. Sherbourne. The MOS 36-Item Short-Form Health Survey (SF-36®): I. conceptual framework and item selection. *Med Care*, 30(6):473–483, 1992.

[WW87]   S.E. Williams and J.B. Watson. Speaking proficiency variations according to method of alaryngeal voicing. *Laryngoscope*, 97(6):737–739, 1987.

[WWS92]   A. Wingfield, S.C. Wayland, and E.A. Stine. Adult age differences in the use of prosody for syntactic parsing and recall of spoken sentences. *Journal of Gerontology*, 47(5):P350–P356, 1992.

[YAD98]   B. Yegnanarayana, C. d'Alessandro, and V. Darsinos. An interactive algorithm for decomposition of speech signals into periodic and aperiodic components. *IEEE Trans. on Speech and Audio Processing*, 6(1):1–11, 1998.

[YSAN03]   H. Yamaguchi, R. Shrivastav, M.L. Andrews, and S. Niimi. A comparison of voice quality ratings made by Japanese and American listeners using the GRBAS scale. *Folia Phoniatr Logop*, 55(3):147–157, 2003.

[YSL05]   C. Yang, F.K. Soong, and T. Lee. Static and Dynamic Spectral Features: Their Noise Robustness and Optimal Weights for ASR. In *Proc. Int. Conf. on Acoustics, Speech, and Signal Processing (ICASSP)*, volume I, pages 241–244, Philadelphia, PA (USA), 2005.

[ZB92]   P. Zwirner and G.J. Barnes. Vocal tract steadiness: a measure of phonatory and upper airway motor control during phonation in dysarthria. *J Speech Hear Res*, 35(4):761–768, 1992.

[Zei01]   V. Zeißler. Verbesserte linguistische Gewichtung in einem Spracherkenner. Diploma thesis, Lehrstuhl für Mustererkennung (Chair for Pattern Recognition), Universität Erlangen–Nürnberg, Erlangen (Germany), 2001.

[Zei07]   V. Zeißler. Robuste Erkennung der prosodischen Phänomene und der emotionalen Benutzerzustände in einem multimodalen Dialogsystem. PhD thesis, Lehrstuhl für Mustererkennung (Chair for Pattern Recognition), Universität Erlangen–Nürnberg, Erlangen (Germany), 2007. To appear.

[Zel06]   M. Zeller. Automatic Speech Recognition Using a Reverberation Model in the Feature Domain. Diploma thesis, Chair of Multimedia Communications and Signal Processing, Universität Erlangen–Nürnberg, Erlangen (Germany), 2006.

[Zen86]   H.-P. Zenner. The postlaryngectomy telephone intelligibility test (PLTT). In I.F. Herrmann, editor, *Speech Restoration via Voice Prosthesis*, pages 148–152. Springer, Berlin, Heidelberg, 1986.

[Zen93]   H.-P. Zenner, editor. *Praktische Therapie von Hals-Nasen-Ohren-Krankheiten*. Schattauer, Stuttgart (Germany), 1993.

[ZMLS91]   R.J. Zijlstra, H.F. Mahieu, J.T. van Lith-Bijl, and H.K. Schutte. Aerodynamic properties of the low-resistance Groningen button. *Arch Otolaryngol Head Neck Surg*, 117(6):657–661, 1991.

[Zor06]   D. Zorn. Characterization of Speech Disorders Using the Sammon Transform. Diploma thesis, Lehrstuhl für Mustererkennung (Chair for Pattern Recognition), Universität Erlangen–Nürnberg, Erlangen (Germany), 2006.

[ZP86]   H.-P. Zenner and H. Pfrang. Ein einfacher Sprachverständlichkeitstest zur Beurteilung der Stimmrehabilitation des Laryngektomierten. *Laryngo-Rhino-Otologie*, 65(5):271–276, 1986.

Appendix A

Reading Material

A.1 The Text "The North Wind and the Sun"

The following text is the German "The North Wind and the Sun" text which was read by the test persons for this thesis. The wording equals the variant that is used in the Department of Phoniatrics and Pedaudiology at the University of Erlangen-Nuremberg. The version used for the *bas16* group (Chapter 4.5) of laryngeal speakers by the Bavarian Archive for Speech Signals [BAS] was slightly different as remarked in the footnotes.

Einst stritten sich Nordwind und Sonne, wer von ihnen beiden wohl der Stärkere wäre, als ein Wanderer, der in einen warmen Mantel gehüllt war, des Weges daher kam.[1] Sie wurden einig, daß derjenige für den Stärkeren gelten sollte, der den Wanderer zwingen würde, seinen Mantel auszuziehen.[2] Der Nordwind blies mit aller Macht, aber je mehr er blies, desto fester hüllte sich der Wanderer in seinen Mantel ein. Endlich gab der Nordwind den Kampf auf. Nun wärmte[3] die Sonne die Luft mit ihren freundlichen Strahlen, und schon nach wenigen Augenblicken zog der Wanderer seinen Mantel aus. Da mußte der Nordwind zugeben, daß die Sonne von ihnen beiden der Stärkere war.

The same text in machine-readable notation (words as in the recognizer dictionary) with segmental markers as defined in Table 7.16:

```
einst stritten sich IC2 Nordwind und Sonne SM2 wer von ihnen bei
den IC2 wohl der St"arkere w"are SC2 als ein Wanderer SC2 der in einen
warmen Mantel geh"ullt war SC2 des Weges daherkam SM3 sie wurden einig
SM2 da"s derjenige IC2 f"ur den St"arkeren gelten sollte SC2 der den
Wanderer IC2 zwingen w"urde SC2 seinen Mantel auszuziehen SM3 der
Nordwind IC2 blies mit aller Macht SM3 aber je mehr er blies SM2 desto
fester IC2 h"ullte sich der Wanderer IC2 in seinen Mantel ein SM3
endlich IC2 gab der Nordwind IC2 den Kampf auf SM3 nun w"armte die
Sonne IC2 die Luft IC2 mit ihren freundlichen Strahlen SM3 und schon
IC2 nach wenigen Augenblicken IC2 zog der Wanderer IC2 seinen Mantel
aus SM3 da mu"ste der Nordwind zugeben SM2 da"s die Sonne IC2 von
ihnen beiden IC2 der St"arkere war ;
```

---

[1]BAS version: "daherkam"
[2]BAS version: "abzunehmen"
[3]BAS version: "erwärmte"

A.2   The Reading Sheets for the PLTT

Figure A.1 and A.2 show a PLTT sheet to be read at the telephone (Chapter 7.4). As this version appeared to be impractical for the patients, a new version with bigger lettering was designed (Figure A.3). The text "The North Wind and the Sun" was read from a separate sheet then.

[Therapeut(in): Für das automatische Telefonsystem bitte UNBEDINGT die Bogennummer um die 5-stellige Patientennummer – mit führenden Nullen – ergänzen! Bogen mit Name und Alter ausgefüllt bitte zurück an ●●●●●●●●●●●●●●●●●●] Bogen erzeugt: 25. Oktober 2005 10:44

Name: _____   Alter (Jahre, Monate): _____

Bogennummer: _ _ _ _ _ 001

Sehr geehrte Patientin, sehr geehrter Patient,

bitte lesen Sie sich den folgenden Text einmal durch, bevor Sie anrufen, damit Sie mit dem Ablauf vertraut sind. Führen Sie dann die Anweisungen bitte genau aus. Vielen Dank für Ihre Mitarbeit.

Ihre Abteilung für Phoniatrie und Pädaudiologie des Universitätsklinikums Erlangen

---

1. *Rufen Sie bitte die Telefonnummer 09131 / ●●● ●●● ●● an.*

2. *Sie hören dann die Stimme des automatischen Aufnahmeprogramms. Hören Sie dieser Stimme bitte einfach zu. Wenn Sie dazu aufgefordert werden, geben Sie bitte über die Tasten Ihres Telefons die Bogennummer, die oben auf diesem Blatt zu finden ist, ein. Die Nummer wird dann noch einmal automatisch vorgelesen. Wenn die Nummer falsch ist, kann sie nochmals eingegeben werden. Wenn sie richtig ist, drücken Sie bitte die #-Taste („Rautetaste") an Ihrem Telefon.*

3. *Nun beginnt die Aufnahme. Wenn Sie dazu aufgefordert werden, sagen Sie bitte etwa zwei bis drei Sekunden lang*
   „aaah" .

4. *Warten Sie die nächste Ansage ab; lesen Sie danach folgenden Text vor:*

   Einst stritten sich Nordwind und Sonne, wer von ihnen beiden wohl der Stärkere wäre, als ein Wanderer, der in einen warmen Mantel gehüllt war, des Weges daherkam. Sie wurden einig, daß derjenige für den Stärkeren gelten sollte, der den Wanderer zwingen würde, seinen Mantel auszuziehen. Der Nordwind blies mit aller Macht, aber je mehr er blies, desto fester hüllte sich der Wanderer in seinen Mantel ein. Endlich gab der Nordwind den Kampf auf. Nun wärmte die Sonne die Luft mit ihren freundlichen Strahlen, und schon nach wenigen Augenblicken zog der Wanderer seinen Mantel aus. Da mußte der Nordwind zugeben, daß die Sonne von ihnen beiden der Stärkere war.

5. *Drücken Sie bitte die #-Taste („Rautetaste") an Ihrem Telefon.*   ⟹

1

Figure A.1: Original reading sheet for the PLTT (front side)

6. *Lesen Sie nach der nächsten Ansage bitte folgende Wörter und Sätze vor:*

**Haar, Scherz, Bild, Mord, Dolch, Nuß,
Wuchs, Glied, Zeit, Rost, Bahn, Bart,
Garn, Maus, Kreis, Wert, Blech, Stoß,
Schweiß, Reif, Fink, Wahl.**

**Doris will draußen Schnee fegen.
Öffnet doch gleich beide Türen!
Erste Stunde Deutsch, dann Englisch.
Darf ich Deine Schleife binden?
Vor'm Essen Deine Hände waschen!
Sonntags trinken viele Männer Bier.**

7. *Drücken Sie bitte die #-Taste („Rautetaste") an Ihrem Telefon. Das Aufnahmeprogramm verabschiedet sich von Ihnen, dann können Sie auflegen.*

2

Figure A.2: Original reading sheet for the PLTT (back side)

[Therapeut(in): Für das automatische Telefonsystem (09131 / ••• ••• ••) bitte UNBEDINGT die
Bogennummer um die 5-stellige Patientennummer – mit führenden Nullen – ergänzen!
Vor den Listen auf diesem Bogen gehaltenen Vokal („aaaaa“) und Nordwind-Text lesen lassen!
Bogen ausgefüllt bitte zurück an •••••••••••••••••••••••] Bogen erzeugt: 3. November 2005 10:12

Name, Vorname: _____   **Bogennummer:** _ _ _ _ _ 119

Geburtsdatum: _____   Aufnahmedatum: _____

Star, Tee, Dienst, Fink, Sekt, Schild,
Zelt, Wahl, Rang, Lohn, Stier, Haar,
Schaf, Blick, Busch, Pfeil, Lust, Floh,
Boot, Axt, Fall, Schreck.

Diese zarten Blumen welken rasch.

Diese Wohnung liegt zu hoch.

Nervöse Menschen brauchen viel Ruhe.

Diese Durchsage ist ohne Gewähr.

Mein Dackel pariert auf's Wort.

Wer weiß dort genau Bescheid?

Figure A.3: Second version of the reading sheet for the PLTT; the text "The North Wind and the Sun" ("Nordwind und Sonne") was now read from a separate sheet.

Appendix B

Human Evaluation Results

This appendix contains the human evaluation results for the *laryng41* data (see Chapter 4.4.3). For the abbreviations of the rating criteria, see Table 4.12.

file	quality					hoarse					effort				
	K	L	R	S	U	K	L	R	S	U	K	L	R	S	U
m000011s01	2	2	3	3	3	3	2	1	2	1	2	2	3	3	3
m000012s01	3	3	3	4	4	2	2	1	1	1	3	3	3	4	4
m000013s01	2	2	2	3	3	2	2	1	2	2	2	2	2	3	3
m000014s01	4	3	4	4	3	1	1	2	1	4	4	3	4	4	3
m000017s01	3	4	3	4	3	1	1	1	1	1	3	4	3	4	3
m000018s01	4	3	3	4	4	1	1	1	1	1	4	3	3	4	4
m000019s01	2	1	1	1	1	4	4	5	4	4	2	1	1	1	1
m000052s01	2	2	1	2	2	3	4	3	3	2	2	2	1	2	2
m000054s01	2	2	2	2	3	2	3	2	2	3	2	2	2	2	3
m000055s01	4	4	3	3	3	1	1	1	2	1	4	4	3	3	3
m000057s01	3	3	3	3	3	3	2	2	2	2	3	3	3	3	3
m000058s01	1	1	2	1	2	2	4	2	4	3	1	1	2	1	2
m000059s01	3	4	4	4	4	1	1	1	1	1	3	4	4	4	4
m000060s01	2	2	2	1	2	3	2	3	4	3	2	2	2	1	2
m000061s01	2	1	2	2	3	2	2	2	4	2	2	1	2	2	3
m000062s01	1	1	1	1	2	4	4	4	4	3	1	1	1	1	2
m000063s01	2	2	3	2	3	4	2	4	3	2	2	2	3	2	3
m000064s01	1	1	1	1	3	4	4	4	4	2	1	1	1	1	3
m000067s01	2	2	2	1	3	4	3	3	2	1	2	2	2	1	3
m000069s01	3	3	3	3	4	1	1	2	2	2	3	3	3	3	4
m000073s01	4	3	3	4	4	1	1	4	1	3	4	3	3	4	4
m000074s01	2	1	1	1	1	2	3	2	4	3	2	1	1	1	1
m000304s01	3	3	2	4	4	1	2	1	1	1	3	3	2	4	4
m000305s01	3	3	2	2	3	2	2	3	3	2	3	3	2	2	3
m000306s01	2	2	1	1	1	3	4	4	4	4	2	2	1	1	1
m000307s01	2	2	1	2	3	2	3	3	3	2	2	2	1	2	3
m000329s01	2	3	2	2	2	2	3	3	3	3	2	3	2	2	2
m000437s01	3	4	4	4	3	2	1	2	1	2	3	4	4	4	3
m000467s01	3	2	3	2	2	3	4	4	4	3	3	2	3	2	2
m000500s01	3	3	1	2	3	2	2	3	4	3	3	3	1	2	3
m000504s01	1	1	1	2	2	4	3	3	3	2	1	1	1	2	2
m000506s01	4	4	4	4	3	2	2	1	1	2	4	4	4	4	3
m000507s01	2	1	2	2	2	4	4	3	2	4	2	1	2	2	2
001257.nw-nah.01	3	2	2	2	2	2	2	4	3	2	3	2	2	2	2
001264.nw-nah.02	2	2	4	3	2	2	2	1	2	2	2	2	4	3	2
001265.nw-nah.01	4	2	4	3	3	1	1	1	2	2	4	2	4	3	3
001266.nw-nah.02	3	3	4	4	3	4	2	4	1	4	3	3	4	4	3
001274.nw-nah.01	3	1	1	1	2	4	4	5	4	2	3	1	1	1	2
001275.nw-nah.01	2	2	2	2	2	3	2	3	3	2	2	2	2	2	2
001279.nw-nah.01	3	3	2	2	2	2	3	3	3	2	3	3	2	2	2
001280.nw-nah.02	1	1	1	1	1	5	4	4	5	3	1	1	1	1	1

Table B.1: Evaluation results by 5 experts for the *laryng41* speaker group

file	penetr K	L	R	S	U	proso K	L	R	S	U	brsense K	L	R	S	U
m000011s01	3	2	4	4	2	2	3	4	4	2	2	3	3	3	3
m000012s01	4	3	3	5	3	3	4	4	4	4	4	4	3	2	5
m000013s01	2	2	2	3	3	2	3	2	2	2	2	2	2	1	3
m000014s01	4	4	4	5	4	4	3	4	5	4	2	3	4	4	5
m000017s01	3	3	2	4	2	4	3	4	4	2	4	4	4	4	4
m000018s01	4	2	3	4	4	3	3	4	4	4	4	3	4	2	3
m000019s01	3	3	4	2	3	2	2	1	2	2	2	2	2	1	2
m000052s01	3	3	2	2	3	3	2	1	1	2	3	1	2	1	2
m000054s01	2	2	2	3	4	2	3	2	3	3	2	2	4	2	4
m000055s01	5	3	3	4	3	4	4	4	4	4	2	3	4	3	4
m000057s01	3	2	3	2	3	3	3	5	4	4	4	4	4	3	5
m000058s01	3	2	2	2	3	2	1	2	3	2	1	1	2	1	3
m000059s01	4	4	5	5	4	4	4	5	4	4	4	5	5	3	5
m000060s01	2	2	1	1	3	3	3	3	2	3	3	2	3	1	4
m000061s01	2	2	2	3	3	3	2	3	2	3	2	2	3	3	2
m000062s01	2	2	2	2	4	1	1	2	1	2	1	1	2	1	2
m000063s01	3	3	3	3	3	3	2	3	2	4	3	2	3	2	4
m000064s01	2	2	3	2	2	3	2	3	3	4	3	2	4	1	4
m000067s01	2	2	3	2	3	2	2	3	3	4	2	3	3	1	3
m000069s01	3	2	3	2	3	3	3	4	4	4	4	3	4	3	4
m000073s01	3	3	4	4	3	3	3	2	3	4	2	3	2	3	4
m000074s01	2	2	2	3	2	2	1	2	2	2	2	1	2	2	2
m000304s01	4	2	2	3	3	2	3	4	3	4	4	2	3	1	4
m000305s01	4	2	4	2	3	3	3	4	2	4	4	4	4	3	5
m000306s01	3	3	2	3	3	2	2	1	1	2	3	2	1	1	2
m000307s01	3	2	2	3	3	2	2	3	3	2	2	1	2	1	3
m000329s01	3	4	3	3	4	4	3	4	3	3	3	2	4	3	3
m000437s01	4	4	4	5	5	3	4	4	4	3	3	3	4	2	4
m000467s01	4	4	5	4	2	3	3	2	2	2	3	1	2	1	1
m000500s01	3	3	3	3	3	3	3	1	2	2	3	2	1	2	2
m000504s01	3	3	3	3	3	3	2	2	3	2	1	1	2	2	2
m000506s01	4	5	4	4	4	4	4	4	4	4	4	4	4	4	5
m000507s01	3	3	3	3	2	2	2	2	3	2	2	1	3	1	2
001257.nw-nah.01	2	2	2	2	3	3	3	2	2	3	2	3	4	1	2
001264.nw-nah.02	3	2	3	3	3	3	3	4	4	3	3	3	4	2	2
001265.nw-nah.01	4	3	4	4	3	4	4	5	3	4	4	4	5	4	4
001266.nw-nah.02	4	4	4	5	4	4	3	4	4	4	4	4	5	4	4
001274.nw-nah.01	3	3	1	2	4	4	1	1	2	2	2	1	2	1	2
001275.nw-nah.01	2	4	4	3	3	2	3	4	3	3	2	2	4	2	4
001279.nw-nah.01	3	3	3	3	3	3	2	3	3	3	2	2	3	2	2
001280.nw-nah.02	1	2	2	1	2	1	2	1	1	2	2	1	3	2	2

Table B.2: Evaluation results by 5 experts for the *laryng41* speaker group (continued)

file	noise					tone					change				
	K	L	R	S	U	K	L	R	S	U	K	L	R	S	U
m000011s01	3	2	4	4	2	2	3	4	4	2	2	3	3	3	3
m000012s01	4	3	3	5	3	3	4	4	4	4	4	4	3	2	5
m000013s01	2	2	2	3	3	2	3	2	2	2	2	2	2	1	3
m000014s01	4	4	4	5	4	4	3	4	5	4	2	3	4	4	5
m000017s01	3	3	2	4	2	4	3	4	4	2	4	4	4	4	4
m000018s01	4	2	3	4	4	3	3	4	4	4	4	3	4	2	3
m000019s01	3	3	4	2	3	2	2	1	2	2	2	2	2	1	2
m000052s01	3	3	2	2	3	3	2	1	1	2	3	1	2	1	2
m000054s01	2	2	2	3	4	2	3	2	3	3	2	2	4	2	4
m000055s01	5	3	3	4	3	4	4	4	4	4	2	3	4	3	4
m000057s01	3	2	3	2	3	3	3	5	4	4	4	4	4	3	5
m000058s01	3	2	2	2	3	2	1	2	3	2	1	1	2	1	3
m000059s01	4	4	5	5	4	4	4	5	4	4	4	5	5	3	5
m000060s01	2	2	1	1	3	3	3	3	2	3	3	2	3	1	4
m000061s01	2	2	2	3	3	3	2	3	2	3	2	2	3	3	2
m000062s01	2	2	2	2	4	1	1	2	1	2	1	1	2	1	2
m000063s01	3	3	3	3	3	3	2	3	2	4	3	2	3	2	4
m000064s01	2	2	3	2	2	3	2	3	3	4	3	2	4	1	4
m000067s01	2	2	3	2	3	2	2	3	3	4	2	3	3	1	3
m000069s01	3	2	3	2	3	3	3	4	4	4	4	3	4	3	4
m000073s01	3	3	4	4	3	3	3	2	3	4	2	3	2	3	4
m000074s01	2	2	2	3	2	2	1	2	2	2	2	1	2	2	2
m000304s01	4	2	2	3	3	2	3	4	3	4	4	2	3	1	4
m000305s01	4	2	4	2	3	3	3	4	2	4	4	4	4	3	5
m000306s01	3	3	2	3	3	2	2	1	1	2	3	2	1	1	2
m000307s01	3	2	2	3	3	2	2	3	3	2	2	1	2	1	3
m000329s01	3	4	3	3	4	4	3	4	3	3	3	2	4	3	3
m000437s01	4	4	4	5	5	3	4	4	4	3	3	3	4	2	4
m000467s01	4	4	5	4	2	3	3	2	2	2	3	1	2	1	1
m000500s01	3	3	3	3	3	3	3	1	2	2	3	2	1	2	2
m000504s01	3	3	3	3	3	3	2	2	3	2	1	1	2	2	2
m000506s01	4	5	4	4	4	4	4	4	4	4	4	4	4	4	5
m000507s01	3	3	3	3	2	2	2	2	3	2	2	1	3	1	2
001257.nw-nah.01	2	2	2	2	3	3	3	2	2	3	2	3	4	1	2
001264.nw-nah.02	3	2	3	3	3	3	3	4	4	3	3	3	4	2	2
001265.nw-nah.01	4	3	4	4	3	4	4	5	3	4	4	4	5	4	4
001266.nw-nah.02	4	4	4	5	4	4	3	4	4	4	4	4	5	4	4
001274.nw-nah.01	3	3	1	2	4	4	1	1	2	2	2	1	2	1	2
001275.nw-nah.01	2	4	4	3	3	2	3	4	3	3	2	2	4	2	4
001279.nw-nah.01	3	3	3	3	3	3	2	3	3	3	2	2	3	2	2
001280.nw-nah.02	1	2	2	1	2	1	2	1	1	2	2	1	3	2	2

Table B.3: Evaluation results by 5 experts for the *laryng41* speaker group (continued)

file	intell					overall				
	K	L	R	S	U	K	L	R	S	U
m000011s01	2	2	3	4	4	4.4	3.0	4.8	8.0	6.2
m000012s01	3	4	4	5	5	6.1	8.0	6.7	9.4	8.0
m000013s01	2	2	2	3	3	3.2	3.6	2.7	5.5	5.3
m000014s01	4	4	4	5	4	8.0	7.8	7.6	9.6	7.9
m000017s01	4	3	2	5	4	7.2	8.5	7.4	9.5	5.8
m000018s01	3	3	4	5	5	7.5	8.5	7.7	8.0	8.2
m000019s01	2	1	2	1	2	2.2	0.5	1.6	0.5	1.8
m000052s01	2	2	1	2	3	2.8	2.3	1.5	3.1	2.3
m000054s01	2	2	2	2	3	2.5	3.1	2.5	4.6	5.4
m000055s01	3	3	4	4	3	7.9	6.6	6.5	8.6	5.8
m000057s01	3	3	2	3	3	5.3	7.0	3.8	6.1	5.7
m000058s01	1	1	2	2	3	1.8	0.5	2.8	2.6	4.8
m000059s01	3	4	4	5	4	6.5	10.0	7.5	9.6	8.2
m000060s01	2	2	2	1	2	4.9	2.7	2.5	1.8	5.7
m000061s01	2	2	1	2	2	3.5	1.5	3.2	2.9	5.0
m000062s01	1	1	1	1	2	1.1	1.1	1.9	0.0	3.4
m000063s01	2	2	1	2	3	4.9	3.0	4.0	2.8	4.8
m000064s01	2	1	2	1	3	4.2	1.9	3.1	1.7	6.1
m000067s01	1	2	1	1	2	1.9	2.5	2.9	2.5	5.0
m000069s01	3	3	3	3	4	6.4	6.8	5.5	6.2	8.4
m000073s01	3	3	2	4	4	6.6	7.0	5.6	8.2	8.5
m000074s01	2	1	1	1	2	3.3	1.1	1.1	1.6	3.4
m000304s01	3	3	2	4	4	5.6	6.6	4.2	7.9	7.7
m000305s01	4	3	4	2	3	7.1	7.5	6.6	5.0	6.3
m000306s01	2	2	1	1	2	3.9	2.8	1.6	1.6	3.2
m000307s01	2	2	1	2	2	4.0	2.6	2.1	3.4	5.5
m000329s01	2	3	2	3	3	5.0	5.2	3.6	5.0	4.5
m000437s01	3	4	4	5	4	6.9	8.6	7.5	8.5	6.0
m000467s01	2	2	2	2	2	4.0	3.2	7.0	3.0	3.3
m000500s01	2	3	1	2	2	5.0	6.9	1.0	4.8	5.4
m000504s01	1	1	1	2	2	1.5	1.2	2.3	2.8	2.5
m000506s01	5	5	4	5	5	8.5	9.8	6.6	9.5	8.1
m000507s01	1	2	1	2	2	1.5	1.9	2.5	5.2	5.1
001257.nw-nah.01	2	2	2	2	2	2.1	4.1	2.0	2.6	4.2
001264.nw-nah.02	2	2	1	3	2	5.0	3.8	1.8	5.5	3.7
001265.nw-nah.01	3	2	2	3	4	5.5	4.1	7.0	6.6	7.0
001266.nw-nah.02	3	4	3	4	2	7.1	7.3	5.3	9.4	6.4
001274.nw-nah.01	2	2	2	1	3	4.5	0.9	1.2	1.0	3.5
001275.nw-nah.01	1	2	2	2	3	1.4	2.7	2.9	1.9	5.7
001279.nw-nah.01	2	3	2	3	3	5.3	6.8	3.5	4.7	5.5
001280.nw-nah.02	1	1	1	1	1	0.8	1.0	0.3	0.1	2.2

Table B.4: Evaluation results by 5 experts for the *laryng41* speaker group (continued)

Appendix C

Recognition Results for Gaussianized Features

This appendix contains the detailed recognition results for the EMBASSI-based recognizers with gaussianized features derived from MFCC. The description of the experiments and the results for MFCC can be found in Chapter 6.2.5.

Table C.1, C.2 and C.3 contain the recognition results for the gaussianized Root Cepstrum Coefficients. Table C.4, C.5 and C.6 give an overview about the results on gaussianized μ-law features vs. gaussianized MFCC.

EMB-base, root cepstrum features (gaussianized)								
mic. dist.	lang. model	$n=4$	$n=5$	$n=6$	$n=7$	$n=8$	$n=9$	MFCC
close-talk	4-gram	89.1	91.9	93.9	94.0	**94.5**	94.2	94.3
close-talk	0-gram	44.2	55.3	63.4	66.6	66.3	64.7	**66.8**
1 m	4-gram	73.9	85.6	89.6	89.4	89.0	87.1	**90.1**
1 m	0-gram	23.3	36.9	46.9	48.3	47.0	45.1	**49.4**
2.5 m	4-gram	62.3	72.8	78.6	78.1	78.7	79.4	**83.4**
2.5 m	0-gram	17.8	21.5	29.5	27.3	31.1	32.5	**36.3**

Table C.1: Word accuracy for *EMB-base* recognizers (root cepstrum features, gaussianized) with different root parameters n on test data with different microphone distances; the best results in each line are printed in boldface.

EMB-12, root cepstrum features (gaussianized)								
mic. dist.	lang. model	$n=4$	$n=5$	$n=6$	$n=7$	$n=8$	$n=9$	MFCC
close-talk	4-gram	87.4	90.8	91.3	91.1	90.2	90.3	**91.4**
close-talk	0-gram	42.9	48.2	51.2	53.7	53.5	54.5	**56.0**
1 m	4-gram	80.5	87.2	90.7	91.2	91.7	90.5	**93.5**
1 m	0-gram	36.9	47.5	52.6	55.2	55.3	56.8	**57.6**
2.5 m	4-gram	73.8	83.3	87.1	87.1	85.6	86.5	**88.3**
2.5 m	0-gram	28.6	39.1	43.8	47.8	48.7	**49.9**	49.0

Table C.2: Word accuracy for *EMB-12* recognizers (root cepstrum features, gaussianized) with different root parameters n on test data with different microphone distances; the best results in each line are printed in boldface.

EMB-2, root cepstrum features (gaussianized)								
mic. dist.	lang. model	$n=4$	$n=5$	$n=6$	$n=7$	$n=8$	$n=9$	MFCC
close-talk	4-gram	89.2	93.9	93.9	**94.7**	94.2	93.6	94.5
close-talk	0-gram	46.6	64.2	65.8	67.1	66.9	65.2	**69.1**
1 m	4-gram	78.9	87.7	92.7	93.1	**94.1**	92.6	93.8
1 m	0-gram	32.7	50.6	57.6	57.3	**59.1**	56.3	58.8
2.5 m	4-gram	71.6	83.7	86.3	87.4	86.9	86.7	**87.9**
2.5 m	0-gram	25.0	39.5	44.6	47.3	47.7	47.7	**50.4**

Table C.3: Word accuracy for *EMB-2* recognizers (root cepstrum features, gaussianized) with different root parameters n on test data with different microphone distances; the best results in each line are printed in boldface.

EMB-base, μ-law features (gaussianized)								
mic. dist.	lang. model	$\mu = 10^4$	$\mu = 10^5$	$\mu = 10^6$	$\mu = 10^7$	$\mu = 10^8$	$\mu = 10^9$	MFCC
close-talk	4-gram	94.0	94.2	93.8	94.0	93.9	**94.3**	**94.3**
close-talk	0-gram	**68.2**	68.1	67.3	**68.2**	66.9	67.1	66.8
1 m	4-gram	89.7	89.0	90.5	90.7	**90.9**	**90.9**	90.1
1 m	0-gram	**51.8**	49.5	50.8	49.9	50.5	50.9	49.4
2.5 m	4-gram	84.2	83.3	84.0	84.2	85.7	**86.3**	83.4
2.5 m	0-gram	37.4	36.9	36.1	35.2	37.8	**38.0**	36.3

Table C.4: Word accuracy for *EMB-base* recognizers (μ-law features, gaussianized) with different values for μ on test data with different microphone distances; the best results in each line are printed in boldface.

EMB-12, μ-law features (gaussianized)								
mic. dist.	lang. model	$\mu = 10^4$	$\mu = 10^5$	$\mu = 10^6$	$\mu = 10^7$	$\mu = 10^8$	$\mu = 10^9$	MFCC
close-talk	4-gram	91.4	**91.6**	90.9	91.1	91.2	91.3	91.4
close-talk	0-gram	53.8	55.4	54.3	54.4	55.0	54.3	**56.0**
1 m	4-gram	93.3	92.6	92.9	92.7	92.5	**93.5**	**93.5**
1 m	0-gram	57.4	56.8	56.2	56.8	56.7	56.0	**57.6**
2.5 m	4-gram	86.5	87.7	86.5	87.2	86.3	85.8	**88.3**
2.5 m	0-gram	47.7	**49.9**	48.6	49.0	49.0	48.7	49.0

Table C.5: Word accuracy for *EMB-12* recognizers (μ-law features, gaussianized) with different values for μ on test data with different microphone distances; the best results in each line are printed in boldface.

EMB-2, μ-law features (gaussianized)								
mic. dist.	lang. model	$\mu = 10^4$	$\mu = 10^5$	$\mu = 10^6$	$\mu = 10^7$	$\mu = 10^8$	$\mu = 10^9$	MFCC
close-talk	4-gram	94.8	94.5	94.5	94.3	94.4	**95.1**	94.5
close-talk	0-gram	67.5	68.1	68.3	68.1	68.3	**69.2**	69.1
1 m	4-gram	**94.0**	93.8	93.7	93.3	93.4	93.3	93.8
1 m	0-gram	57.6	58.0	59.4	59.7	**59.8**	59.6	58.8
2.5 m	4-gram	87.0	87.7	87.4	**88.3**	86.9	87.0	87.9
2.5 m	0-gram	49.2	50.3	49.1	50.0	49.9	50.0	**50.4**

Table C.6: Word accuracy for *EMB-2* recognizers (μ-law features, gaussianized) with different values for μ on test data with different microphone distances; the best results in each line are printed in boldface.

Appendix D

Evaluation Environment for Voice Analysis

This chapter describes how to perform automatic speech evaluation with the programs written for this thesis. The recognition and evaluation environment is installed in a root directory with an arbitrary name. The full path of this root directory has to be announced to the Linux shell by assigning it to the environment variable $MSPBASE.[1] A *tcsh* shell is recommended for working. The $MSPBASE directory contains the following subdirectories:

- Evaluation: The programs for the statistical evaluation are located here (see Appendix D.3).

- Perl5lib: It contains the Perl library for the Perl scripts. The shell variable $PERL5LIB might have to be set to this directory.

- Projects: The data to be evaluated have to be stored here (see Appendix D.1 for details).

- Recognizers: The speech recognizers for the automatic recognition are stored here (see Appendix D.2).

D.1   The Projects Directory

First, the data to be analyzed must be provided. For each group of recordings, a different project name *<project>* can be assigned. The following steps have to be performed by the user then:

1. Create a new directory $MSPBASE/Projects/*<project>*.

2. Copy the audio files in raw format (no headers) to the directory
   $MSPBASE/Projects/*<project>*/DATA/SSG/.
   The DATA directory will later contain the feature files computed by the speech recognizers in a subdirectory called UFV (see Appendix D.3.1).

3. Provide a file called *<project>*.list containing the file names of the audio files without path. Store this file in the project directory.

4. A file *<project>*.textref must contain the text reference for the audio files, i.e. the text the readers should read. The format of the file must be like the transliterations (see below) for

---

[1]"MSP" stands for "Medical Speech Processing".

the recognition system of the Chair of Pattern Recognition, Erlangen. This means that for each recording one single line must be given containing the file name, a tabulator sign as delimiter, and the text terminated by a semicolon. Be aware that the words of the text have to be written exactly as in the vocabulary list of the particular recognizer. Otherwise too many "recognition errors" will occur. Punctuation in the text is not permitted.

5. Another essential file is the transliteration of the audio files, i.e the text the readers really uttered. It can differ from the text reference they actually should read (see above). This file is called *<project>*.trl.

These files allow recognition experiments already (see Chapter 7.1). For the computation of the human-machine correlation, some more files are needed. When the audio files were evaluated by a group of raters, a rater group name *<raters>* can be defined.

- In the file *<project>.<raters>*.scores, the evaluation of the sound files by the raters is stored. For each evaluation of one file by one rater, one line is specified. The first entry of this line must be the rater ID and the second the file name. After that an arbitrary number of numerical scores may follow. Two entries are usually separated by a comma. Spaces as delimiters may also be tolerated by many evaluation scripts, but it is recommended to use commas.

- The optional file *<project>.<raters>*.crits contains descriptions for the entries of the score file. These might be the names of the rating criteria, for instance. Each criterion name gets one line in the criteria file. Remember that the first two entries in the scores file are the rater ID and the name of the audio file.

Additional files may be provided in the project directory for different purposes:

- *<project>*.segments contains segmental information of the read texts following the definitions in [BKK+98] (see also Chapter 7.3.4).

- For the prosodic analysis, a configuration file with an arbitrary name, e.g. prosconfig95+G, can be located in this directory. It contains the parameters for compute_merkmale which is called by prosfeat.pl (see Appendix D.3.5).

D.2   The Recognizers Directory

The evaluation scripts search for the speech recognizers in the Recognizers directory. Like each "project", each recognizer gets a name *<recognizer>* for its identification. The recognizer itself is then stored in the directory $MSPBASE/Recognizers/*<recognizer>*/. The essential files there are defined by the local configuration file rcfile.*<lang.mod.>*.ufv where *<lang.mod.>* is a code for the language model of the recognizer, e.g. "uni" for a unigram model. This code can be arbitrarily chosen. The ".ufv" suffix denotes that UFV feature files are used for recognition. The "rcfile" defines the names of 5 files that must be available in the recognizer directory by the parameters File_Sprachmodell, File_HMM-Parameter, File_Orthographie_Lexikon, File_Gausseq_parameter, File_Polygramm. Further essential files in this directory are:

- fex4param: It must contain the parameters of the fex4 call which was also used for feature extraction during the recognizer training. These parameters will be used by recog.pl (see Appendix D.3.1) for the feature extraction of the test data.

- mean.start: It contains a pre-computed average feature vector that will also be used during feature extraction of the test data.

Essential subdirectories (or links to similar directories) in this directory are:

- Perl5lib: It is usually a symbolic link to the Perl library in the Projects directory (see Appendix D.1).

- bin: Here are the programs that are necessary for recognition.

D.3 The Evaluation Directory

The Evaluation directory is the location of the scripts for the speech recognition and statistical evaluation of the results. They can be found in the Scripts subdirectory. In the Prosody subdirectory, the configuration files and programs of the prosody module (Appendix D.3.5) are stored.

The evaluation of some test data (when prepared following Appendix D.1) is described in the following sections. Note that all script calls were tested while the Evaluation directory was the working directory. They should work, however, anywhere else without any difference. For more details concerning the usage, see the synopsis of the respective scripts.

D.3.1 Automatic Speech Recognition

The speech recognition on the test audio files is the first step of the evaluation of human-machine correlation. It is done by

recog.pl *<project>* *<recognizer>* *<lang.mod.>*

and evaluates the results versus a transliteration (TRL) and a text reference file (Appendix D.1). All files are searched for in the file tree defined by the $MSPBASE shell variable. The script computes the features of the audio files for the given recognizer and writes them to
$MSPBASE/Projects/*<project>*/DATA/UFV/*<recognizer>*/ ,
further on called "results directory". The recognition results are written to
$MSPBASE/Projects/*<project>*/Results/.
The following files are created there:

- *<project>*.*<recognizer>*.*<lang.mod.>*.result:
recognized word sequence for all audio files of the *<project>*

- *<project>*.*<recognizer>*.*<lang.mod.>*.listresult:
file ID and recognized word sequence for all audio files of the *<project>*

- *<project>*.*<recognizer>*.*<lang.mod.>*.prot:
protocol of the recognizer run

- *<project>*.ref:
  it is equal to the transliteration file *<project>*.trl in the *<project>* directory, without
  file IDs, however

- *<project>*.*<recognizer>*.*<lang.mod.>*.evalseg:
  the total word accuracy (WA) for the *<project>*, evaluated by the given *<recognizer>*

- *<project>*.*<recognizer>*.*<lang.mod.>*.result.wa:
  single word accuracies for each file of *<project>*, evaluated by the given *<recognizer>*

- *<project>*.*<recognizer>*.*<lang.mod.>*.result.listwa:
  the file IDs and single word accuracies (WA) for each file of *<project>*, evaluated by the
  given *<recognizer>*

If the files concerning the word accuracy have the infix "textref", then they were computed against
the text reference, not against the transliteration of the speech data. Both result files are created
automatically at the same time.

D.3.2   Correlation between a Recognizer and Human Raters

The correlation for a *<project>* between the word accuracy of a given *<recognizer>* and a group
of *<raters>* is computed in this way:

doc-rec_all.pl *<project>* *<recognizer>* *<lang.mod.>* *<raters>* *<rater_list>*
                <integer_boundaries> *<max_categ>*

The *<raters>* define the file with the human ratings, i.e. this is the part of a file name (see
Appendix D.1) in the *<project>* directory. The *<rater_list>* is a list of rater IDs in that file.
In this way, it is possible to compute the correlation for one single rater only or for the average
of more than one rater. The "all" in the script name means that the computation is made for all
rating criteria. The results are stored in the results directory in the file

<project>.*<recognizer>*.*<lang.mod.>*.*<raters>*.*<rater_list>*.corr

where the single raters of *<rater_list>* are separated by dashes. The file contains the correlation
between the word accuracy and *<rater_list>*'s score for the current criterion, the weighted multi-
rater κ by Davies and Fleiss (see Chapter 3.2.3) and optionally Krippendorff's α (switch -a;
see Chapter 3.3). The *<integer_boundaries>* are a list of numbers denoting which interval of
the float-range word accuracy is converted to which integer score. The highest integer number
occurring in the study has to be specified as *<max_categ>*.

   The result file gets the infix "textref" when the word accuracy was computed with the text
reference instead of the transliteration. Both files are created automatically at the same time.

D.3.3   Correlation among Human Raters

The correlation within a rater group can be computed like this:

doc-doc_run.pl *<project>* *<raters>* *<rater_list>* *<max_categ>*

Like in the previous section, the *<raters>* define the file where the human ratings are stored,
i.e. this is the part of a file name. The *<rater_list>* is a list of rater IDs in that file. Thus it is possible to compute the inter-rater correlation for a selected group of raters from the rating file. This

particular script computes the inter-rater correlation and κ values for rater pairs in *<rater_list>*, for one rater vs. all the others, and κ for the entire *<rater_list>*. It does this for all rating criteria. The results are stored in the results directory in the files

   <project>.<raters>.<rater_list_1st_part>-<rater_list_2nd_part>.corr

where the single raters of the parts of *<rater_list>* are separated by underscores. The respective file contains the correlation between the mentioned parts of *<rater_list>* for the current criterion, the weighted multi-rater κ by Davies and Fleiss (see Chapter 3.2.3) and optionally Krippendorff's α (switch -a; see Chapter 3.3). The highest integer score number occurring in the study has to be specified as *<max_categ>*.

D.3.4   Computing "Word Hypotheses Graphs" (WHGs)

The "word hypotheses graphs" (WHGs, see Chapter 5.5.2) contain – in contrast to the usual recognizer output – also the time information at which timestamp which word was assumed to occur in the speech file. They are created by forced time alignment, i.e. the word sequence is a priori known and has to be mapped to the speech file. The WHGs are necessary for the computation of prosodic features (Appendix D.3.5) and time statistics (Appendix D.3.6).

   alignlst.pl *<project> <recognizer> <apn_file> <cch_file> <mean_file>*

does the WHG computation by using the acoustic-phonetical network (*<apn_file>*) and codebook (*<cch_file>*) of a given *<recognizer>*. Both files are expected to be located in the directory of the *<recognizer>*. A *<mean_file>* with a mean feature vector for initialization is also needed. The relative path from $MSPBASE on has to be specified for this file; usually it will be
   Recognizers/*<recognizer>*/mean.start .
The WHGs are written to
   $MSPBASE/Projects/*<project>*/Results/WHG/*<recognizer>*/
for the case of alignment with the transliteration of the audio files and to
   $MSPBASE/Projects/*<project>*/Results/WHG/*<recognizer>*.textref/
for the case of alignment with the text reference. They have the same file name as the original audio files.

   Note: Words in the text reference or transliteration that are not in the recognizer's vocabulary will cause errors!

D.3.5   Computing Prosodic Features

The prosodic features are computed in two steps. First the basic features are created:

   prosbase.pl *<project>*

This has to be repeated in order to get also period-base timestamps instead of F_0 values:

   prosbase.pl -p *<project>*

In the results directory of *<project>*, another subdirectory called Prosody is created. All prosodic features are stored there. The second step is the creation of the final features:

   prosfeat.pl *<project> <recognizer> <config_file>*

They are written to
   $MSPBASE/Projects/*<project>*/Results/Prosody/Prosfeat/*<recognizer>*/*<config_file>*/ .

English name	German name	English name	German name
Pause–beforeWord	PausenStilleVorWort	EnMaxWord	EnergieMaxWort
Pause–afterWord	PausenStilleNachWort	EnMeanWord	EnergieMittelWort
PauseFill-beforeWord	PausenGefuellteVorWort	F0RegCoeffWord	F0RegKoeffWort
PauseFill-afterWord	PausenGefuellteNachWort	F0MseRegWord	F0MseRegWort
DurNormWord	DauerLenNormWort	F0MaxWord	F0MaxWort
DurAbsWord	DauerLenAbsWort	F0MinWord	F0MinWort
DurAbsSylWord	DauerLenAbsSilbeWort	F0MeanWord	F0MittelWort
DurTauLocWord	DauerTauLenLokalWort	F0OnWord	F0OnsetWort
EnRegCoeffWord	EnergieRegKoeffWort	F0OffWord	F0OffsetWort
EnMseRegWord	EnergieMseRegWort	F0OnPosWord	F0OnsetPosWort
EnTauLocWord	EnergieTauEneLokalWort	F0OffPosWord	F0OffsetPosWort
EnNormWord	EnergieEneNormWort	F0MinPosWord	F0MinPosWort
EnAbsWord	EnergieEneAbsWort	F0MaxPosWord	F0MaxPosWort
EnMaxPosWord	EnergieMaxPosWort	F0MeanGWord	F0MittelGlobalWort

Table D.1: List of all local prosodic features in English and German (original name in the prosody module)

The <config_file> is expected to be in the home directory of the project (see Appendix D.1). The script prosfeat.pl uses the text reference of the audio files only. The use of the transliteration can be forced by the option -t.

Note: In both cases the features will be written to the same directory, i.e. a new call will overwrite older results!

Table D.1 and Table D.2 show the feature names used in this thesis and the original German names from the prosody module for local and global prosodic features, respectively.

D.3.6   Further Evaluation Scripts

The following scripts are available in $MSPBASE/Evaluation/Scripts/, but they are not fully integrated in the evaluation environment. This means that that their command line parameters are not simply a <project> or <recognizer> name, but a full path to the respective files or directories. On the other hand, this allows their use for computations outside the environment. For more details, see the synopsis of the respective scripts (sometimes option -h is necessary to display it). Table D.3 contains the number codes and abbreviations for the rating criteria that were used during the experiments for Chapter 7. The codes are needed as parameters for some of the scripts.

For word and pause statistics:

- pausstat.pl: counts non-verbals and pauses in recognizer output or transliteration (TRL)

- segxtrct.pl: takes a list of files created by whgvsseg.pl and computes new statistical time measures from these files

- whgvsseg.pl: compares pauses in WHG to reference text segmentation with prosodic markers

English name	German name
MeanJitter	Mittelwert_jitter
StandDevJitter	Streuung_jitter
MeanShimmer	Mittelwert_shimmer
StandDevShimmer	Streuung_shimmer
#+Voiced	Anzahl_SH_Bereiche
#−Voiced	Anzahl_SL_Bereiche
Dur+Voiced	Laenge_SH_Bereiche
Dur−Voiced	Laenge_SL_Bereiche
DurMax+Voiced	Max_Laenge_SH_Bereich
DurMax−Voiced	Max_Laenge_SL_Bereich
RelNum+/−Voiced	Verhaeltnis_Anz_SH_SL_Bereiche
RelDur+/−Voiced	Verhaeltnis_Laenge_SH_SL
RelDur+Voiced/Sig	Verhaeltnis_Laenge_SH_Laenge_Signal
RelDur−Voiced/Sig	Verhaeltnis_Laenge_SL_Laenge_Signal
StandDevF0	Standartabweichung_F0

Table D.2: List of all global prosodic features in English and German (original name in the prosody module; the 't' in "Standartabweichung" is a historical spelling error)

- whgvsseg_all.pl: computes the number and duration of wanted and unwanted pauses in the WHGs for a given file list

- wordpaus.pl: pause and word statistics from WHG files

- wordSyllPm.pl: syllable and word statistics for audio files

For prosodic analysis:

- pros-crit_all.pl: correlation between human rating and prosodic features

- prosname.pl: adds prosodic feature names to "anonymous" files with correlation values

Statistic measures:

- alphkrip.pl: front-end for Krippendorff's alpha computation (see Chapter 3.3)

- kappflei.pl: computes multi-rater κ according to Davies and Fleiss (see Chapter 3.2.4)

- makeFeatStat.pl: computes histograms

Tools for basic data manipulation and evaluation:

- doc-crit.pl: computes the correlation between the integer scores for different criteria from a group of <*raters*>

no.	criterion	abbreviation	German abbrev.
2	quality of the substitute voice	quality	1
3	hoarseness	hoarse	Rau
4	speech effort	effort	Anstr
5	voice penetration	penetr	Durchdr
6	prosody	proso	Proso
7	match of breath and sense units	brsense	Atemsinn
8	distortions by insufficient occlusion of tracheostoma	noise	Stör
9	vocal tone	tone	Klang
10	change of voice quality during reading	change	Änderung
11	overall intelligibility	intell	Verst
12	overall quality score	overall	Gesamt

Table D.3: Rating criteria for tracheoesophageal voices and their abbreviations in the text and in the original clinics data; the first column contains the internal numbers assigned to the criteria in the program environment (0 and 1 are reserved for rater and file name, respectively).

- doc-doc.pl: combines two files with raters' judgments for later analysis of intra- or inter-rater correlation;
  Note: It extracts **all** entries that were evaluated by both specified raters or rater groups, i.e. it should be applied with care to judgment files that contain more than the desired speaker group.

- doc-doc_all.pl: takes two files with raters' judgments and computes correlation, weighted κ, and Krippendorff's α for corresponding criteria between two lists of raters

- doc-rec.pl: combines raters' judgments and word accuracies for later computation of correlation, etc.

- docxtrct.pl: extracts given criteria for given files from a file with raters' judgments

- rank.pl: takes a file with two numerical columns and converts the entries to their respective rank within the column (needed for Spearman's ρ; see Chapter 3.1)

- wa2score.pl: converts word accuracies (or similar values) to integer scores according to given conversion intervals

- whgvsf0.pl: computes wordwise F_0 values from framewise F_0 values

- whgvsf0_all.pl: computes wordwise F_0 values from framewise F_0 values for a list of files

Appendix E

German Translation of Introduction and Summary

E.1 Titel

Automatische Bewertung tracheoösophagealer Ersatzstimmen

E.2 Inhaltsverzeichnis

E.3 Einleitung

In 20 bis 40 Prozent aller Fälle von Kehlkopfkrebs muss eine totale Laryngektomie, d.h. die Entfernung des gesamten Kehlkopfes, durchgeführt werden [TMF01]. Für den Patienten bedeutet dies den Verlust der natürlichen Stimme und damit auch des wichtigsten Kommunikationsträgers. Für alle betroffenen Personen stellt dies ein herausragendes Stigma dar [DSK94]. In Abhängigkeit von der onkologischen Therapie können verschiedene Methoden der Stimmrehabilitation angewandt werden. Einige davon bedienen sich selten verwendeter chirurgischer Methoden, der ösophagealen Stimme und elektrischer Hilfsmittel. Neben diesen ist die Verwendung sog. Shunt-Ventile („Stimmprothesen") zur Anbahnung einer Ersatzstimme in den USA und auch in Deutschland in den letzten 25 Jahren immer beliebter geworden; für Deutschland war dabei eine Verzögerung um etwa ein Jahrzehnt zu beobachten [AS92, HAA$^+$90, Rob84].

Gegenwärtig wird die Stimmrehabilitation mit Shunt-Ventilen als Stand der Technik betrachtet [BHIB03, Blo00]. Doch obwohl die Sprachrehabilitation grundlegend verbessert wurde, bleiben weitere Probleme mit der Laryngektomie verbunden, wie der Verlust der nasalen Funktion (Riechen, Anfeuchtung des Luftstroms), schwacher Hustenstoß, Schluckbeschwerden und Veränderungen der Lungenfunktion. Nach dem Einsetzen des Shunt-Ventils müssen die Patienten eine Therapie durchlaufen, um wieder sprechen zu lernen. Von Zeit zu Zeit wird die Ersatzstimme durch den Therapeuten evaluiert, um den Behandlungsfortschritt zu dokumentieren. Diese Arbeit stellt Methoden für die objektive, automatische Stimm- und Sprachevaluierung vor. Sie basiert auf einer Kooperation des Lehrstuhls für Mustererkennung der Universität Erlangen-Nürnberg (Technische Fakultät) mit zwei anderen Forschungsinstitutionen derselben Universität.

Die erste ist die Abteilung für Phoniatrie und Pädaudiologie des Klinikums der Universität[1], die den Partner für die Analyse von Ersatzstimmen darstellte. Die andere, für das Gebiet der Erkennung von verhallter Sprache, war der Lehrstuhl für Multimediakommunikation und Signalverarbeitung[2].

E.3.1 Die Notwendigkeit objektiver Evaluierung

Die Evaluierung der Ersatzstimme durch den Patienten und andere Personen erfolgt in erster Linie subjektiv. Dies gilt auch für den Therapeuten, da die verfügbaren technischen Mittel zur objektiven Stimmanalyse, wie das Göttinger Heiserkeitsdiagramm (Kap. 2.5.4), noch nicht an Ersatzstimmen angepasst wurden. Dies bedeutet, dass das medizinische Personal sich auf seine Erfahrung verlassen muss. In dieser Arbeit wird die Korrelation zwischen subjektiver Bewertung durch Menschen und objektive, automatische Bewertungsmethoden untersucht.

Die Erfahrung der Bewerter hat sehr großen Einfluss auf die Übereinstimmung zwischen den Bewertern („inter-rater agreement"). Beruflicher Hintergrund und Erfahrung oder Wissen über die Krankengeschichte können eine große Inter-Rater-, aber auch Intra-Rater-Variabilität bedingen [FPB+05]. Fachpersonal wird, besonders wenn es eng zusammenarbeitet, eine wesentlich höhere Übereinstimmung auf denselben Bewertungskriterien erzielen als Halbprofessionelle, wie z.b. Logopädenschüler oder gar naive Hörer [MMB+06, DRF+96]. Manchmal wird die Inter-Rater-Variation durch eine „erzwungene" Einigung der Bewerter umgangen, bevor der Endwert weiterverarbeitet wird [PJ01]. Dies erfordert jedoch die Einbindung mehrerer Experten, was genau das Gegenteil der gewünschten schnellen und kostengünstigen Evaluierung darstellt.

Für die Entwicklung automatischer Verfahren müssen zunächst subjektive Auswertungsdaten als Referenz erfasst werden. Dies gilt für die Bewertung von Sprachkriterien, wie z.B. der Verwendung von Prosodie durch den Patienten, aber auch für akustische Parameter wie die Intensität der Stimme oder die maximale Tonhaltedauer. Der Vergleich verschiedener früherer Studien zu diesem Thema ist jedoch fast unmöglich, da viele Forschungsgruppen aufgrund niedriger Patientenzahlen nur eine sehr beschränkte Menge an Daten zur Verfügung hatten. In der Literatur finden sich viele Beiträge, die auf Sprechergruppen einstelliger Größe basieren. Viele Forscher entwerfen ihre eigenen Bewertungskriterien für Sprach- und Stimmqualität (vgl. Kap. 2), was es sehr schwer macht, Entsprechungen zwischen ihnen zu finden. Die Sprachdaten für die Auswertung sind ebenfalls sehr unterschiedlich. Um Stimmparameter zu messen, verwenden viele Studien nur gehaltene Vokale, andere verwenden Wörter oder Sätze. Die Analyse dieser Daten wird noch schwieriger dadurch, dass die Forscher unterschiedliche Messgrößen erfassen. Während z.b. die Tonhaltedauer ein sehr gängiges Maß ist, ziehen manche Gruppen Parameter wie die Dauer eines beliebig gewählten Satzes oder sogar die „Intensität in Millimetern" einer analogen Ausgabe vor, was sehr schwer zu reproduzieren sein dürfte. Um die Variabilität in Sprechergruppen zu reduzieren und einen Eindruck davon zu erhalten, welche Sprachqualität bei Ersatzstimmen möglich ist, schlugen Bellandese u.a. vor, dass eine Studie zu diesem Thema nur Sprecher einbeziehen sollte, die als exzellent bewertet worden waren [BLG01]. Das Ergebnis einer solchen Studie kann jedoch nicht auf nicht-exzellente Sprecher verallgemeinert werden und würde kaum die Suche nach wirklich objektiven Analysemethoden unterstützen.

Der Versuchsaufbau von Bewertungsstudien ist ebenfalls sehr wichtig für ihre Allgemeingültigkeit. Zum Beispiel sollte bei Verständlichkeitstests die Menge des den Hörern präsentierten

---

[1]http://www.phoniatrie.uni-erlangen.de
[2]http://www.lnt.de/lms

Materials groß genug sein, um zu verhindern, dass dieselben Daten mehr als einmal vorgespielt werden, um einen Lerneffekt bei den Zuhörern zu verhindern. In einer Studie mit 50 College-Studenten als Hörer wurde die Verständlichkeit von normalen und tracheoösophagealen (TE) Ersatzstimmen (Kap. 2.2.5) in verrauschter Umgebung verglichen [MFP+98]. Die Testpersonen waren ein Normalsprecher und ein TE-Sprecher, die ein Satzpaar aus einem Standardtext vorlasen [Fai60]. Das Hintergrundgeräusch war vielstimmiges „Plappern" aus dem Test „Speech Perception in Noise" (SPIN, [KSE77]). Die Testaufnahmen wurden den Hörern vorgespielt, und zwar einmal ohne Störung und danach mit eingespieltem Hintergrundgeräusch in verschiedenen Intensitäten. Während jedes Durchlaufs sollten die Hörer beurteilen, wie verständlich die Aufnahme war. Obwohl die Studie interessante Ergebnisse erzielte, wurde die Auswertung wohl hochgradig durch die Tatsache beeinflusst, dass alle Hörer dieselben beiden Sätze des jeweiligen Sprechers immer wieder hörten. Es erscheint sehr unwahrscheinlich, dass die Ergebnisse unabhängige oder sogar „objektive" Maße repräsentieren.

Die angegebenen Beispiele zeigen, dass in der Tat eine kompakte Menge automatisch berechenbarer, objektiver Evaluierungskriterien in der Sprachtherapie benötigt wird, umsomehr als einzelne Forscher eine „objektive" Bewertung lediglich als den Durchschnittswert aus mehreren subjektiven Bewertungen oder die Einigung auf einen Wert definieren. Bei der großen Zahl von Studien auf kleinen Datenstichproben dürfte dies keine konsistente und gültige Definition sein. Die Vereinheitlichung der Stimmbewertung muss bereits zum Zeitpunkt der Datenerhebung beginnen. Diese Prozedur ist jedoch abhängig vom Ziel der Sprachtherapie, wie der nächste Abschnitt zeigt.

E.3.2 Auf das Screening in „natürlichen" Situationen gerichtet

Zum Zwecke der umfassenden Dokumentation einer Stimme hat die European Laryngological Research Group (ELRG) fünf grundlegende Elemente der Stimmbewertung definiert [DBC+01]:

- Videostroboskopie

- akustische Analyse

- aerodynamische Messungen

- perzeptive Bewertungen

- Selbstbewertung, d.h. Bewertung durch den/die Patient(in) selbst

Die körperlich unangenehmste Erfassung für den Patienten ist die Videostroboskopie, da sie das Einführen eines Endoskops in den Mund und die Aufnahme der Glottis oder – im Falle der Ersatzstimmen – der Pseudoglottis beinhaltet (siehe Kap. 2.2.2).

Das Ziel für die Zukunft der Stimmdokumentation muss die größtmögliche Reduktion der Anstrengung oder gar Schmerzen für den Patienten sein. Ein anderer wichtiger Punkt ist die Verminderung des psychischen Drucks auf den Patienten. In einer für die Testperson idealen Situation könnte der Patient frei sprechen und hätte nicht den Eindruck, beobachtet oder kontrolliert zu werden. Für den Fall der perzeptiven Bewertungen versucht diese Arbeit, einige Lösungen anzugeben. Im Idealfall würde der Patient ohne Sprechgarnitur, d.h. Kopfhörer mit Mikrofon, sprechen. Wenn die Aufnahme mit einem Raummikrofon gemacht wird, ist sich die Testperson der laufenden Evaluierung wesentlich weniger stark bewusst. Spracherkennung in verhallter

Umgebung ist daher ein wichtiges Thema in dieser Arbeit. Weiterhin sollte der Proband spontan sprechen können, d.h. zwischen Patient und Therapeut wird ein normaler Dialog geführt, der aufgenommen wird und als Grundlage für die spätere Analyse dient. Völlig freies Sprechen ist jedoch für die automatische Evaluierung aus verschiedenen Gründen nicht geeignet, wie z.b. das Out-of-vocabulary-Problem oder schwankende Wortdauern, wenn verschiedene Sprecher unterschiedliche Wörter benutzen. Aus diesem Grund wurde von den Testsprechern ein phonetisch reicher Standardtext mit einem festgelegten Vokabular vorgelesen und danach analysiert. Dies stellt dennoch eine große Verbesserung im Vergleich mit den eingeführten objektiven Verfahren dar, welche auf die Auswertung eines gehaltenen Vokals beschränkt sind. Typische Merkmale der objektiven Analyse werden automatisch aus der Frequenz (z.b. Jitter) oder Amplitude (z.b. Shimmer) von Teilen des Sprachsignals berechnet, oder sie werden aus zeitabhängigen Messgrößen gewonnen, wie etwa die Dauer von Wörtern und Sätzen oder die maximale Tonhaltedauer [BLG01, PFKB89, Rob84]. Die Position der Formanten [CMG01] und die Stimmeinschwingzeit [RCK86, SKA00, SC02] werden ebenfalls in Betracht gezogen. Während die Berechnung der akustischen Parameter, wie Jitter, Shimmer etc., automatisch abläuft, wird die Dauer eines Textes oder einer Phrase oft immer noch durch Anhören bestimmt.

Im Falle der Lautdauer war die grafische Darstellung des Stimm- oder Sprachsignals auf einem Monitor und die anschließende Messung der gewünschten Dauer per Hand zu Beginn der 1990er Jahre immer noch üblich. Der Personalaufwand ist in solchen Experimenten sehr hoch, besonders wenn mehrere Bewerter eingesetzt werden, um ein gewisses Maß an Objektivität zu erzielen [GW83].

Um Sprachqualität in einer realen Kommunikationssituation objektiv zu bewerten, ist die Analyse ganzer Wörter und Sätze nötig, da die Verständlichkeit der Ersatzstimme ein wesentliches Kriterium für ihre Bewertung durch die Patienten selbst und durch Experten darstellt [AS92, MFP+98, SKA00]. Besonders ist hier die Kommunikation über das Telefon betroffen [MZ96, MMG93, ZP86], da durch die Bandbeschränkung des Telefonkanals die Stimme noch stärker beeinträchtigt wird und es keine Möglichkeit gibt, die Kommunikation durch Mimik oder Handgesten zu unterstützen.

Die Analyse von Telefonanrufen ist ein Aspekt, der die Situation für die Patienten erleichtern könnte. Das Telefon ist ein wesentlicher Bestandteil des sozialen Lebens. Laryngektomierte sind oft älter als 70 oder sogar 80 Jahre (siehe Kap. 4.4), und es ist für sie notwendig, ein Kommunikationsmittel zu besitzen, welches nicht das Verlassen des Hauses erfordert. Und wenn diese Menschen Hilfe irgendwelcher Art benötigen, werden sie wahrscheinlich das Telefon benutzen, um einen Arzt oder ihre Verwandten anzurufen. Ein anderer Aspekt, der beachtet werden muss, ist die Tatsache, dass ihre Kontaktpersonen häufig auch ältere Menschen sind, was zu Problemen beim Zuhörer führen kann [Cla85]. Deshalb spiegelt die Stimmevaluierung über das Telefon eine für den Patienten wichtige Kommunikationssituation wider. Eine objektive Bewertung der Verständlichkeit von Telefonsprache als Teil einer klinischen Bewertung der Stimmrehabilitation wäre für die betroffenen Personen sehr vorteilhaft, und sie wäre ein Schritt hin zu einer globalen Bewertung der Sprache nach der Laryngektomie.

Perzeptuelle Stimmevaluierung ist in erster Linie subjektiv, da sie von menschlichen Experten durchgeführt wird. Außerdem setzen die Experimente, die in der Literatur beschrieben sind, ein gewisses Maß an Hörerfahrung mit Ersatzstimmen voraus [DDRS98], was zunächst nicht der Alltagssituation des Patienten entspricht. Die subjektiven und objektiven Verfahren zur Erfassung der Stimmfunktion, die derzeit in der Sprachtherapie verwendet werden, entsprechen meist nicht dem Standard der technisch möglichen Stimm- und Sprachanalyse. Im Rahmen dieser Arbeit wurde untersucht, wie solche Methoden eingesetzt werden können, um ein objektives Hilfsmittel zur Bewertung von Ersatzstimmen bereitzustellen. Der nächste Abschnitt gibt einen Überblick über die Ansätze, die untersucht wurden.

E.3.3 Beitrag dieser Arbeit zur Forschung

In dieser Arbeit wird der Schritt von der automatischen Analyse von Vokalaufnahmen zu Textaufnahmen vollzogen. Die neuen Verfahren erfordern lediglich einen Standardrechner und ein Mikrofon. Sie sind auch für die internetbasierte Verarbeitung entworfen. Es wurde untersucht,

- ob automatische Maße gewonnen werden können, die tracheoösophageale Ersatzstimmen objektiv beschreiben und evaluieren können,

- ob die objektiven Parameter gut mit den Bewertungskriterien menschlicher Bewerter korrelieren

- und ob die objektive Auswertung auch über das Telefon oder bei Verwendung eines Raummikrofons möglich ist.

Die Spracherkenner für die Experimente mit TE-Sprechern wurden mit Normalsprechern trainiert, da es für die Auswertung wichtig war, dass das System einen naiven Hörer simuliert, also eine Person, die nie zuvor TE-Sprache gehört hat. Dies entspricht der Situation, mit der die Patienten im täglichen Leben konfrontiert werden. Dennoch wurde die Interpolation der akustischen Modelle mit TE-Sprache untersucht.

Menschliche Bewertungskriterien in der Sprachtherapie sind üblicherweise unter anderem Verständlichkeit, Stimmklang, Stimmqualität und Prosodiefähigkeit. Die Korrelation zwischen derartigen menschlichen „Noten" und der Wortakkuratheit des Spracherkenners wurde für eine Stichprobe von TE-Sprachaufnahmen bestimmt. Sie wurde auch für automatisch generierte, prosodische Merkmale berechnet, die z.B. die Stimmeinschwingzeit oder Wort- und Pausendauern repräsentieren.

Für einige Experimente wurde besonders die Verständlichkeitsbewertung betrachtet, da sie das wichtigste Kriterium der Stimmbewertung durch menschliche Hörer darstellt. Eine automatisierte Version des Postlaryngektomie-Telefontests (PLTT) wird vorgestellt. Der Test wurde ursprünglich für menschliche Hörer entwickelt, um die Kommunikationssituation am Telefon darzustellen. Zusätzlich wurden die Wortakkuratheit und die prosodischen Merkmale mittels der sog. Leave-one-speaker-out-Multikorrelations-/Regressionsanalyse verarbeitet, um diejenigen Maße zu bestimmen, die das Verständlichkeitskriterium am besten repräsentieren.

Für Sprachtherapeuten kann eine grafische Darstellung pathologischer Sprache sehr hilfreich sein. Die Sammon-Transformation führt eine topologieerhaltende Dimensionsreduktion auf den Eingabedaten durch. Sie minimiert eine „Spannungsfunktion" zwischen der Topologie der niederdimensionalen Sammon-Karte und den hochdimensionalen originalen Sprachdaten. In dieser Arbeit wird die Fähigkeit der Sammon-Karten, menschliche Bewertungskriterien darzustellen, untersucht.

Für die Spracherkennung in verhallter Umgebung kamen Korpora normaler Sprache zum Einsatz, welche synchron aufgenommene Nahbesprechungs- und Raummikrofonaufnahmen enthalten. Verschiedene Ansätze wurden getestet, um die Erkennungsergebnisse von verhallten Testdaten zu verbessern. Im Gegensatz zu den meisten anderen Studien wurde die Testumgebung während der Trainingsphase als nicht bekannt angenommen, d.h. die Testdaten waren in einer anderen Umgebung aufgenommen als alle Trainingsdaten. Um einen „universellen" Erkenner für Nahbesprechungs- und verhallte Testdaten zu erhalten, wurden die Trainingsmengen teilweise oder ganz unter Zuhilfenahme vieler verschiedener Raumcharakteristiken künstlich verhallt. Mel-Frequenz-Cepstrum-Koeffizienten (MFCC) kamen in den Baseline-Erkennern als Merkmale zum Einsatz. Allerdings kann die logarithmische Komprimierung der Filterbankkoeffizienten bei verrauschten Daten nachteilig sein. Aus diesem Grund wurden alternative Merkmale getestet. Das Root-Cepstrum und die „μ-law-Merkmale", die auf einem Komprimierungsverfahren aus dem Bereich der Telekommunikation basieren, ersetzen den Logarithmus durch andere Funktionen, die diese Probleme umgehen sollen.

Da keine Raummikrofonaufnahmen von Laryngektomierten verfügbar waren, wurden Root-Cepstrum und μ-law-Merkmale auf künstlich verhallter TE-Sprache getestet, um eine Therapiesitzung zu simulieren, in der keine Sprechgarnitur (Headset) verwendet wird. Diese Merkmale wurden auch auf simulierten Telefondaten getestet.

Synchrone Aufnahmen der Testdaten wurden durch Delay-and-sum-Beamforming als Vorverarbeitungsschritt kombiniert, um ein neues Signal mit niedrigerem Rauschanteil zu erzeugen. Diese Testmenge wurde mit Spracherkennern verarbeitet, die wiederum unterschiedliche Merkmale und künstlich verhallte Trainingsdaten verwenden.

E.3.4 Übersicht

Diese Arbeit ist wie folgt aufgeteilt:

Kapitel 2 führt verschiedene Möglichkeiten zur Anbahnung einer Ersatzstimme ein, wie z.B. operative Methoden oder die ösophageale Stimme. Der Schwerpunkt liegt auf tracheoösophagealen (TE) Stimmen. Die Eigenschaften einiger Stimmrehabilitationsmethoden werden verglichen, und subjektive Evaluierungsverfahren, die in der Sprachtherapie zum Einsatz kommen, werden vorgestellt. Objektive Messgrößen für die Stimmqualität werden zusammen mit kommerziellen Anwendungen im Detail diskutiert.

Kapitel 3 beschreibt Maße, die benutzt werden, um die Übereinstimmung zwischen menschlichen Bewertern oder zwischen einem Bewerter und der maschinellen Evaluierung eines Sprachsignals zu bestimmen. Konkret werden die Korrelationskoeffizienten von Pearson und Spearman mit Cohens κ und dessen Erweiterungen verglichen, und Krippendorffs α wird als mächtige Alternative vorgestellt.

Informationen über die Sprachkorpora, die für die Experimente in dieser Arbeit verwendet wurden, sind in Kapitel 4 zu finden. Das EMBASSI-Korpus und die Müdigkeitsstichprobe sind in verschiedenen Signalqualitäten verfügbar und wurden deshalb für die Verbesserung der Spracherkennung in verhallter Umgebung eingesetzt. Teile des VERBMOBIL-Korpus dienten als Trainingsdaten für alle Spracherkenner. Für die Erkennung der laryngektomierten Testsprecher wurden auch menschliche Bewertungen als Referenz für die automatische Auswertung erhoben. Die entsprechenden Details sind ebenfalls in diesem Kapitel aufgeführt.

Ein wichtiger Aspekt bei der Arbeit am Spracherkennungssystem war die Suche nach Merkmalen, die robuster gegen Hall sind als Mel-Frequenz-Cepstrum-Koeffizienten, um die automatische Erkennung von Raummikrofonaufnahmen zu verbessern. Die Adaption von Hidden-Markov-Modellen an TE-Sprache wurde durchgeführt, um die Erkennungsergebnisse für Ersatzstimmen zu verbessern. Die grafische Darstellung von Sprachdaten, basierend auf der Lautmodellanpassung, und die prosodische Analyse waren weitere unverzichtbare Aspekte für die

Evaluierung. Die theoretischen Grundlagen dieser Verfahren sind in Kapitel 5 zu finden. In Kapitel 6 sind die Ergebnisse der Spracherkennung in verhallter Umgebung zusammengestellt. Dies beinhaltet Experimente mit künstlich verhallten Trainingsdaten, um so viele unbekannte Testumgebungen wie möglich abzudecken. Die Verbesserung der Ergebnisse durch modifizierte MFCC als Merkmale wird ebenso beschrieben wie die Kombination von Signalen von mehr als einem Mikrofon (Beamforming), um Störgeräusche in den entsprechenden Testsignalen zu eliminieren.

Die Experimente zur automatischen Bewertung von Ersatzstimmen werden in Kapitel 7 beschrieben. Die Übereinstimmung zwischen menschlicher Bewertung und den automatisch erhobenen Messgrößen wird im Detail für das Verständlichkeitskriterium dargestellt, welches am besten durch die Wortakkuratheit des Spracherkenners repräsentiert wird, und für die prosodische Analyse von TE-Sprachdaten. Die Verständlichkeit am Telefon wird mithilfe der automatischen Version des Postlaryngektomie-Telefontests ermittelt. Die Auswirkungen von Hall in den Testsignalen und von der Erkenneradaption auf die Erkennungsergebnisse werden ebenso erläutert. Abschließend wird die grafische Darstellung von Ersatzstimmen durch die Sammon-Transformation präsentiert.

Wesentliche Erkenntnisse anderer Forschungsgruppen und ihre Vergleichbarkeit mit dieser Arbeit werden in Kapitel 8 zusammengefasst und diskutiert. Zukünftige Experimente und mögliche Erweiterungen der Evaluierungsverfahren werden in Kapitel 9 angesprochen. Kapitel 10 fasst die gesamte Arbeit zusammen.

E.4 Zusammenfassung

In 20 bis 40 Prozent aller Fälle von Kehlkopfkrebs muss eine totale Laryngektomie, d.h. die Entfernung des gesamten Kehlkopfes, durchgeführt werden. Nach der Operation bleiben die Luftröhre (Trachea) und die Speiseröhre (Ösophagus) voneinander getrennt. Für den Patienten bedeutet dies den Verlust der natürlichen Stimme und damit auch des wichtigsten Kommunikationsträgers. Die moderne Chirurgie erlaubt die Anbahnung einer Ersatzstimme, die von Zeit zu Zeit durch den Therapeuten zum Zwecke der Dokumentation des Therapiefortschritts evaluiert werden muss. Diese Evaluierung ist subjektiv. Sie ist deshalb abhängig von der Erfahrung des jeweiligen Experten und von anderen Faktoren. In dieser Arbeit wurde untersucht, wie automatische Verfahren verwendet werden können, um eine objektives Hilfsmittel zur Bewertung von Ersatzstimmen bereitzustellen.

Es gibt viele Methoden zur Wiederherstellung der Stimme. Bei der ösophagealen Ersatzstimme dient ein Teil des Ösophagus als Pseudoglottis, und der Magen kann als Luftreservoir verwendet werden. Jedoch kann es einige Monate oder sogar Jahre dauern, bevor Laryngektomierte dazu fähig sind, diese Art der Stimme zu kontrollieren. Mit Hilfe unterschiedlicher chirurgischer Methoden wurde versucht, die Umlenkung der Luft beim Ausatmen von der Luftröhre in den Rachen (Pharynx) durch Fisteln oder auf ähnliche Weise zu ermöglichen. Jedoch war die Aspirationsrate sehr hoch, weshalb die meisten dieser Ansätze heute nicht mehr zur Anwendung kommen. Die Stimmfunktion des Kehlkopfes kann auch durch einen Tongenerator ersetzt werden. In den meisten Fällen wird dieser elektrisch betrieben und folglich als Elektrolarynx bezeichnet. Das Gerät wird entweder an die Außenseite des Halses oder den Mundboden gehalten, oder es wird im Mund platziert. Die Qualität dieser Stimmen ist häufig jedoch nicht zufriedenstellend, da sie sehr „roboterhaft" und monoton klingt.

Bei einer beliebten Methode der Stimmrehabilitation wird ein sog. Shunt-Ventil („Stimmprothese") zwischen Trachea und pharyngoösophagealem (PE) Segment eingebracht, das die tracheoösophageale (TE) Ersatzstimme ermöglicht. Das Ventil erlaubt beim Ausatmen die Umlenkung der Luft in das PE-Segment, wo die Ersatzstimmgebung stattfindet. Der Ursprung der Stimme ist derselbe wie bei der ösophagealen Stimme, aber das Shunt-Ventil erlaubt es den betroffenen Personen, wieder das gesamte Lungenvolumen zum Sprechen zu nutzen. Zudem ist die Zeit des Lernens, mit einer TE-Stimme zu sprechen, wesentlich kürzer. Für über 90% der laryngektomierten Personen bedeutet das Shunt-Ventil eine sofortige Wiederherstellung ihrer Stimmfunktion, und 65% der Patienten benutzen die TE-Stimme dauerhaft. Alle Patienten, die für diese Arbeit rekrutiert wurden, waren mit einem Shunt-Ventil vom Typ Provox® ausgestattet, das 1988 am Niederländischen Krebsinstitut entwickelt wurde.

Es gibt etablierte subjektive Verfahren zur Analyse der Qualität von pathologischen Stimmen. Es ist jedoch möglich, dass verschiedene Therapeuten ihrer Erfahrung entsprechend eine Stimme unterschiedlich bewerten (Inter-Rater-Diskrepanz), und auch ein einzelner Bewerter kann eine andere Meinung haben, wenn er eine Stimme einige Zeit später erneut hört (Intra-Rater-Diskrepanz). Dies wird durch automatische Verfahren vermieden. Sie sind deterministisch und objektiv, liefern auf denselben Daten stets das gleiche Resultat, und sie können als Referenz dienen, die von der individuellen „Karriere" eines bestimmten Experten unabhängig ist. Eingeführte Methoden für die objektive Auswertung analysieren jedoch lediglich Aufnahmen von gehaltenen Vokalen, um Unregelmäßigkeiten in der Stimme zu finden. Dies entspricht keiner realen Kommunikationssituation. Die Untersuchung von Sprache ist für das tägliche Leben des Patienten wichtiger. Da die automatische Verarbeitung völlig freier Rede sehr schwierig ist, lasen die Testpersonen im Rahmen dieser Arbeit einen Standardtext vor. Dieser Text wurde dann mit Verfahren der automatischen Spracherkennung analysiert.

Wenn eine automatische Methode und die menschliche Bewertung verglichen werden sollen, dann muss der Grad der Übereinstimmung innerhalb der Expertengruppe und zwischen den menschlichen und automatisch berechneten Resultaten bestimmt werden. Neben Pearsons Korrelationskoeffizient r wurden hierzu weitere Maße, die in der Medizin und den Sozialwissenschaften verwendet werden, eingesetzt. Zwei Ursachen der Übereinstimmung sind zu unterscheiden. Die eine ist die Übereinstimmung durch Kompetenz, d.h. sie resultiert aus der Erfahrung der Bewerter mit den jeweiligen Patienten und ihren (Sprach-)Daten. Der andere Anteil ist durch eine bestimmte Anzahl gleicher Bewertungen, die bereits zufällig möglich sind, bedingt und wird deshalb als erwartete Übereinstimmung bezeichnet. Folglich ist ein Übereinstimmungsmaß erforderlich, das nur den Anteil durch Kompetenz widerspiegelt, und eine Art „Zufallskorrektur" muss erfolgen. Erweiterungen von Cohens κ, wie κ_{DF} nach Davies und Fleiss, leisten dies für eine beliebige Zahl von Bewertern und Bewertungskategorien. Krippendorffs α ist sogar in der Lage, mit dem Problem fehlender Bewertungen in den Daten umzugehen. Beide Maße wurden für den Vergleich der menschlichen und automatischen Bewertungen verwendet.

Die Sprachdaten für die Experimente im Rahmen dieser Arbeit wurden mehreren Sprachkorpora entnommen. In einer Sprachtherapiesitzung sollte es dem Patienten nicht bewusst sein, dass er aufgezeichnet wird, da dies den Eindruck des Kontrolliertwerdens erwecken kann. Aus diesem Grund war eines der Ziele die Verbesserung der Spracherkennungsergebnisse in verhallter Umgebung. Die Experimente wurden allerdings nicht mit Stichproben von pathologischer Sprache durchgeführt, da keine Sprachkorpora vorhanden waren, die groß genug gewesen und mit Raummikrofonen aufgenommen worden wären. Das EMBASSI-Korpus wurde für Pilotexperimente zu diesem Thema benutzt. Wenn ein Erkenner in vielen verschiedenen Umgebungen zufriedenstellend arbeiten soll, dann sollten als Trainingsdaten Aufnahmen zur Verfügung stehen, die in einer Vielzahl unterschiedlicher Räumlichkeiten aufgenommen wurden. Durch die künstliche Verhallung von Nahbesprechungsdaten mit vordefinierten Raumimpulsantworten kann dieses Problem umgangen werden. Ausgesuchte Resultate wurden mit der Müdigkeitsstichprobe und dem VERBMOBIL-Korpus verifiziert. Für das Erkennertraining wurden die ursprünglichen Nahbesprechungssignale teilweise oder vollständig durch ihre künstlich verhallten Versionen ersetzt. Die VERBMOBIL-Erkenner wurden mit der originalen und der künstlich verhallten VERBMOBIL-Testmenge, den Nahbesprechungsaufnahmen der Müdigkeitsstichprobe und deren entsprechenden Raummikrofonaufnahmen ausgewertet.

Das VERBMOBIL-Korpus war auch die Grundlage für das Erkennertraining bei der Ersatzstimmanalyse. Die Testdaten für diese Experimente waren Aufnahmen von 41 TE-Sprechern sowie von 18 älteren und 16 jüngeren Normalsprechern als Kontrollgruppen. Jede Testperson las den Standardtext „Der Nordwind und die Sonne" vor, der alle Phoneme der deutschen Sprache enthält. Er besteht aus 108 Wörtern und wird in der Sprachtherapie eingesetzt. Eine menschliche Referenzbewertung für die TE-Sprachdaten wurde von fünf Sprachpathologieexperten erhoben. Elf Kriterien, wie z.B. „Verständlichkeit", „Sprechanstrengung" und „Rauigkeit", wurden anhand von fünfstufigen Likert-Skalen bewertet, d.h. eine aus fünf benannten Alternativen musste ausgewählt werden. Die Gesamtqualität wurde auf einer visuellen Analogskala mit Werten zwischen 0,0 und 10,0 angegeben. Zwischen einigen der Kriterien wurde eine hohe Übereinstimmung beobachtet, z.B. für die Verständlichkeit zur Gesamtqualität ($r = +0,96$). Dies zeigt die Relevanz der Verständlichkeit für den perzeptiven Gesamteindruck von TE-Sprache. Stimmklang ($r = +0,96$) und die Fähigkeit zur Prosodie ($r = +0,88$) scheinen weitere wichtige Aspekte für menschliche Hörer zu sein.

Verschiedene Verfahren wurden getestet, um die Erkennungsergebnisse der verhallten Testdaten zu verbessern. Das erste war die Anwendung der künstlich verhallten Trainingsdaten. Es wurde angenommen, dass die Testumgebung während der Trainingsphase nicht bekannt ist. Aus diesem Grund wurden zwölf verschiedene Raumimpulsantworten verwendet, um die Nahbesprechungsdaten des Baseline-Spracherkenners zu verhallen. Die Resultate zeigten, dass es möglich ist, sowohl Nahbesprechungs- als auch verhallte Testdaten zufriedenstellend zu verarbeiten, wenn die Trainingsmenge aus Nahbesprechungs- und künstlich verhallten Signalen zusammengestellt wird. Auf der Müdigkeitsstichprobe stieg die durchschnittliche Wortakkuratheit von klaren und natürlich verhallten Signalen von 68,2% auf dem Nahbesprechungserkenner bis auf 76,8% auf einem Erkenner, dessen eine Hälfte der Trainingsmenge aus künstlich verhalltem Material bestand. Alle Erkenner waren HMM-basiert.

Die zweite Änderung am Ausgangssystem betraf die Merkmalsextraktion. Als Merkmale für die Spracherkennung wurden ursprünglich Mel-Frequenz-Cepstrum-Koeffizienten (MFCC) verwendet. Die logarithmische Komprimierung der Filterbankkoeffizienten kann jedoch auf gestörten Daten nachteilig sein. Folglich wurden alternative Merkmale untersucht. Das Root-Cepstrum ersetzt den Logarithmus durch eine Wurzelfunktion, und die „μ-law-Merkmale" benutzen stattdessen eine Kompandierungsfunktion, die niedrige Werte erhöht und hohe Werte staucht. Das Root-Cepstrum erreichte nur annähernd die Ergebnisse der Standard-MFCC, aber manche Verbesserungen mit μ-law-Merkmalen auf den EMBASSI-Daten waren signifikant. Auf der Müdigkeitsstichprobe erreichte die durchschnittliche Wortakkuratheit auf klaren und natürlich verhallten Signalen 77,2%. Obwohl dies nur wenig besser ist als mit MFCC, können die μ-law-Merkmale für die Erkennung von Raummikrofonaufnahmen empfohlen werden.

Die Gauß-Normierung der Merkmale war für einige der Root-Cepstrum-Merkmale vorteilhaft, aber im Allgemeinen trat eine Erhöhung der Wortakkuratheit nicht häufig genug auf, um das Verfahren als zuverlässig für andere Daten erachten zu können. Für den dritten Ansatz wurde nicht der Erkenner verändert, sondern die Testdaten. Da von den EMBASSI- und Müdigkeitsdaten einige synchrone Aufnahmen vorhanden waren, wurden diese Signale durch Delay-and-sum-Beamforming kombiniert, um ein neues Signal mit weniger Rauschanteil zu erzeugen. In der Tat stieg für den VERBMOBIL-Baseline-Erkenner (MFCC-Merkmale) die Wortakkuratheit auf dem verhallten Teil der Müdigkeits-Testmenge von 47,8% auf 63,1%. Wiederum hatten eine künstlich verhallte Trainingsmenge und μ-law-Merkmale einen positiven Effekt auf die Resultate. Die beste erzielte Wortakkuratheit lag bei 77,4%, als alle Trainingsdaten verhallt waren.

Alle Ergebnisse in Betracht ziehend, kann folgendes Fazit gezogen werden: Für ein Aufnahmeszenario in einem Raum mit verteilten Mikrofonen, wobei die Testumgebung in der Trainingsphase nicht bekannt ist, sollte ein Erkenner mit Nahbesprechungsaufnahmen und künstlich verhallten Signalen trainiert werden. Er sollte Beamforming als Vorverarbeitungsschritt und μ-law-Merkmale anstelle von MFCC verwenden.

Die Spracherkenner für die Experimente mit TE-Sprechern wurden vom Baseline-VERB-MOBIL-Erkenner abgeleitet. Sie wurden mit jungen, normal sprechenden Personen trainiert, weil nicht genügend Trainingsdaten von den älteren Personen oder laryngektomierten Sprechern vorhanden waren. Zudem war es wichtig, dass das System einen naiven Hörer simuliert, d.h. jemanden, der nie zuvor TE-Sprache gehört hat, weil dies die Situation ist, mit der die Patienten in ihrem täglichen Leben konfrontiert werden. Für die Aufnahmen der TE-Sprecher war die durchschnittliche Wortakkuratheit auf einem polyphonbasierten Erkenner 36,9%. Es wurde erwartet, dass das robustere Training von Monophonmodellen einen positiven Effekt auf die Erkennung von Ersatzstimmen hat. Dies konnte jedoch nicht beobachtet werden. Obwohl die automatische Erkennung so schlechte Resultate erzielte, war die Korrelation mit den menschlichen Bewertungen hoch. Der Grund dafür ist, dass das entscheidende Maß nicht der Durchschnitt der Erkennungsrate ist, sondern deren Wertebereich. Verständlichkeit, Stimmklang, Qualität der Ersatzstimme und der Gebrauch von Prosodie während des Sprechens zeigten die höchste Korrelation zur Wortakkuratheit ($|r| \geq 0{,}7$). Dies bestätigt auch die Beobachtung, dass diese Kriterien in hohem Maße miteinander in den menschlichen Bewertungsergebnissen korrelieren. Die Korrelation zwischen dem durchschnittlichen Bewerter und der Wortakkuratheit des polyphonbasierten Erkenners für das Verständlichkeitskriterium war $|r| = 0{,}88$.

Zur Verbesserung der Erkennung wurden die akustischen Modelle der VERBMOBIL-basierten Erkenner auch mit TE-Sprachaufnahmen interpoliert. Es wurde jedoch keine positive Auswirkung auf die Korrelation zwischen Wortakkuratheit und menschlicher Bewertung beobachtet. Aus diesem Grund kann die zeitraubende Anpassung vernachlässigt werden.

Die Wortakkuratheit ist ein sehr gutes Maß für Verständlichkeit. Es gibt jedoch Bewertungskriterien, die nicht durch die Zahl richtig verstandener oder erkannter Wörter ausgedrückt werden können. Um adäquate automatische Gegenstücke für sie zu finden, wurde ein Prosodiemodul angewendet. Prosodische Merkmale werden aus der Analyse von stillen Pausen, gefüllten Pausen, der Signalenergie, Wort- und Silbendauern und der Sprachgrundfrequenz F_0 gewonnen. Die Analyse prosodischer Merkmale zeigte Maße auf, die eine hohe Korrelation zu den menschlichen Bewertungskriterien aufweisen. TE-Sprache ist üblicherweise langsamer als normale Sprache, und die Anzahl stimmhafter Abschnitte ist stark verringert. Dies beeinflusst viele Merkmale, die die Stimmein- und Stimmausschwingzeit erfassen, aber auch Wort- und Pausendauern. Diese Merkmale zeigen Korrelationen von bis zu $|r| = 0{,}76$ zu Kriterien wie Verständlichkeit,

Gesamtqualität, Sprechanstrengung oder zur Übereinstimmung von Atem- und Sinneinheiten. Das Kriterium „Stimmklang" wird durch Energiemaße dargestellt. Wegen der hohen Irregularität von Ersatzstimmen ist es nicht einfach, korrekte F_0-Werte zu ermitteln. Dies könnte der Grund dafür sein, dass F_0-Merkmale die Bewertungskriterien nicht sehr gut abbildeten.

Als die Wortakkuratheit der Spracherkenner und die prosodischen Merkmale gemeinsam mit Leave-one-speaker-out-Multikorrelations-/Regressionsanalyse verarbeitet wurden, wurde wiederum die Wortakkuratheit als dasjenige Maß bestimmt, das Verständlichkeit am besten darstellt. Beim Postlaryngektomie-Telefontest (PLTT), der entwickelt wurde, um die Kommunikationssituation am Telefon abzubilden, war jedoch die Korrelation zum menschlichen PLTT-Resultat für die Worterkennungsrate besser ($r \approx 0{,}9$, polyphonbasierter Erkenner).

Da keine Raummikrofondaten von Laryngektomierten vorhanden waren, wurden das Root-Cepstrum und die μ-law-Merkmale auf künstlich verhallten TE-Sprachsignalen getestet, um eine Therapiesitzung zu simulieren, in der kein Headset benutzt wird. Die μ-law-Merkmale erzielten konsistent bessere Erkennungsresultate und bewiesen folglich, dass sie auch bei pathologischer Sprache eine Alternative zum klassischen MFCC-Ansatz darstellen.

Für Sprachtherapeuten könnte es sehr nützlich sein, eine grafische Darstellung pathologischer Sprache zu erhalten. Die Sammon-Transformation führt eine topologieerhaltende Reduktion der Datendimension durch. Sie minimiert eine „Spannungsfunktion" zwischen der Topologie der niederdimensionalen Sammon-Karte und den hochdimensionalen Originaldaten. Letztere Topologie wird durch ein Abstandsmaß zwischen Äußerungen oder Sprechern definiert. In einer Sammon-Karte von TE-Sprechern und normal sprechenden Kontrollgruppen wurden alle Sprechergruppen voneinander getrennt. In einer Karte, die nur TE-Sprecher enthielt, erreichten die Positionen der einzelnen Sprecher Korrelationen von bis zu $r = 0{,}74$ zur Wortakkuratheit und von $|r| \approx 0{,}7$ für Bewertungskriterien wie Verständlichkeit und Stimmklang.

Trotz der guten Resultate, die in dieser Arbeit erzielt wurden, gibt es einige Aspekte, die in Zukunft bearbeitet werden müssen. Ein Standardtext repräsentiert keine reale Kommunikationssituation, aber er stellt eine viel genauere Näherung von flüssiger, spontaner Sprache dar als ein einzelner, gehaltener Vokal. Dieser Kompromiss ist notwendig, da die Auswertung völlig freier Rede umfangreiche Änderungen an allen Bestandteilen des Analysesystems erfordern würde. Das Out-of-vocabulary-Problem (OOV) wurde noch nicht untersucht, da die Zahl der Lesefehler in den vorhandenen Aufnahmen sehr klein war. Für eine zukünftige klinische Anwendung müssen jedoch die zwei Arten von Fehlern – durch das Vorlesen und durch die Erkennung – voneinander getrennt werden. Zusätzlich sollten die Auswertungsergebnisse durch eine Langzeitstudie bestätigt werden. Die Verfahren, die in dieser Arbeit beschrieben werden, können nicht nur für Patienten nach totaler Laryngektomie vorteilhaft sein. Sie werden im Rahmen eines neuen Forschungsprojekts zur Bewertung der Stimme nach Larynxteilresektion erweitert und verbessert werden.

Index